Nurses'
Drug
Reference

NDR

Nurses'
Drug
Reference

Little, Brown and Company

Library of Congress Catalog Card No. 77–6563

ISBN 0–316–10973–8

Printed in the United States of America

Editor

Stewart M. Brooks, M.S.

Chairman, Science Curriculum, Newton-Wellesley Hospital School of Nursing, Newton Lower Falls, Massachusetts

Contributors

Anna T. Manseau, M.Ed., R.N.

Coordinator, First-Year Program, Newton-Wellesley Hospital School of Nursing, Newton Lower Falls, Massachusetts

William R. Principe, M.S., R.Ph.

Director of Pharmacy Services, Newton-Wellesley Hospital, Newton Lower Falls, Massachusetts

Medical Consultant

Edward C. Dyer, M.D.

Instructor in Pediatric Nurse Practitioner Program, Northeastern University; Associate Pediatrician, Massachusetts General Hospital, Boston, Massachusetts

Editorial Assistant

Natalie Paynton-Brooks, B.A.

Assistant in Science, Newton-Wellesley Hospital School of Nursing, Newton Lower Falls, Massachusetts

Contents

Foreword

The pharmaceutical industry has contributed greatly to modern medicine, but the number and variety of its products and the multiplicity of names present very real problems in the learning and practice of drug therapeutics. Clearly, there is a need for a reference source tailored to nursing—one that not only complements an appropriate text in the classroom but also serves as a guide "on the floor." NDR supplies this need in a concise and palatable manner within the framework of three carefully designed sections.

Section 1 is the classification of over a thousand drugs within an all-inclusive spectrum of action, use, and chemical category, ranging alphabetically from adrenergic blocking agents to vitamins. Section 2, the body of NDR, presents alphabetically 555 monographs on standard and commonly used drugs and provides complete cross-referencing between thousands of brand names and generic designations. Section 3 presents supportive information on key topics of theoretical and practical concern and includes an extensive glossary of pharmacological and pharmaceutical terms. The special notes that preface Section 1 and Section 2 should be read carefully to insure proper use of NDR.

S. M. B.

Nurses' Drug Reference

Section 1
Classification
of Drugs

Drug Combinations

Drug combinations are indicated by slashes. In all instances the drug named first belongs to the class under discussion. The other drugs in the combination may or may not belong to the class. For example, in the combination magnesium hydroxide/ aluminum hydroxide (under Antacids), both constituents are antacids, whereas in the combination magnesium hydroxide/aluminum hydroxide/simethicone, the last constituent is an antiflatulent.

Brand Names (Trademarks)

The listing of two or more brand names following a generic designation implies nothing beyond the fact that the same drug or active ingredient is involved.

Adrenergic-blocking agents

See ANTIADRENERGICS.

Adrenergics

Adrenergics are agents that produce effects similar to those caused by stimulation of the sympathetic nervous system. They serve as antihypotensives, vasoconstrictors, decongestants, bronchodilators, vasodilators, and mydriatics. The drug of choice for a particular indication depends on whether the desired action involves predominantly alpha receptors or beta receptors. Stimulants of alpha receptors cause vasoconstriction of arterioles in the skin and splanchnic areas (resulting in a rise in blood pressure), dilatation of the pupil, and relaxation of the gastrointestinal tract. Stimulants of beta receptors cause vasodilatation of arterioles of the skeletal muscles, relaxation of the bronchioles, and increased heart contraction and heart rate. Adrenergics include the natural neurohormones—epinephrine, norepinephrine, and dopamine—as well as a number of synthetic congeners.

Prominent adrenergics include:
 dopamine hydrochloride (Intropin®)
 ephedrine sulfate (I-sedrin®)
 epinephrine (Adrenalin®)
 epinephrine bitartrate (Epitrate®, Medihaler-Epi®)
 ethylnorepinephrine hydrochloride (Bronkephrine®)
 isoproterenol hydrochloride (Isuprel®)
 isoproterenol sulfate (Medihaler-Iso®, Norisodrine®)
 levarterenol bitartrate (Levophed®)
 metaproterenol sulfate (Alupent®, Metaprel®)
 metaraminol bitartrate (Aramine®)
 methoxamine hydrochloride (Vasoxyl®)
 naphazoline hydrochloride (Privine®)
 nylidrin hydrochloride (Arlidin®)
 oxymetazoline hydrochloride (Afrin®)
 phenylephrine hydrochloride (Neo-Synephrine®)
 phenylephrine hydrochloride/isoetharine mesylate
   (Bronkometer®)
 propylhexedrine (Benzedrex®)
 pseudoephedrine hydrochloride (Novafed®, Sudafed®)
 terbutaline sulfate (Brethine®, Bricanyl®)
 tetrahydrozoline hydrochloride (Tyzine®, Visine®)
 xylometazoline hydrochloride (Otrivin®)

Allergens

See BIOLOGICALS.

Amebicides

See ANTIPROTOZOALS.

Amino acids

See PARENTERAL ALIMENTATION.

Ammonia detoxicants

See ELECTROLYTE SOLUTIONS AND WATER-BALANCE AGENTS.

Analeptics

See RESPIRATORY STIMULANTS.

Analgesics

Analgesics are agents that relieve pain without producing loss of consciousness and reflex activity. Narcotic analgesics (opiates and synthetic congeners) are used in the management of moderate to severe pain; nonnarcotic agents are used in the management of mild to moderate pain. Typically, analgesics act upon the brain, but some medications are specific to particular conditions (e.g., gout and migraine); in these medications the mechanism is peripheral and highly selective.

Prominent narcotic analgesics include:
alphaprodine hydrochloride (Nisentil®)
anileridine (Leritine®)
aspirin/codeine (Ascodeen-30®)
codeine phosphate
codeine sulfate
fentanyl citrate (Sublimaze®)
fentanyl citrate/droperidol (Innovar®)
hydromorphone hydrochloride (Dilaudid®)
meperidine hydrochloride (Demerol®)
methadone hydrochloride (Dolophine®)
morphine sulfate
opium alkaloids (Pantopon®)
opium/belladonna suppositories
oxycodone/APC (Percodan®)
oxycodone hydrochloride/acetaminophen (Percocet™-5, Tylox™)
oxymorphone hydrochloride (Numorphan®)

Prominent nonnarcotic analgesics include:
acetaminophen (Datril®, Liquiprin®, Nebs®, Phenaphen®, Tempra®, Tylenol®, Valadol®)

acetaminophen/allobarbital (Dialog®)
aspirin (acetylsalicyclic acid)
aspirin/caffeine (Anacin®)
aspirin/aluminum glycinate/magnesium carbonate (Bufferin®)
aspirin/phenacetin/caffeine (APC, aspirin compound)
 (Empirin® Compound)
aspirin/phenacetin/caffeine/butalbital (Fiorinal®)
aspirin/salicylamide/acetaminophen/caffeine (Excedrin®)
choline salicylate (Arthropan®)
ethoheptazine (Zactane®)
ethoheptazine/aspirin/meprobamate (Equagesic®)
mefenamic acid (Ponstel®)
pentazocine hydrochloride (Talwin® Hydrochloride)
pentazocine hydrochloride/aspirin (Talwin® Compound)
pentazocine lactate (Talwin® Lactate)
propoxyphene hydrochloride (Darvon®, Dolene®)
propoxyphene hydrochloride/acetaminophen (Dolene® AP,
 Wygesic®)
propoxyphene hydrochloride/aspirin (Darvon® with A.S.A.)
propoxyphene hydrochloride/aspirin compound (Darvon®
 Compound, Darvon® Compound-65, Dolene® Compound)
propoxyphene napsylate (Darvon-N®)
propoxyphene napsylate/acetaminophen (Darvocet-N® 100)
propoxyphene napsylate/aspirin (Darvon-N® with A.S.A.®)
sodium bicarbonate/citric acid/aspirin (Alka-Seltzer® Effervescent Pain Reliever and Antacid)

Analgesics specific to gout include:
allopurinol (Zyloprim®)
colchicine
probenecid (Benemid®)
probenecid/colchicine (ColBENEMID®)
sulfinpyrazone (Anturane®)

Analgesics specific to migraine include:
ergotamine tartrate (Ergostat™, Gynergen®)
ergotamine tartrate/caffeine (Cafergot®)
ergotamine tartrate/caffeine/belladonna alkaloids/pentobarbital
 sodium (Cafergot® P-B)
ergotamine tartrate/caffeine/cyclizine hydrochloride (Migral®)
methysergide maleate (Sansert®)

Analgesics specific to rheumatoid arthritis, osteoarthritis, and certain
related conditions include:
aurothioglucose (Solganal®)
fenoprofen calcium (Nalfon®)
gold sodium thiomalate (Myochrysine®)
ibuprofen (Motrin®)

indomethacin (Indocin®)
naproxen (Naprosyn®)
oxyphenbutazone (Oxalid®, Tandearil®)
phenylbutazone (Azolid®, Butazolidin®)
phenylbutazone/aluminum hydroxide/magnesium trisilicate
     (Azolid®-A, Butazolidin® Alka)
tolmetin sodium (Tolectin®)

Analgesic specific to the urinary tract:
     phenazopyridine hydrochloride (Pyridium®)

Androgens

Androgens are male sex hormones. Those used clinically include testosterone, the most potent natural hormone, and its derivatives and synthetic congeners. Basic therapeutic indications include hypogonadism, eunuchoidism, and cryptorchidism (in the last case, androgens are used alone or along with gonadotropins). Other uses include the male climacteric and breast cancer. Certain androgens of low androgenicity (anabolic steroids) are used for their protein-sparing action in osteoporosis, presurgical and post-surgical care, burns, and uremia, and as adjuvant therapy in certain types of refractory anemia.

Prominent androgens include:
     fluoxymesterone (Halotestin®)
     methandrostenolone (Dianabol®)
     methyltestosterone (Android®, Metandren®, Oreton® Methyl, Testred®)
     nandrolone decanoate (Deca-Durabolin®)
     nandrolone phenpropionate (Durabolin®)
     oxymetholone (Anadrol®-50)
     stanozolol (Winstrol®)
     testosterone cypionate (Depo®-Testosterone)
     testosterone enanthate (Delatestryl®)
     testosterone enanthate/estradiol valerate (Deladumone®)
     testosterone propionate (Oreton® Propionate)

Anesthetics

Anesthetics produce insensibility to pain. Those that produce surgical anesthesia are referred to as general anesthetics, and those that produce local insensibility are referred to as local anesthetics. General anesthetics are administered by inhalation or intravenously (depending on the physical state of the agent); local anesthetics are administered topically or by injection (e.g., by infiltration, nerve block, or spinal).

Prominent general anesthetics include:
- cyclopropane
- ether (ethyl ether)
- fluroxene (Fluoromar®)
- halothane (Fluothane®)
- ketamine hydrochloride (Ketaject®, Ketalar®)
- methohexital sodium (Brevital®)
- methoxyflurane (Penthrane®)
- nitrous oxide
- thiamylal sodium (Surital®)
- thiopental sodium (Pentothal®)
- trichloroethylene (Trilene®)
- vinyl ether (Vinethene®)

Prominent local anesthetics include:
- antipyrine/benzocaine (Auralgen®/glycerin)
- antipyrine/benzocaine/phenylephrine (Tympagesic®)
- benzocaine (Americaine®)
- bupivacaine hydrochloride (Marcaine®)
- butethamine hydrochloride (Monocaine®)
- calamine lotion, phenolated
- chloroprocaine hydrochloride (Nesacaine®)
- cocaine hydrochloride
- cyclomethycaine sulfate (Surfacaine®)
- dibucaine (Nupercainal®)
- dibucaine hydrochloride (Nupercaine®)
- dimethisoquin hydrochloride (Quotane®)
- diperodon (Diothane®)
- dyclonine hydrochloride (Dyclone®)
- ethyl chloride
- eugenol
- hexylcaine hydrochloride (Cyclaine®)
- lidocaine hydrochloride (Xylocaine®)
- mepivacaine hydrochloride (Carbocaine®)
- pramoxine hydrochloride (Tronothane®)
- prilocaine hydrochloride (Citanest®)
- procaine hydrochloride (Novocain®)
- proparacaine hydrochloride (Alcaine®, Ophthaine®)
- tetracaine hydrochloride (Pontocaine®)

Anorectics

See CEREBRAL STIMULANTS.

Antacids

Antacids are agents used in the treatment of hyperacidity (hyperchlorhydria) and peptic ulcer. Some act by direct neutralization of hydrochloric acid and some by hydrogen-ion adsorption; other antacids act by combined adsorption, buffering, and partial neutralization. Agents that inhibit the formation of hydrochloric acid, such as anticholinergics (see) and H_2 receptor antagonists (see p. 19), are not generally considered antacids.

Prominent antacids include:
aluminum carbonate gel (Basaljel®)
aluminum glycinate/magnesium carbonate (Di-Alminate®)
aluminum hydroxide gel (Amphojel®)
aluminum hydroxide/magnesium trisilicate (Gelusil®)
aluminum hydroxide/magnesium trisilicate/magnesium hydroxide (Gelusil-M®)
aluminum phosphate (Phosphaljel®)
calcium carbonate/glycine (Titralac®)
dihydroxyaluminum aminoacetate (Alglyn®, Alzinox®, Robalate®)
magaldrate (Riopan®)
magnesia, milk of (magnesia magma, magnesium hydroxide)
magnesium hydroxide/aluminum hydroxide (Aludrox®, Creamalin®, Maalox®)
magnesium hydroxide/aluminum hydroxide/calcium carbonate (Camalox®)
magnesium hydroxide/aluminum hydroxide/simethicone (Maalox® Plus, Mylanta®, Mylanta®-II)
sodium bicarbonate (baking soda)
sodium bicarbonate/citric acid/aspirin (Alka-Seltzer® Effervescent Pain Reliever and Antacid)

Anthelmintics

Anthelmintics are drugs used in the treatment of worm infestations (helminthiases).

Prominent anthelmintics include:
For filariasis:
diethylcarbamazine citrate (Hetrazan®)
For hookworm:
bephenium hydroxynaphthoate (Alcopara®)
hexylresorcinol
mebendazole (Vermox®)
tetrachloroethylene
thiabendazole (Mintezole®)

8

For pinworm:
    piperazine citrate (Antepar®)
    pyrantel pamoate (Antiminth®)
    pyrvinium pamoate (Povan®)
    thiabendazole (Mintezole®)
For roundworm (ascariasis):
    bephenium hydroxynaphthoate (Alcopara®)
    hexylresorcinol
    mebendazole (Vermox®)
    piperazine citrate (Antepar®)
    pyrantel pamoate (Antiminth®)
    thiabendazole (Mintezol®)
For schistosomiasis:
    antimony potassium tartrate (tartar emetic)
    niridazole (Ambilhar®)
    stibophen (Fuadin®)
For tapeworm:
    niclosamide (Yomesan®)
    quinacrine hydrochloride (Atabrine®)
For threadworm:
    thiabendazole (Mintezol®)
For trichinosis:
    thiabendazole (Mintezol®)
For whipworm:
    hexylresorcinol
    mebendazole (Vermox®)
    thiabendazole (Mintezol®)

Antiadrenergics

Antiadrenergics are agents that inhibit sympathetic function (hence, the expressions *sympatholytics, adrenolytics,* and *adrenergic blocking agents*). Alpha-adrenergic blocking agents are used in the treatment of hypertension, peripheral vascular disease, and certain forms of shock, and in the diagnosis of pheochromocytoma. Beta-adrenergic blocking agents are used in the control of cardiac arrhythmias, hypertension, and certain forms of angina pectoris.

Prominent antiadrenergics include:
    guanethidine sulfate (Ismelin®)
    isoxsuprine hydrochloride (Vasodilan®)
    methyldopa (Aldomet®)
    phenoxybenzamine hydrochloride (Dibenzyline®)
    phentolamine hydrochloride (Regitine® Hydrochloride)
    phentolamine mesylate (Regitine® Mesylate)
    propranolol hydrochloride (Inderal®)
    reserpine (Serpasil®)

Antialcoholics

The classic antialcoholic is disulfiram (Antabuse®), an agent that interacts with alcohol to produce flushing, a throbbing headache, dyspnea, tachycardia, hypotension, syncope, dizziness, blurred vision, and confusion. Severe reactions may result in death. Disulfiram is used as an aid in the management of selected chronic alcoholic patients who have a strong desire to remain in a state of enforced sobriety.

Antiallergics

See ANTIHISTAMINES.

Antianemics

See HEMATINICS.

Antiarrhythmics

See CARDIACS.

Antiarthritics

See ANALGESICS; CORTICOSTEROIDS.

Antiasthmatics

Antiasthmatics are agents used in the management of bronchial asthma. There are four major classes: methylated xanthines (theophylline and its analogues), adrenergics, corticosteroids, and cromolyn sodium. The first two classes are bronchodilators; corticosteroids have a beneficial anti-inflammatory effect on mucosal edema and abnormal mucus; cromolyn sodium is a prophylactic medication that acts by preventing leakage of bronchoconstricting mediators (namely histamine) from mast cells and basophils. Xanthines are used alone or in combination with ephedrine, expectorants, and sedatives.

Prominent xanthine preparations include:
aminophylline (theophylline ethylenediamine) (Aminodur® Dura-Tabs®, Somophyllin®)
aminophylline/guaifenesin/ephedrine/phenobarbital (Mudrane®-GG)
dyphylline (Dilor®)
oxtriphylline (Choledyl®)
oxtriphylline/guaifenesin (Brondecon®)
theophylline (Aerolate®, Elixophyllin®, Theolair™)
theophylline/ephedrine/hydroxyzine (Marax®)
theophylline/ephedrine/phenobarbital (Tedral®)
theophylline/guaifenesin (Quibron®)

Prominent adrenergics include:
   ephedrine sulfate (I-sedrin®) (also available in combination with
      xanthine preparations; see above)
   epinephrine (Adrenalin®)
   epinephrine bitartrate (Medihaler-Epi®)
   ethylnorepinephrine hydrochloride (Bronkephrine®)
   isoproterenol hydrochloride (Isuprel®)
   isoproterenol sulfate (Medihaler-Iso®, Norisodrine®)
   metaproterenol sulfate (Alupent®, Metaprel®)
   phenylephrine hydrochloride/isoetharine mesylate
      (Bronkometer®)
   terbutaline sulfate (Brethine®, Bricanyl®)

Prominent aerosol steroids include:
   beclomethasone dipropionate (Vanceril®)
   dexamethasone (Decadron®, Deronil®, Dexone™,
      Gammacorten®, Hexadrol®)
   triamcinolone (Aristocort®, Kenacort®)

Prominent systemic steroids include:
   hydrocortisone sodium succinate (Solu-Cortef®)
   methylprednisolone (Medrol®)
   prednisone (Deltasone®, Meticorten®)

Cromolyn is available as:
   cromolyn sodium (Aarane®, Intal®)

Antibiotics

Antibiotics are agents produced by microorganisms that inhibit or
destroy other microorganisms. Those used therapeutically to treat
infection include natural products and their chemical derivatives
and synthetic substitutes. Antibiotics act by one of three mechanisms—inhibition of cell wall synthesis, inhibition of protein synthesis, or interference with the function of the plasma (cellular)
membrane.

Penicillin
Penicillin refers to penicillin G, the fundamental molecule, and its
derivatives and semisynthetic congeners. Penicillin prevents bacteria
from forming new cell wall material (eventually leading to their destruction) and thus is typically bactericidal. Specific infections yield-
ing to penicillin include gonorrhea, syphilis, meningococcal meningitis, gas gangrene, and necrotizing ulcerative gingivitis (Vincent's
infection). Sensitive bacteria include *Streptococcus pyogenes, Streptococcus pneumoniae,* and certain strains of *Staphylococcus aureus.*
So-called broad-spectrum penicillins are also effective against a number of gram-negative pathogens, including *Hemophilus influenzae,
Klebsiella pneumoniae, Escherichia coli,* and *Proteus* species.

Prominent penicillins include:
  amoxicillin (Amoxil®, Larotid®)
  ampicillin (Alpen®, Amcil®, Omnipen®, Penbritin®,
    Pencin®, Polycillin®, Principen®)
  carbenicillin disodium (Geopen®, Pyopen®)
  carbenicillin indanyl sodium (Geocillin®)
  cloxacillin sodium (Tegopen®)
  dicloxacillin sodium (Dynapen®, Pathocil®, Veracillin®)
  methicillin sodium (Celbenin®, Staphcillin®)
  nafcillin sodium (Unipen®)
  oxacillin sodium (Bactocill®, Prostaphlin®)
  penicillin G benzathine (Bicillin®, Bicillin® L-A)
  penicillin G benzathine/penicillin G procaine (Bicillin® C-R)
  penicillin G potassium (Pentids®, Pfizerpen G®)
  penicillin G procaine (Cysticillin®, Duracillin® A.S.,
    Wycillin®)
  penicillin G sodium
  penicillin V (Pen-Vee®, V-Cillin®)
  penicillin V potassium (Compocillin®-VK, Ledercillin® VK,
    Pen-Vee® K, SK-Penicillin VK™, V-Cillin® K, Veetids®)
  ticarcillin disodium (Ticar®)

Tetracyclines
Tetracyclines are natural and semisynthetic broad-spectrum antibiotics derived from *Streptomyces aureofaciens* and related strains. Indications include infections caused by a variety of pathogens, including gram-positive and gram-negative bacteria, chlamydiae, and rickettsiae.

Prominent tetracyclines include:
  chlortetracycline hydrochloride (Aureomycin®)
  demeclocycline hydrochloride (Declomycin®)
  doxycycline (Vibramycin®)
  methacycline hydrochloride (Rondomycin®)
  minocycline hydrochloride (Minocin®, Vectrin®)
  oxytetracycline (Terramycin®)
  tetracycline/amphotericin B (Mysteclin-F®)
  tetracycline hydrochloride (Achromycin®, Achromycin® V,
    Cyclopar®, Panmycin®, Sumycin®, Tetracyn®)
  tetracycline hydrochloride/nystatin (Achrostatin® V)
  tetracycline phosphate complex (Tetrex®)

Erythromycin
Erythromycin refers to the fundamental molecule (erythromycin), derived from *Streptomyces erythreus,* and its pharmaceutical derivatives. Its antibacterial spectrum is similar to that of penicillin. For the most part, erythromycin is used when pathogens are penicillin-resistant or when the patient is allergic to penicillin.

Prominent erythromycins include:
- erythromycin (Erythrocin®, Ilotycin®)
- erythromycin, enteric-coated (E-Mycin®)
- erythromycin estolate (Ilosone®)
- erythromycin ethylsuccinate (E.E.S. 400™, Erythrocin® Ethyl Succinate-I.M., Pediamycin®)
- erythromycin gluceptate (Ilotycin® Gluceptate)
- erythromycin lactobionate (Erythrocin® Lactobionate)
- erythromycin stearate (Bristamycin®, Erythrocin® Stearate, Ethril®, Pfizer-E®)

Cephalosporins
Cephalosporins are a family of semisynthetic antibiotics that are effective against both gram-positive and gram-negative organisms. For the most part, they are used in patients who are allergic to penicillin and in patients with penicillin-resistant infections.

Prominent cephalosporins include:
- cefazolin (Ancef®, Kefzol®)
- cephalexin (Keflex®)
- cephaloglycin (Kafocin®)
- cephaloridine (Loridine®)
- cephalothin sodium (Keflin® Neutral)
- cephapirin sodium (Cefadyl®)
- cephradine (Anspor®, Velosef®)

Chloramphenicol
Chloramphenicol is a broad-spectrum antibiotic originally derived from *Streptomyces venezuelae* and now produced synthetically. It is the drug of choice in typhoid fever and rickettsial infections.

Prominent preparations in use include:
- chloramphenicol (Chloromycetin®)
- chloramphenicol palmitate (Chloromycetin® Palmitate)
- chloramphenicol sodium succinate (Chloromycetin® Sodium Succinate)

Antifungal Antibiotics
Antifungal antibiotics are used systemically and topically to treat mycoses.

Prominent antifungal antibiotics include:
- amphotericin B (Fungizone®)
- candicidin (Candeptin®, Vanobid®)
- griseofulvin (Fulvicin-U/V®, Grifulvin V®, Grisactin®, Gris-PEG®)
- nystatin (Mycostatin®, Nilstat®)

Miscellaneous Antibiotics
A number of antibiotics are available that have special indications or that serve as alternative therapy when penicillin and the tetracyclines are without effect.

Miscellaneous antibiotics include:
amikacin sulfate (Amikin™)
bacitracin (Baciquent®)
clindamycin hydrochloride (Cleocin®)
clindamycin palmitate hydrochloride (Cleocin® Pediatric)
clindamycin phosphate (Cleocin® Phosphate)
colistimethate sodium (Coly-Mycin® M Parenteral)
colistin sulfate (Coly-Mycin® S Oral and Otic)
cycloserine (Seromycin®)
gentamicin sulfate (Garamycin®)
kanamycin sulfate (Kantrex®)
lincomycin hydrochloride (Lincocin®)
neomycin sulfate (Mycifradin®, Neobiotic®)
paromomycin sulfate (Humatin®)
polymyxin B sulfate (Aerosporin®)
spectinomycin hydrochloride (Trobicin®)
streptomycin sulfate
tobramycin sulfate (Nebcin®)
troleandomycin (TAO®)
vancomycin hydrochloride (Vancocin®)
viomycin sulfate (Viocin®)

Anticholinergics

Anticholinergics are drugs that inhibit parasympathetic function. Typically, they relax smooth muscle, inhibit secretion of exocrine glands, dilate the pupil, and cause paralysis of accommodation. For the most part, anticholinergics are used as mydriatics, cycloplegics, and antispasmodics; they are also used to treat patients with gastric and duodenal ulcers. Pharmaceutically, anticholinergics include the belladonna alkaloids (atropine, scopolamine, and hyoscyamine) and their derivatives and synthetic substitutes. Those used as gastrointestinal antispasmodics are often combined with sedatives and tranquilizers.

Prominent anticholinergics include:
adiphenine hydrochloride (Trasentine®)
atropine sulfate
belladonna alkaloids (Bellafoline®, Prydon®)
belladonna alkaloids/phenobarbital (Belladenal®, Donnatal®)
belladonna alkaloids/phenobarbital/simethicone (Kinesed®)
belladonna tincture
benztropine mesylate (Cogentin®)

clidinium bromide/chlordiazepoxide hydrochloride (Librax®)
cyclopentolate hydrochloride (Cyclogyl®)
dicyclomine hydrochloride (Bentyl®)
echothiophate iodide (Phospholine Iodide®)
ethopropazine hydrochloride (Parsidol®)
glycopyrrolate (Robinul®)
hexocyclium methylsulfate (Tral®)
homatropine methylbromide (Homapin®)
hyoscyamine sulfate (Levsin®)
isopropamide iodide (Darbid®)
isopropamide iodide/prochlorperazine (Combid®)
mepenzolate bromide (Cantil®)
methantheline bromide (Banthīne®)
methixene hydrochloride (Trest®)
methscopolamine bromide (Pamine®)
pipenzolate bromide (Piptal®)
pralidoxime chloride (Protopam®)
procyclidine hydrochloride (Kemadrin®)
propantheline bromide (Pro-Banthīne®)
scopolamine hydrobromide (hyoscine)

Anticoagulants

Anticoagulants prevent or depress pathological intravascular clotting by inhibiting coagulation. They are used in the treatment of venous thrombosis, pulmonary embolism, acute arterial embolism of the extremities, and disseminated intravascular coagulation. Anticoagulants are used prophylactically to prevent recurrent embolism secondary to intracardiac thrombi and recurrent venous thromboses in thrombophilic individuals; they also reduce thromboembolic complications in selected postoperative and postpartum patients. In myocardial infarction, anticoagulation reduces reinfarction and mortality. Frequent assessment of the clotting mechanism is necessary during treatment to ensure that effective therapy is maintained while the risk of hemorrhage is minimized. The chief anticoagulants include heparin, which has prompt action and is the agent of choice in acute thromboembolic disorders, and vitamin K antagonists, which act more slowly and are usually preferred for long-term treatment.

Prominent anticoagulants include:
acenocoumarol (Sintrom®)
anisindione (Miradon®)
dicumarol (bishydroxycoumarin)
diphenadione (Dipaxin®)
ethyl biscoumacetate (Tromexan®)
heparin sodium injection (Lipo-Hepin®, Liquaemin®, Panheprin®)

phenprocoumon (Liquamar®)
sodium warfarin (Coumadin®, Panwarfarin®)
wrokinase* (Abbokinase®)

Anticonvulsants

Anticonvulsants are agents used in the treatment of epilepsy and other convulsive disorders. Their precise mode and site of action are still uncertain but presumably the motor cortex is involved. Further, a given anticonvulsant may be effective in one form of epilepsy and ineffective in another.

Prominent anticonvulsants include:
carbamazepine (Tegretol®)
clonazepam (Clonopin®)
ethosuximide (Zarontin®)
ethotoin (Peganone®)
magnesium sulfate injection
mephenytoin (Mesantoin®)
mephobarbital (Mebaral®)
metharbital (Gemonil®)
methsuximide (Celontin®)
paramethadione (Paradione®)
phenacemid (Phenurone®)
phenobarbital (Luminal®)
phenobarbital/phenytoin sodium/methamphetamine
   hydrochloride (Phelantin®)
phensuximide (Milontin®)
phenytoin sodium (Dilantin®)
primidone (Mysoline®)
trimethadione (Tridione®)
valproic acid (Depakene®)

Antidepressants

See PSYCHOTROPICS.

Antidiabetics

Antidiabetics are agents used in the treatment and control of diabetes mellitus, which in most cases results from the inadequate production and secretion of insulin by the beta cells of the islets of Langerhans. These agents include several types of insulin (from two species, pork and beef) and several oral hypoglycemics. Oral hypoglycemics include the sulfonylureas, which stimulate pancreatic insulin release; these agents appear to be most effective in mild cases of diabetes without ketosis and infection. The commercial insulins include short-acting insulin (regular insulin), and intermediate and long-acting insulins,

*Effects dissolution of clot.

namely, protamine zinc insulin (PZI), isophane insulin (NPH), globin zinc insulin, and the lente group of insulins (insulin zinc suspensions). The duration of action for each type of insulin relates to its rate of absorption from the site of injection. Lente insulins contain no sensitizing substances (such as protamine and globin).

Prominent oral hypoglycemics include:
acetohexamide (Dymelor®)
chlorpropamide (Diabinese®)
tolazamide (Tolinase®)
tolbutamide (Orinase®)

Antidiarrheals

Antidiarrheals are agents used to control diarrhea. For the most part, they act through either adsorption of toxic substances, inhibition of gastrointestinal motility, or suppression of enteropathic organisms. Often they are used in combination.

Prominent preparations include:
colistin sulfate (Coly-Mycin® S Oral Suspension)
bismuth subsalicylate (Pepto-Bismol®)
diphenoxylate hydrochloride/atropine sulfate (Colonil™, Lomotil®)
furazolidone (Furoxone®)
kaolin/pectin (Kaopectate®)
kaolin/pectin/belladonna alkaloids (Donnagel®)
kaolin/pectin/opium (Parepectolin®)
Lactobacillus acidophilus/L. bulgaricus (Lactinex®)
loperamide hydrochloride (Imodium®)
mepenzolate bromide/phenobarbital (Cantil®-PHB)
neomycin sulfate (Mycifradin®, Neobiotic®)
opium, deodorized tincture of (DTO)
paregoric (camphorated tincture of opium)
thiphenamil hydrochloride (Trocinate®)

Antidiuretics

See PITUITARY HORMONES.

Antidotes

See EMETICS; HEAVY METAL ANTAGONISTS.

Antiemetics

Antiemetics are agents used in the relief and treatment of nausea and vomiting and vertigo. The mechanism of action mainly involves the inhibition of vestibular function and/or the suppression of the vomiting center or reflex.

Prominent antiemetics include:
> benzquinamide hydrochloride (Emete-con®)
> buclizine hydrochloride (Bucladin®-S)
> diphenidol (Vontrol®)
> doxylamine succinate/pyridoxine hydrochloride (Bendectin®)
> prochlorperazine (Compazine®)
> promethazine hydrochloride (Phenergan®)
> thiethylperazine (Torecan®)
> triflupromazine (Vesprin®)
> trimethobenzamide hydrochloride (Tigan®)

Antiemetics used primarily in management of motion sickness include:
> cyclizine hydrochloride (Marezine®)
> dimenhydrinate (Dramamine®)
> meclizine hydrochloride (Antivert®, Bonine®)

Antiflatulents

Antiflatulents are medicinals used to prevent or relieve flatulence; these include digestive enzymes, panthenol, and defoaming agents. Panthenol, a coenzyme A precursor, improves gastrointestinal muscle tone; defoaming agents lower the surface tension of gas bubbles, thereby causing them to coalesce and be eliminated more easily via eructation.

Prominent antiflatulents include:
> dexpanthenol (Ilopan®)
> lipase/amylase/protease/hemicellulase/bile constituents
>   (Festal®)
> magnesium hydroxide/aluminum hydroxide/simethicone
>   (Mylanta®)
> pepsin/pancreatin/cellulase/glutamic acid/ox bile extract
>   (Kanulase®)
> simethicone (Mylicon®)
> simethicone/pancreatin (Phazyme®)

Antifungals

Antifungals suppress the growth or reproduction of fungi and are used against fungal (mycotic) infections. These agents include a wide variety of local anti-infectives (see), certain antibiotics (see), and a few special (nonantibiotic) systemic agents, such as flucytosine (Ancobon®).

Antiglaucomatous agents

Antiglaucomatous agents are used in the management of glaucoma. They include carbonic anhydrase inhibitors (see), miotics (see), and topical adrenergics (see); adrenergics are contraindicated in narrow-angle glaucoma. Intravenous mannitol (Osmitrol®), IV urea (Urea-phil®), and oral glycerol (Osmoglyn®) are used in the emergency reduction of intraocular pressure.

Antigonadotropics

Antigonadotropics are agents that inhibit the output or action of gonadotropins. They include the oral contraceptives (p. 37) and the drug danazol (Danocrine®). By depressing the output of both follicle-stimulating hormone (FSH) and luteinizing hormone (LH), danocrine is useful in selected cases of endometriosis.

Antihemorrhoidals

Antihemorrhoidals are topical preparations formulated to provide relief of itching and pain in anorectal disorders (such as hemorrhoids, pruritus ani, anal fissure, and acute proctitis) and relief of local pain following anorectal surgery. These agents, which are employed alone or (more commonly) in combination, include local anesthetics, astringents, antipruritics, emollients, protectants, and corticosteroids. A representative formulation (Rectal Medicone®-HC Suppositories) contains benzocaine, hydrocortisone acetate, menthol, oxyquinoline sulfate, peruvian balsam, and zinc oxide.

Antihistamines

The characteristic action of all antihistamines is their ability to block the action of histamine. Differences among them relate to sedation, antiemetic and other CNS effects, and anticholinergic and local anesthetic properties. Based on their action at receptor sites they fall into two categories—H_1 receptor antagonists and H_2 receptor antagonists. H_1 receptor antagonists (H_1 blocking agents), the conventional antihistamines, are useful for treating seasonal hay fever, allergic rhinitis, perennial vasomotor rhinitis, urticaria, certain allergic dermatoses, and pruritus. They provide little benefit in the common cold (although they may help control rhinorrhea) and provide no benefit in bronchial asthma or systemic anaphylaxis. H_2 receptor antagonists are useful in the treatment of peptic ulcer, in which condition they reduce pain and promote healing by inhibiting the secretion of gastric acid.

Prominent antihistamines in current use include the H_2 antagonist cimetidine (Tagament®) and the following H_1 antagonists:
  bromodiphenhydramine (Ambodryl®)
  brompheniramine maleate (Dimetane®)
  brompheniramine/phenylephrine/phenylpropanolamine hydro-
    chloride (Dimetapp®)
  chlorpheniramine maleate (Chlor-Trimeton®, Teldrin®)
  cyproheptadine hydrochloride (Periactin®)
  dexbrompheniramine maleate (Disomer®)

dexbrompheniramine maleate/dextro-isoephedrine sulfate
(Drixoral®)
dexchlorpheniramine maleate (Polaramine®)
dimethindene maleate (Forhistal®, Triten®)
diphenhydramine hydrochloride (Benadryl®)
doxylamine succinate (Decapryn®)
methapyrilene fumarate (Histadyl® Fumarate)
methapyrilene hydrochloride (Histadyl®)
promethazine hydrochloride (Phenergan®)
pyrrobutamine compound (Co-Pyronil™)
trimeprazine tartrate (Temaril®)
tripelennamine hydrochloride (Pyribenzamine®)
triprolidine hydrochloride (Actidil®)
triprolidine hydrocholride/pseudoephedrine hydrochloride
(Actifed®)

Antihyperlipemics

See ANTILIPEMICS.

Antihypertensives

Antihypertensives are agents used to lower blood pressure. Although
the precise mechanism of action is uncertain for most of these drugs,
they achieve their effect through vasodilatation, in some cases by direct
action on the arterioles and in others by sympathetic inhibition. The
uncertainty about the mechanism of action especially applies to the
thiazides and related diuretics, which are the "first approach" medicinals in the management of hypertension. One view is that these agents
rid the tissues of sodium and thereby render the arterioles less reactive
to neurohormonal vasoconstriction. Hypotensive diuretics are used
alone in mild forms of the disease and in conjunction with sympathetic
inhibitors (or arteriolar relaxants) in moderate to severe cases.

Prominent antihypertensive diuretics include:
bendroflumethiazide (Naturetin®)
chlorothiazide (Diuril®)
chlorthalidone (Hygroton®)
furosemide (Lasix®)
hydrochlorothiazide (Esidrix®, HydroDIURIL®,
Oretic®)
methychlothiazide (Enduron®)
spironolactone (Aldactone®)
triamterene (Dyrenium®)

Prominent nondiuretic antihypertensives include:
clonidine hydrochloride (Catapres®)
cryptenamine tannate (Unitensin®)
deserpidine (Harmonyl®)

diazoxide (Hyperstat®)
guanethidine sulfate (Ismelin®)
hydralazine hydrochloride (Apresoline®, Dralzine™)
methyldopa (Aldomet®)
pargyline hydrochloride (Eutonyl®)
prazosin (Minipres®)
rauwolfia serpentina (Raudixin®)
rescinnamine (Moderil®)
reserpine (Serpasil®)
sodium nitroprusside (Nipride®)
trimethaphan camsylate (Arfonad®)

Prominent antihypertensive combinations include:
clonidine hydrochloride/chlorthalidone (Combipres®)
guanethidine sulfate/hydrochlorothiazide (Esimil®)
hydralazine hydrochloride/hydrochlorothiazide (Apresazide™)
hydralazine hydrochloride/reserpine/hydrochlorothiazide
   (Ser-Ap-Es®)
methyldopa/hydrochlorothiazide (Aldoril®)
pargyline hydrochloride/methyclothiazide (Eutron®)
reserpine/chlorothiazide (Diupres®)
reserpine/hydrochlorothiazide (Hydropres®)
spironolactone/hydrochlorothiazide (Aldactazide®)
triamterene/hydrochlorothiazide (Dyazide®)

Antihypoglycemics

See HYPERGLYCEMICS.

Anti-infectives, local

Local anti-infectives include a wide range of medicinals and chemical compounds. Some are applied to the skin and mucous membranes to prevent or treat infection; others are used to disinfect inanimate objects. Depending upon their action or intended use, local anti-infectives are loosely categorized as antiseptics, disinfectants, germicides, fungicides, and scabicides and pediculicides.

Standard local anti-infectives include:
antibiotics:
   bacitracin (Baciquent®)
   chloramphenicol (Chloromycetin®)
   erythromycin (Erythrocin®)
   neomycin sulfate (Mycifradin®)
   neomycin sulfate/hydrocortisone acetate (Neo-Cortef®)
   polymyxin B sulfate (Aerosporin®)
   polymyxin B sulfate/bacitracin (Polycin®, Polysporin®)
   polymyxin B sulfate/bacitracin/neomycin sulfate
      (Neosporin®)

polymyxin B sulfate/bacitracin/neomycin sulfate/hydro-
cortisone acetate (Cortisporin®)
tetracycline hydrochloride (Achromycin®)
sulfonamides:
mafenide acetate cream (Sulfamylon®)
silver sulfadiazine (Silvadene®)
sulfacetamide sodium (Sodium Sulamyd®)
sulfisoxazole diolamine (Gantrisin®)
miscellaneous antiseptic-disinfectants:
acetic acid (e.g., VōSoL® Otic Solution)
acetic acid/aluminum acetate (Otic Domeboro® Solution)
alcohol (ethanol, ethyl alcohol)
benzalkonium chloride (Zephiran®)
benzoyl peroxide
boric acid
chlorhexidene gluconate (Hibiclens®)
hexachlorophene detergent (pHisoHex®)
hydrogen peroxide
idoxuridine (Dendrid®, Herplex®, Stoxil®)
iodine tincture
iodochlorhydroxyquin (Vioform®)
iodoform
isopropyl alcohol
mercocresols (Mercresin®)
mercuric oxide, yellow
mercury, ammoniated
nitrofurazone (Furacin®)
poloxamer iodine (Prepodyne®)
potassium permanganate
povidone-iodine (Betadine®)
silver nitrate
sodium hypochlorite solution, diluted (Dakin's solution)
thimerosal (Merthiolate®)
thymol iodide
zinc peroxide
zinc sulfate
fungicides:
acrisorcin (Akrinol®)
amphotericin B (Fungizone®)
benzoic acid/salicylic acid (Whitfield's ointment)
calcium undecylenate (Caldesene®)
candicidin (Candeptin®, Vanobid®)
carbol-fuchsin solution (Castellani's paint)
chlordantoin (Sporostacin®)
clotrimazole (Lotrimin®)
coparaffinate (Iso-Par®)
gentian violet (crystal violet)
haloprogin (Halotex®)

miconazole nitrate (MicaTin®, Monistat®)
nystatin (Mycostatin®, Nilstat®)
nystatin/neomycin sulfate/gramicidin/triamcinolone
  acetonide (Mycolog®)
propionate compound (Propion Gel®)
sodium propionate, sodium caprylate, zinc caprylate
  (Sopronol®)
sodium thiosulfate
sodium thiosulfate/salicylic acid/2-propanol (Tinver®)
tolnaftate (Tinactin®)
undecylenic acid/zinc undecylenate (Desenex®)
scabicide-pediculicides:
  benzyl benzoate compound
  benzyl benzoate lotion
  crotamiton (Eurax®)
  gamma benzene hexachloride (Gamene®, Kwell®)
  pyrethrins/piperonyl butoxide (RID™)

Anti-inflammatory agents (general)

Anti-inflammatory agents are used in the treatment of inflammation and in conditions characterized by the inflammatory process
(e.g., rheumatic arthritis and osteoarthritis). They encompass a
wide pharmacologic spectrum, including salicylates (p. 5), phenyl-
butazones (p. 6), corticosteroids (p. 37), and anti-inflammatory enzymes (below).

Anti-inflammatory enzymes

Anti-inflammatory enzymes are systemic proteolytic agents that presumably cause the depolymerization of fibrin and modify the permea-
bility of venules and lymphatics. In conjunction with other measures,
they are helpful in inflammation and edema resulting from postoperative tissue reactions and accidental trauma.

Prominent anti-inflammatory enzymes include:
  bromelains (Ananase®)
  papain (Papase®)
  trypsin/chymotrypsin (Chymoral®)

Antileprotics

Antileprotics are agents used in the treatment of leprosy.

Prominent antileprotics include:
  dapsone (DDS) (Avlosulfon®)
  glucosulfone sodium (Promin®)
  sulfoxone sodium (Diasone®)

Antilipemics

Antilipemics are used together with diet and other measures in the control of hyperlipidemia. For the most part, they act by interfering with either the absorption or the synthesis of cholesterol.

Prominent antilipemics include:
    cholestyramine (Questran®)
    clofibrate (Atromid-S®)
    colestipol (Colestid®)
    dextrothyroxine sodium (Choloxin®)
    niacin (nicotinic acid)
    probucol (Lorelco®)
    sitosterols (Cytellin®)

Antimalarials

See ANTIPROTOZOALS.

Antimaniacals

See PSYCHOTROPICS.

Antinauseants

See ANTIEMETICS.

Antineoplastics

Antineoplastics inhibit the maturation and proliferation of malignant cells; these drugs have distinct mechanisms of action that vary at different drug concentrations and have different effects on different types of normal cells and cancer cells. Typically, antineoplastics cause more extensive injury to certain cancer cells than to the normal tissues. Biochemical mechanisms of action that are known to be involved include inhibition of nucleic acid synthesis (antimetabolites), modification of DNA structure and function (alkylating agents and antibiotics), inhibition of protein synthesis (L-asparaginase), mitotic inhibition (vincristine and vinblastine), and cell membrane interference (steroid compounds). For the most part, antineoplastics are highly toxic, and patients must be monitored closely during therapy.

Prominent alkylating agents include:
    busulfan (Myleran®)
    chlorambucil (Leukeran®)
    cyclophosphamide (Cytoxan®)
    mechlorethamine hydrochloride (nitrogen mustard)
      (Mustargen®)
    melphalan (Alkeran®)
    pipobroman (Vercyte®)
    thiotepa

Prominent antibiotics include:
   bleomycin sulfate (Blenoxane®)
   dactinomycin (actinomycin D) (Cosmegen®)
   daunorubicin
   doxorubicin hydrochloride (Adriamycin®)
   mithramycin (Mithracin®)
   mitomycin (Mutamycin®)

Prominent antimetabolites include:
   cytarabine (Cytosar®)
   dacarbazine (DTIC-Dome®)
   floxuridine (FUDR)
   fluorouracil (5-FU) (Efudex®, Fluoroplex®, Fluorouracil
      Roche®)
   mercaptopurine (6-MP) (Purinethol®)
   methotrexate
   procarbazine hydrochloride (Matulane®)
   tamoxifen citrate (Nolvadex®)
   thioguanine (Thioguanine, Tabloid® Brand)

Prominent corticosteroids include:
   dexamethasone (Decadron®)
   hydrocortisone sodium succinate (Solu-Cortef®)
   methylprednisolone sodium succinate (Solu-Medrol®)
   prednisolone (Meticortelone®)
   prednisone (Deltasone®, Meticorten®)
   triamcinolone (Kenacort®)

Prominent hormones include:
   androgens:
         dromostanolone propionate (Drolban®)
         fluoxymesterone (Halotestin®)
         testolactone (Teslac®)
   estrogens:
         chlorotrianisene (Tace®)
         diethylstilbestrol (DES, stilbestrol)
         diethylstilbestrol diphosphate (Stilphostrol®)
         estradiol (Progynon®)
         estradiol benzoate
         estrogens, conjugated (Premarin®)
         estrogens, esterified (Amnestrogen®, Evex®, Femogen®,
            Menest®)
         ethinyl estradiol (Estinyl®)
         polyestradiol phosphate (Estradurin®)
   progestogens:
         hydroxyprogesterone caproate (Delalutin®)
         medroxyprogesterone acetate (Provera®)
         megestrol acetate (Megace®)

Prominent radioisotopes include:
  gold Au 198 (Aureotope®)
  sodium iodide I 131 (Oriodide®)
  sodium phosphate P 32 (Phosphotope®)

Miscellaneous antineoplastic agents include:
  asparaginase (Elspar®)
  carmustine (BCNU)
  hydroxyurea (Hydrea®)
  lomustine (CCNU) (Cee Nu®)
  mitotane (Lysodren®)
  quinacrine hydrochloride (Atabrine®)
  vinblastine sulfate (Velban®)
  vincristine sulfate (Oncovin®)

Antiparkinsonics

Antiparkinsonics are autonomic and neurohormonal agents used specifically in the management of Parkinson's disease.

Prominent antiparkinsonics include:
  amantadine hydrochloride (Symmetrel®)
  benztropine mesylate (Cogentin®)
  biperiden hydrochloride (Akineton®)
  cycrimine hydrochloride (Pagitane®)
  diphenhydramine (Benadryl®)
  ethopropazine hydrochloride (Parsidol®)
  levodopa (Bendopa®, Dopar®, Larodopa®)
  levodopa/carbidopa (Sinemet®)
  orphenadrine hydrochloride (Disipal®)
  procyclidine hydrochloride (Kemadrin®)
  trihexyphenidyl hydrochloride (Artane®, Tremin®)

Antiprotozoals

Antiprotozoals are drugs used in the treatment of infections caused by protozoa, namely malaria, amebiasis, trichomonas vaginitis, and trypanosomiasis.

Prominent antimalarials (plasmodicides) include:
  amodiaquine hydrochloride (Camoquin®)
  chloroquine hydrochloride (Aralen® Hydrochloride)

chloroquine phosphate (Aralen® Phosphate)
hydroxychloroquine sulfate (Plaquenil®)
primaquine phosphate
pyrimethamine (Daraprim®)
quinine sulfate

Prominent antiamebials (amebicides, antiamebics) include:
arsthinol (Balarsen®)
carbarsone
chloroquine phosphate (Aralen® Phosphate)
diiodohydroxyquin (Diodoquin®)
emetine hydrochloride
metronidazole (Flagyl®)
paromomycin (Humatin®)

Prominent antitrichomonals (trichomonacides) include:
furazolidone/nifuroxime (Tricofuron®)
metronidazole (Flagyl®)
oxyquinoline sulfate (Triva® Combination)
polyoxyethylene nonyl phenol/sodium edetate/sodium dioctyl
sulfosuccinate (Vagisec®)
povidone-iodine (Betadine®)

Prominent antitrypanosomals include:
pentamidine (Lomidine®)
suramin (Antrypol®, Germanin®, Naphuride®)

Prominent antitoxoplasmosis agents include:
pyrimethamine (Daraprim®)
sulfadiazine

Antipruritics

Antipruritics are agents used topically and systemically to allay itching. For the most part they can be categorized as local anesthetics, antihistamines, corticosteroids, or tranquilizers.

Prominent topical preparations include:
benzocaine (Americaine®)
benzyl alcohol/benzocaine (Foille®)
benzyl alcohol/menthol/camphor (Topic®)
calamine lotion, phenolated
cyclomethycaine sulfate (Surfacaine®)
dibucaine hydrochloride (Nupercaine®)
dimethisoquin hydrochloride (Quotane®)

dyclonine hydrochloride (Dyclone®)
menthol preparations (Derma Medicone®, Rhulicream®,
    Solarcaine®)
oatmeal, colloidal (Aveeno®)
pramoxine hydrochloride (Tronothane®)
starch

Prominent systemic preparations include:
cholestyramine (Questran®)
cyproheptadine hydrochloride (Periactin®)
methdilazine hydrochloride (Tacaryl®)
trimeprazine tartrate (Temaril®)

Antipsoriatics

Antipsoriatics encompass the various agents and preparations used in the treatment of psoriasis. These include coal tar, anthralin (Anthra-Derm®, Lasan® Unguent), keratolytics (see), topical and systemic corticosteroids (see), and the photosensitizing agent methoxsalen (Oxsoralen®). (Methoxsalen is used in conjunction with ultraviolet A light.)

Antipsychotics

See PSYCHOTROPICS.

Antipyretics

Antipyretics are agents that relieve or reduce fever. The most commonly used are aspirin, acetaminophen, and phenacetin (see ANALGESICS).

Antiseptics

See ANTI-INFECTIVES, LOCAL.

Antispasmodics

Antispasmodics relieve spasms of the smooth muscle in the arteries, bronchi, intestine, bile duct, ureters, and sphincters. Therapeutic indications include myocardial infarction, angina pectoris, embolism, peripheral vascular disease, neurogenic bladder, and ureteral, biliary, and gastrointestinal colic. For the most part, antispasmodics include anticholinergics (see), adrenergic vasodilators (see), and direct muscle relaxants.

Standard direct muscle relaxants include:
dioxyline phosphate (Paveril®)
ethaverine hydrochloride (Cebral®, Eta-Lent®, Ethaquin®, Isovex-100®)
flavoxate hydrochloride (Urispas®)
oxybutynin chloride (Ditropan®)
papaverine hydrochloride (Cerespan®, Pavabid®, Pavakey®, Vasospan®)
thiphenamil hydrochloride (Trocinate®)

Antithyroids

Antithyroids (goitrogens) are agents that interfere with the formation of thyroid hormones; they are used in the treatment of hyperthyroidism. For the most part, the category includes iodine (regular and radioactive) and thiouracil derivatives.

Prominent antithyroids include:
iodine solution, strong (Lugol's solution)
methimazole (Tapazole®)
propylthiouracil (PTU)
sodium iodide I 131 (Oriodide®, Theriodide®)

Antitoxins

See BIOLOGICALS.

Antituberculotics

Antituberculotics are agents used in the treatment of tuberculosis. They include antibiotics and miscellaneous anti-infectives, and they act chiefly by preventing the multiplication of the tubercle bacilli *(Mycobacterium tuberculosis)*.

The major antituberculotics include:
aminosalicylic acid (PAS) (Pamisyl®, Rezipas®)
capreomycin sulfate (Capastat®)
cycloserine (Seromycin®)
ethambutol hydrochloride (Myambutol®)
ethionamide (Trecator®-SC)
isoniazid (INH) (Nydrazid®)
pyrazinamide (PZA) (Aldinamide®)
rifampin (Rifadin®, Rimactane®)
rifampin/isoniazid (Rifamate™, Rimactazid®)
streptomycin sulfate
viomycin sulfate (Viocin®)

Antitussives and expectorants

Antitussives and expectorants are the basic ingredients of most cough preparations (see); antitussives act on the cough center to suppress the cough reflex, and expectorants promote or facilitate secretion or expulsion of mucus from the respiratory passageways.

Prominent antitussives include:
> benzonatate (Tessalon®)
> codeine phosphate
> dextromethorphan hydrobromide
> hydrocodone bitartrate/homatropine methylbromide (Hycodan®)
> levopropoxyphene napsylate (Novrad®)

Prominent expectorants include:
> ammonium chloride
> guaifenesin (Robitussin®)
> hydriodic acid syrup
> potassium iodide solution (SSKI)
> terpin hydrate

Antivenins

See BIOLOGICALS.

Antivertigo agents

See ANTIEMETICS.

Antivirals

Antivirals are agents that destroy viruses or suppress their replication. Those of note at present include: idoxuridine (Dendrid®, Herplex®, Stoxil®), a local anti-infective; vidabarine (Vira-A®), a local anti-infective; and amantadine hydrochloride (Symmetrel®), used in the prophylaxis and treatment of influenza A respiratory tract illness.

Astringents

Astringents are chemical agents that contract and harden tissues and arrest discharges. They are applied to the skin and mucous membranes of patients with conditions that are improved by this type of action, namely bed sores, weeping ulcers, and similar denuded and bleeding surfaces.

Prominent astringents include:
> aluminum acetate solution, modified (Bluboro® Powder, Domeboro® Powder)
> aluminum acetate solution (Burow's solution)
> aluminum chloride (Drysol™)

aluminum subacetate solution
silver nitrate
witch hazel
zinc sulfate

Ataractics

See PSYCHOTROPICS.

Barbiturates

See SEDATIVE-HYPNOTICS.

Biologicals

Biologicals are preparations of biological origin used in the treatment and prevention of allergies, infectious diseases, and envenomation. Biologicals include allergens, immune serums, antitoxins, vaccines, toxoids, and antivenins. Allergens, which are proteinaceous extracts of various substances, are used to determine the susceptibility of the patient to these agents; allergens are also used to prevent and relieve the conditions caused by hypersensitivity. Immune serums and antitoxins are blood serums of animal or human origin containing high concentrations of antibodies against specific pathogens and/or microbial toxins. They are used to prevent infection in exposed susceptible persons (via passive immunity) as well as to treat infection. Vaccines (preparations of killed or attenuated microorganisms and/or cellular components thereof) and toxoids (neutralized toxins) are used to provoke active, long-term immunity against infection. Antivenins (serums containing venom-neutralizing globulins) are used against the poisonous effects of bites, stings, or effluvia of insects and other arthropods, and of the bites of snakes.

Standard preparations include allergenic extracts of
drugs
dusts
epidermals
foods
inhalants
insects
molds
pollen
poison ivy, poison oak, poison sumac
smuts

Prominent immune serums and antitoxins include:
antirabies serum
antivenin, *Latrodectus mactans* (black widow spider)

antivenin, *Micrurus fulvius* (coral snake)
antivenin, polyvalent crotaline (pit viper)
botulism antitoxin
diphtheria antitoxin
gas gangrene antitoxin, polyvalent
globulin, immune human serum (Gamastan®, Gammagee®, Immu-G®)
globulin, Rh_o (D) immune human (Gamulin® Rh, RhoGAM®)
mumps immune human globulin (Hyparotin®)
pertussis immune human globulin (Hypertussis®)
tetanus antitoxin
tetanus immune human globulin (Ar-Tet®, Homo-Tet®, Hyper-Tet®, IMMU-Tetanus®)

Prominent toxoids include:
diphtheria toxoid
diphtheria toxoid/tetanus toxoid, adsorbed
diphtheria toxoid/tetanus toxoid/pertussis vaccine, absorbed (DTP) (Tri-Immunol®, Triogen®, Tri-Solgen®)
tetanus toxoid, adsorbed

Prominent vaccines include:
BCG vaccine (tuberculosis vaccine)
cholera vaccine
influenza virus vaccine
measles, mumps, and rubella virus vaccine, live (M-M-R®)
measles virus vaccine, live attenuated (Attenuvax®)
mumps virus vaccine, live (Mumpsvax®)
pneumococcal vaccine, polyvalent (Pneumovax®)
poliovirus vaccine, live oral (Diplovax®, Orimune®)
rabies vaccine
Rocky Mountain spotted fever vaccine
rubella and mumps virus vaccine, live (Bivax®)
rubella virus vaccine, live (Cendevax®, Meruvax®)
smallpox vaccine
typhoid vaccine
typhus vaccine
yellow fever vaccine

Blood calcium regulators

Blood calcium regulators are used to maintain the proper level of ionic calcium in the plasma and to treat hypoparathyroidism, rickets, and certain other hypocalcemic conditions. These agents include calcium salts, the parathyroid hormone, calcitonin, and vitamin D. The parathyroid hormone stimulates the release of calcium from bone, whereas calcitonin inhibits bone resorption. Vitamin D stimulates the absorption of calcium and phosphate from the intestine.

Prominent blood calcium regulators include:
calcitonin (Calcimar®)
calcium chloride injection
calcium gluceptate injection
calcium gluconate
dihydrotachysterol (Hytakerol®)
ergocalciferol (vitamin D₂) (Calciferol™, Drisdol®)
ergocalciferol/dibasic calcium phosphate (Dical-D®)
parathyroid injection

Bronchodilators

See ANTIASTHMATICS.

Calcium regulators

See BLOOD CALCIUM REGULATORS.

Carbonic anhydrase inhibitors

Carbonic anhydrase inhibitors limit the production of aqueous humor (the fluid of the anterior cavity of the eye), although they promote the production of urine; both actions result from the inhibition of the enzyme carbonic anhydrase. These agents are useful in the management of glaucoma because the reduced production of aqueous humor leads to lowered intraocular pressure.

Major carbonic anhydrase inhibitors include:
acetazolamide (Diamox®)
dichlorphenamide (Daranide®)
ethoxzolamide (Cardrase®)
methazolamide (Neptazane®)

Cardiacs

Cardiacs are agents that act on the heart; they include digitalis and digitalis-like glycosides, antiarrhythmics, coronary vasodilators, and beta-adrenergic blocking agents. Cardiac glycosides strengthen heart muscle (positive inotropic action) and are used in the treatment of congestive heart failure. Antiarrhythmics alter the heart rate; they are used to re-establish and maintain normal cardiac rhythmicity and excitability. Coronary vasodilators are used in the treatment of angina pectoris. Beta-adrenergic blocking agents are used to treat arrhythmias, angina pectoris, and hypertension.

Standard cardiac glycosides include:
    acetyldigitoxin (Acylanid®)
    deslanoside (Cedilanid®-D)
    digitalis
    digitoxin (Crystodigin®, Digitaline Nativelle®, Purodigin®)
    digoxin (Lanoxin®)
    gitalin (Gitaligin®)
    lanatoside C (Cedilanid®)
    ouabain (G-strophanthin)

Prominent antiarrhythmics include:
    disopyramide phosphate (Norpace®)
    lidocaine hydrochloride (Xylocaine®)
    phenytoin sodium (Dilantin®)
    procainamide hydrochloride (Pronestyl®)
    propranolol hydrochloride (Inderal®)
    quinidine gluconate (Quinaglute®)
    quinidine polygalacturonate (Cardioquin®)
    quinidine sulfate (Quinidex®, Quinora®)

Prominent coronary vasodilators include:
    amyl nitrite
    dipyridamole (Persantine®)
    erythrityl tetranitrate (Cardilate®)
    isosorbide dinitrate (Iso-Bid®, Isordil®, Laserdil®, Sorate®, Sorbitrate®)
    nitroglycerin (glyceryl trinitrate) (Nitro-Bid, Nitroglyn®, Nitrol®, Nitrong®, Nitrospan®, Nitrostat®)
    papaverine hydrochloride (Cerespan®, Vasopan®)
    pentaerythritol tetranitrate (Pentritol®, Peritrate®)

Prominent beta-adrenergic blocking agents include:
    propranolol hydrochloride (Inderal®)

Cathartics

Cathartics are agents that promote defecation. Those with a strong effect are referred to as purgatives and those with a mild effect are referred to as laxatives. The mechanisms of action include fecal softening, lubrication, and peristaltic stimulation; the peristaltic stimulation occurs as a result of either irritation or bulk.

Prominent cathartics include:
    bisacodyl (Dulcolax®)
    carboxymethylcellulose sodium (Dialose®)
    casanthranol (Peristim® Forte)
    cascara sagrada

castor oil
danthron (Dorbane®, Modane®)
dioctyl calcium sulfosuccinate (Surfak®)
dioctyl sodium sulfosuccinate (Colace®, Comfolax®,
    Doxinate®)
dioctyl sodium sulfosuccinate/casanthranol (Peri-Colace®)
glycerin suppositories
magnesia, milk of (magnesia magma, magnesium hydroxide)
magnesium citrate solution (citrate of magnesia)
magnesium sulfate (Epsom salt)
mineral oil (liquid petrolatum) (Agoral®)
psyllium hydrophilic mucilloid (Effersyllium®, Konsyl®,
    Metamucil®)
senna concentrate (Senokot®)
sodium phosphate and biphosphate enema (Fleet® Brand
    Enema)
sodium phosphate and biphosphate oral solution (Fleet® Brand
    Phospho®-Soda)

Cerebral stimulants

Cerebral stimulants act on the higher centers of the brain and possibly
on the limbic system; the amphetamines and their congeners also
exhibit adrenergic activity. Cerebral stimulants are used to treat narcolepsy, minimal brain dysfunction, and hyperkinesis, and to suppress
the appetite in weight control.

Prominent cerebral stimulants include:
    amphetamine sulfate (Benzedrine®)
    deanol acetamidobenzoate (Deaner®)
    dextroamphetamine sulfate (Dexedrine®)
    dextroamphetamine sulfate/amobarbital (Dexamyl®)
    methylphenidate hydrochloride (Ritalin®)
    pemoline (Cylert®)

Cerebral stimulants used exclusively as anorectics include:
    benzphetamine hydrochloride (Didrex™)
    chlorphentermine hydrochloride (Pre-sate®)
    clortermine hydrochloride (Voranil®)
    diethylpropion hydrochloride (Tenuate®, Tepanil®)
    fenfluramine hydrochloride (Pondimin®)
    mazindol (Sanorex®)
    methamphetamine hydrochloride (Fetamin®)
    phenmetrazine hydrochloride (Preludin®)
    phentermine resin (Ionamin®)

Ceruminolytics

Ceruminolytics are agents that dissolve cerumen (earwax) in the external auditory canal.

Prominent preparations include:
    carbamide peroxide 6.5% (Debrox®)
    hydrogen peroxide
    mineral oil (liquid petrolatum)
    triethanolamine polypeptide oleate condensate (Cerumenex®)

Chelating agents

See HEAVY METAL ANTAGONISTS.

Choleretics

Choleretics are agents that stimulate the production of bile by the liver by either cholepoiesis or hydrocholeresis. The most important, bile acids and bile salts, are used to aid digestion (see DIGESTANTS) in hepatic disorders and increase biliary drainage in functional (nonobstructive) disorders of the biliary tract. For the latter purpose, the medicinals of choice are hydrocholeretics.

Prominent hydrocholeretics include:
    dehydrocholic acid (Decholin®)
    dehydrocholic acid/homatropine (Hepahydrin®)
    florantyrone (Zanchol®)
    sodium dehydrocholate (Decholin® Sodium)

Cholinergics

Cholinergics are agents that produce effects similar to those caused by stimulation of the parasympathetic nervous system; some act by simulating acetylcholine and others by inhibiting cholinesterase. For the most part, cholinergics are used in the treatment of intestinal atony, urinary retention, glaucoma, and anticholinergic poisoning, and in the diagnosis and treatment of myasthenia gravis.

Prominent cholinergics include:
    acetylcholine chloride (Miochol®)
    ambenoniun chloride (Mytelase®)
    bethanechol chloride (Urecholine®)
    carbachol (Isopto® Carbachol)
    demecarium bromide (Humorsol®)
    echothiophate iodide (Phospholine Iodide®)
    edrophonium chloride (Tensilon®)
    neostigmine bromide (Prostigmin®)

oxyphencyclimine hydrochloride (Daricon®)
physostigmine salicylate (eserine) (Antilirium®)
pilocarpine hydrochloride (Isopto® Carpine)
pyridostigmine bromide (Mestinon®)

Contraceptives, oral

Oral contraceptives ("the pill") contain synthetic progestogens and estrogens; they are almost 100% effective if taken according to directions. The mechanism of action seems mainly to involve the inhibition of ovulation by the suppression of the pituitary (anterior) output of gonadotropic hormones.

Prominent preparations (listed in the order progestogen/estrogen) include:
ethynodiol diacetate/ethinyl estradiol (Demulen®)
ethynodiol diacetate/mestranol (Ovulen®)
norethindrone/mestranol (Norinyl®, Ortho-Novum®)
norethindrone acetate/ethinyl estradiol (Loestrin®, Norlestrin®)
norethynodrel/mestranol (Enovid-E®)
norgestrel/ethinyl estradiol (Lo/Ovral®)

Contraceptives, topical

Topical contraceptives are spermicides that are used alone or in combination with mechanical devices.

Prominent topical contraceptives include:
dodecaethyleneglycol monolaurate (Ramses® Vaginal Jelly)
nonoxynol 9 (Conceptrol®, Ortho-Creme®, Semicid®)
nonylphenoxypolyoxyethylene ethanol (Because®)
para-diisobutylphenoxypolyethoxyethanol (Preceptin®)
phenylmercuric acetate (Lorophyn®)

Contrast media, radiopaque

See DIAGNOSTICS, roentgenography.

Corticosteroids

Corticosteroids include the hormones of the adrenal cortex and their analogues and congeners. For the most part, they can be categorized as *glucocorticoids,* which mainly affect carbohydrate and protein metabolism, and *mineralocorticoids,* which predominantly affect water and electrolyte metabolism.* Corticosteroids are used as specific re-

---

*All except desoxycorticosterone and fludrocortisone are basically glucocorticoids; fludrocortisone is both a potent mineralocorticoid and glucocorticoid.

placement therapy in adrenocortical insufficiency and for suppression of adrenal overactivity, but they are most commonly used for their anti-inflammatory, antiallergic, and lympholytic properties (in leukemia). Corticosteroids are available both as single entities and as combinations (along with analgesics, antihistamines, antibiotics, antipruritics, local anesthetics, vasoconstrictors, or other supportive additions). Depending on the condition being treated and/or the nature of the preparation, corticosteroids are administered orally, by injection (for systemic and local effect), or topically (in ophthalmic, otic, and dermatologic disorders).

Prominent corticosteroids include:
    beclomethasone dipropionate (Vanceril®)
    betamethasone (Celestone®)
    betamethasone benzoate (Benisone®, Flurobate®)
    betamethasone dipropionate (Diprosone®)
    betamethasone valerate (Valisone®)
    cortisone acetate (Cortone®)
    desonide (Tridesilon®)
    desoximetasone (Topicort®)
    desoxycorticosterone acetate (Doca®, Percorten®)
    desoxycorticosterone pivalate (Percorten® Pivalate)
    dexamethasone (Decadron®, Deronil®, Dexone™, Gammacorten®, Hexadrol®)
    dexamethasone acetate (Decadron-LA®)
    fludrocortisone acetate (Florinef®)
    flumethasone pivalate (Locorten®)
    fluocinolone acetonide (Fluonid®, Synalar®, Synemol®)
    fluocinonide (Lidex®)
    flurandrenolide (Cordran®)
    halcinonide (Halog®)
    hydrocortisone (Cort-Dome®, Cortef®, Cortril®)
    hydrocortisone sodium succinate (Solu-Cortef®)
    meprednisone (Betapar®)
    methylprednisolone (Medrol®)
    paramethasone acetate (Haldrone®)
    prednisolone (Delta-Cortef®, Hydeltra®, Meticortelone®)
    prednisolone acetate (Sterane®)
    prednisolone acetate/sodium sulfacetamide (Metimyd®)
    prednisolone sodium phosphate (Metreton®, Optimyd®)
    prednisolone sodium succinate (Meticortelone® Soluble Sterile Powder)
    prednisone (Deltasone®, Meticorten®)
    triamcinolone (Aristocort®, Kenacort®)
    triamcinolone acetonide (Aristocort® A, Kenalog®)
    triamcinolone hexacetonide (Aristospan®)

Cough-cold preparations

Cough-cold preparations (antitussives, expectorants, decongestants, "cold remedies," and the like) number in the hundreds. Typically, they contain two or more active ingredients from among the following: antitussives and expectorants (see), nasal decongestants (see), antihistamines (see), antipyretics (see), and analgesics (see). For the most part, those without codeine are available without prescription.

Popular cough preparations (with the amount of active ingredients per 5 ml) include:

Actifed-C® Expectorant

codeine phosphate	10	mg
guaifenesin	100	mg
pseudoephedrine hydrochloride	30	mg
triprolidine hydrochloride	2	mg

Ambenyl® Expectorant

ammonium chloride	80	mg
bromodiphenhydramine hydrochloride	3.75	mg
codeine sulfate	10	mg
diphenhydramine hydrochloride	8.75	mg
menthol	500	μg
potassium guaiacolsulfonate	80	mg

Benylin® Cough Syrup

diphenhydramine hydrochloride	12.5	mg

Cerose® Sedative Expectorant

citric acid	60	mg
codeine phosphate	10	mg
fluidextract of ipecac	0.16	minim
glycerol	40	minim
phenindamine tartrate	10	mg
phenylephrine hydrochloride	5	mg
potassium guaiacolsulfonate	80	mg
sodium citrate	180	mg

Cerose®-DM

The same as Cerose® Sedative Expectorant except for dextromethorphan hydrobromide 10 mg instead of codeine

Cheracol®

codeine phosphate	11	mg
guaifenesin	15	mg
white pine and wild cherry bark		

Cheracol® D
  The same as Cheracol® except for
  dextromethorphan hydrobromide
  10 mg instead of codeine

Dimetane® Expectorant

brompheniramine maleate	2	mg
guaifenesin	100	mg
phenylephrine hydrochloride	5	mg
phenylpropanolamine hydro-chloride	5	mg

Dimetane® Expectorant DC
  The same as Dimetane® Expectorant
  plus codeine phosphate 10 mg

Hycomine® Syrup

hydrocodone bitartrate	5	mg
phenylpropanolamine hydro-chloride	25	mg

Hycotuss® Expectorant

guaifenesin	100	mg
hydrocodone bitartrate	5	mg

Novahistine® DH

codeine phosphate	10	mg
phenylpropanolamine hydro-chloride	18.75	mg

Novahistine® Elixir

chlorpheniramine maleate	2	mg
phenylpropanolamine hydro-chloride	18.75	mg

Novahistine® Expectorant

codeine phosphate	10	mg
guaifenesin	100	mg
phenylpropanolamine hydro-chloride	18.75	mg

Phenergan® Expectorant*

citric acid	60	mg
fluidextract of ipecac	0.17	minim
potassium guaiacolsulfonate	44	mg
promethazine hydrochloride	5	mg
sodium citrate	197	mg

Phenergan® VC Expectorant*

citric acid	60	mg
fluidextract of ipecac	0.17	minim
phenylephrine hydrochloride	5	mg

*Available with codeine phosphate (10 mg) or dextromethorphan hydrobromide (7.5 mg).

potassium guaiacolsulfonate	44	mg
promethazine hydrochloride	5	mg
sodium citrate	197	mg
Robitussin®		
guaifenesin	100	mg
Robitussin A-C®		
codeine phosphate	10	mg
guaifenesin	100	mg
Robitussin-CF®		
dextromethorphan hydrobromide	10	mg
guaifenesin	50	mg
phenylpropanolamine hydrochloride	12.5	mg
Robitussin-DM®		
dextromethorphan hydrobromide	15	mg
guaifenesin	100	mg
Robitussin-PE®		
guaifenesin	100	mg
pseudoephedrine hydrochloride	30	mg
terpin hydrate/codeine elixir		
codeine	10	mg
terpin hydrate	85	mg
Triaminic® Expectorant		
guaifenesin	100	mg
pheniramine maleate	6.25	mg
phenylpropanolamine hydrochloride	12.5	mg
pyrilamine maleate	6.25	mg
Triaminicol® Cough Syrup		
ammonium chloride	90	mg
dextromethorphan hydrobromide	15	mg
pheniramine maleate	6.25	mg
phenylpropanolamine hydrochloride	12.5	mg
pyrilamine maleate	6.25	mg
Tussend® Expectorant		
guaifenesin	200	mg
hydrocodone bitartrate	5	mg
pseudoephedrine hydrochloride	30	mg

Popular preparations for the common cold and other upper respiratory illnesses (with the amount of each ingredient per tablet or capsule) include:

Actifed® Tablets		
pseudoephedrine hydrochloride	60	mg
triprolidine hydrochloride	2.5	mg
Cerose® Compound Capsules		
acetaminophen	194	mg
ascorbic acid	25	mg
chlorpheniramine maleate	2	mg
dextromethorphan hydrobromide	10	mg

phenylephrine hydrochloride	7.5	mg
terpin hydrate	64.8	mg
Coricidin® "D" Decongestant Tablets		
aspirin	390	mg
chlorpheniramine maleate	2	mg
phenylpropanolamine hydrochloride	12.5	mg
Dimetapp® Extentabs®		
brompheniramine maleate	12	mg
phenylephrine hydrochloride	15	mg
phenylpropanolamine hydrochloride	15	mg
Emprazil® Tablets		
aspirin	200	mg
caffeine	30	mg
phenacetin	150	mg
pseudoephedrine hydrochloride	20	mg
Novafed® A Capsules		
pseudoephedrine hydrochloride	120	mg
chlorpheniramine maleate	8	mg
Ornade® Spansule® Capsules		
chlorpheniramine maleate	8	mg
isopropamide iodide	2.5	mg
phenylpropanolamine hydrochloride	50	mg
Sinutab® Tablets		
acetaminophen	325	mg
phenylpropanolamine hydrochloride	25	mg
phenyltoloxamine citrate	22	mg
Tuss-Ornade® Spansule® Capsules		
caramiphen edisylate	20	mg
chlorpheniramine maleate	8	mg
isopropamide iodide	2.5	mg
phenylpropanolamine hydrochloride	50	mg

Counterirritants

Counterirritants are topical agents employed to produce local irritation and thereby counter or relieve another, more distressing irritation or pain. Typically they are employed for minor aches and pains, athletic soreness, and temporary relief of minor arthritis and rheumatism.

Prominent counterirritants include:
    camphor
    menthol
    methyl nicotinate
    methyl salicylate

Debridement enzymes

Debridement enzymes are proteolytic enzymes used topically in the chemical debridement of necrotic wounds, abscesses, empyema, fistulas, hematomas, and blood clots. They also help to resolve inflammation. Their basic action is the digestion and liquefaction of dead material.

Prominent agents include:
    collagenase (Santyl®)
    fibrinolysin/desoxyribonuclease (Elase®)
    fibrinolysin/desoxyribonuclease/chloramphenicol
        (Elase-Chloromycetin® Ointment)
    neomycin palmitate/trypsin/chymotrypsin (Biozyme®)
    papain/urea/chlorophyll derivatives (Panafil®)
    streptokinase/streptodornase (Varidase®)
    sutilains (Travase®)

Decongestants

See NASAL DECONGESTANTS.

Deodorants

Medical deodorants are used topically to reduce unpleasant odors in wounds, burns, surface ulcers, cuts, abrasions, and skin irritations; systemically, they are used to reduce fecal and urinary odors in patients with colostomy, ileostomy, or incontinence.

Prominent deodorants include:
    charcoal, activated
    chlorophyll derivatives, oral (Derifil®)
    chlorophyll derivatives, topical (Chloresium®)

Detergents

Medicinal detergents are chemical agents and preparations used for the cleansing and/or disinfection of the skin.

Prominent detergents include:
    cetyl alcohol/sodium lauryl sulfate (Cetaphil®)
    chlorhexidene gluconate (Hibiclens®)
    entsulfon sodium (pHisoDerm®)
    green soap tincture (medicinal soft soap liniment)
    hexachlorophene detergent (pHisoHex®)
    povidone-iodine (Betadine®)
    sodium lauryl sulfoacetate (Lowila® Cake)

Diagnostics

Diagnostics are agents used to signal abnormal function, organic pathological conditions, and specific infections.

Prominent diagnostics (listed under the appropriate disorders or tests) include:

    adrenocortical insufficiency:
        corticotropin (ACTH) (Acthar®)
        cosyntropin (Cortrosyn®)
    allergy (skin tests):
        allergenic extracts
    cardiac output:
        indocyanine green (Cardio-Green®, CG®)
    circulation time:
        sodium dehydrocholate (Decholin® Sodium)
    coccidioidomycosis:
        coccidioidin
    conjunctival lesions:
        fluorescein sodium
    diabetes mellitus:
        tolbutamide sodium (Orinase Diagnostic®)
    diphtheria (susceptibility to):
        diphtheria toxin for Schick test
    gastric function:
        betazole hydrochloride (Histalog®)
        histamine phosphate injection
    glucose tolerance:
        Glucola®
    histoplasmosis:
        histoplasmin
    kidney function:
        mannitol
        indigotindisulfonate sodium (indigo carmine)
        phenolsulfonphthalein (PSP)
    liver function:
        sulfobromophthalein sodium (BSP®, Bromsulphalein®)
    mononucleosis:
        Monospot™
    mumps:
        mumps skin test antigen
    myasthenia gravis:
        edrophonium chloride (Tensilon®)
        neostigmine methylsulfate (Prostigmin®)
    pancreatic function:
        secretin (Secretin–Boots)

parathyroid function:
    parathyroid injection
pheochromocytoma:
    histamine phospate injection
    phentolamine mesylate (Regitine®)
pituitary function:
    metyrapone (Metopirone®)
pregnancy:
    Gravindex™ Slide Test
roentgenography (radiopaque contrast media):
    barium sulfate (Barosperse®, Barotrast®)
    diatrizoate meglumine preparations (Cardiografin®, Cysto-
        grafin®, Gastrografin®, Renografin®, Reno-M-30®,
        Reno-M-60®)
    diatrizoate sodium (Hypaque® Sodium)
    iodipamide meglumine (Cholografin®)
    iodipamide meglumine/diatrizoate meglumine
        (Sinografin®)
    iopanoic acid (Telepaque®)
    iophendylate (Pantopaque®)
    iothalamate meglumine (Conray®)
    ipodate calcium (Oragrafin® Calcium)
    ipodate sodium (Oragrafin® Sodium)
    Lipiodol®
    metrizoate preparations (Isopaque® 280, Isopaque® 440)
    tyropanoate sodium (Bilopaque®)
thyroid function test:
    thyrotropin (Thytropar®)
tuberculosis:
    tuberculin, old
    tuberculin, purified protein derivative (PPD) (Aplisol®,
        Tubersol®)
urine (bacteriuria):
    Microstix®-3
urine (glucose):
    Clinitest®
    Tes-Tape®
urine (phenylketonuria)
    Phenistix®
urine (protein, glucose, ketones, bilirubin, blood, urobilinogen,
    nitrite, pH):
    N-Multistix™
vaginal candidiasis:
    Microstix®-Candida

Dialyzing solutions

Dialyzing solutions are hypertonic solutions employed in intermittent peritoneal dialysis, a simplified technique of extrarenal excretion that employs the peritoneum as the dialyzing membrane. Indications include acute renal failure, barbiturate poisoning (and other dialyzable poisons), intractable edema, hepatic coma, hypercalcemia, azotemia, hyperkalemia, and uremia.

Prominent preparations include:
Dianeal®/Dextrose 1.25%
Dianeal®/Dextrose 4.25%
Dianeal®K/Dextrose 1.5%
Inpersol®/Dextrose 1.5%
Inpersol®/Dextrose 4.25%
Inpersol®-K/Dextrose 1.5%
Peridial®/Dextrose 1.5%
Peridial®/Dextrose 4.25%

Digestants

Digestants promote digestion and constitute replacement therapy in deficiency states. In healthy persons, they are used to diminish intestinal gas. For the most part, digestants include hydrochloric acid, bile salts, and enzymes. (Alcoholic beverages also function as digestants.)

Prominent preparations include:
dehydrocholic acid (Decholin®)
florantyrone (Zanchol®)
glutamic acid hydrochloride (Acidulin®)
hydrochloric acid 10%
ox bile extract (bile salts)
pancreatin (Viokase®)
pancrelipase (Cotazym®, Ilozyme®)
peppermint spirit
pepsin
pepsin/pancreatin/bile salts (Entozyme®)
pepsin/pancreatin/bile salts/belladonna alkaloids/phenobarbital (Donnazyme®)
pepsin/pancreatin/cellulase/glutamic acid/ox bile extract (Kanulase®)

Digitalis

See CARDIACS.

Disinfectants

See ANTI-INFECTIVES, LOCAL.

Diuretics

Diuretics increase the output of urine; they are used to treat edema and hypertension. The mechanism of diuretic action (leading to relief of edema) mainly involves inhibiting electrolyte (namely sodium) reabsorption in the renal tubules or increasing the osmotic pressure of the glomerular filtrate or plasma compartment. The mechanism of the antihypertensive effect is unknown.

Prominent diuretics include:
  acetazolamide (Diamox®)
  bendroflumethiazide (Naturetin®)
  benzthiazide (Exna®)
  chlorothiazide (Diuril®)
  chlorthalidone (Hygroton®)
  ethacrynic acid (Edecrin®)
  furosemide (Lasix®)
  hydrochlorothiazide (Esidrix®, HydroDIURIL®, Oretic®)
  hydroflumethiazide (Diucardin®)
  mannitol injection (Osmitrol®)
  mercaptomerin sodium (Thiomerin®)
  merethoxylline procaine (Dicurin®)
  metolazone (Zaroxolyn®)
  polythiazide (Renese®)
  quinethazone (Hydromox®)
  spironolactone (Aldactone®)
  spironolactone/hydrochlorothiazide (Aldactazide®)
  triamterene (Dyrenium®)
  triamterene/hydrochlorothiazide (Dyazide®)
  trichlormethiazide (Naqua®)
  urea, sterile (Ureaphil®)

Electrolyte solutions and water-balance agents

Electrolyte solutions and water-balance agents are preparations (exclusive of diuretics) used to maintain fluid, electrolyte, and acid-base balance and to correct imbalances. Electrolyte solutions (injections) supply anions and cations (namely acetate, lactate, Na^+, K^+, Ca^{2+}, Cl^-, HCO_3^-, PO_4^{3-}) and water.

Standard preparations include:
  acidifying agents:
    ammonium chloride
    potassium acid phosphate (K-Phos®)
  alkalizing agents:
    sodium bicarbonate
    sodium citrate
    sodium citrate/potassium citrate (Polycitra®)

    sodium lactate
    tromethamine (Tham)
ammonia detoxicants:
    arginine glutamate
    arginine hydrochloride (R-Gene™ 10)
    lactulose syrup (Cephulac®)
plasma extenders:
    albumin, normal human serum (Albuspan®)
    dextran 40 (Rheomacrodex®)
    dextran 70 (Macrodex®)
    plasma protein fraction, human (Plasmanate®,
      Plasmatein®)
potassium-removing resin:
    sodium polystyrene sulfonate (Kayexalate®)
potassium supplements (oral):
    potassium bicarbonate/potassium citrate (K-Lyte®)
    potassium chloride (Kaochlor®, Kay Ciel®, K-Lor®,
      Kaon-Cl Tabs®, Slow-K®)
    potassium gluconate (Kaon®, Kolyum®)
replacement solutions:
    electrolyte solution, oral
      (Pedialyte®)

calcium	4	mEq/L
calories	20.03	ml
chloride	30	mEq/L
dextrose	50	g/L
lactate	28	mEq/L
magnesium	4	mEq/L
potassium	20	mEq/L
sodium	30	mEq/L

    potassic saline injection, lactated
      (Darrow's solution)

chloride	104	mEq/L
lactate	53	mEq/L
potassium	35	mEq/L
sodium	122	mEq/L

    Ringer's injection

calcium	5	mEq/L
chloride	156	mEq/L
potassium	4	mEq/L
sodium	147	mEq/L

    Ringer's injection, lactated

calcium	3	mEq/L
chloride	110	mEq/L
lactate	27	mEq/L
potassium	4	mEq/L
sodium	130	mEq/L

sodium chloride injection (hypo-
tonic)   0.45%
sodium chloride injection (iso-
tonic)   0.9%

Emetics

Emetics induce vomiting by direct action on the vomiting center or
at some point in the reflex arc. They are used as a first-aid measure
when prompt evacuation is essential.

The most effective agents are:
apomorphine hydrochloride
ipecac syrup

Emollient-protectants

Emollients-protectants are topical agents used to soothe and/or protect the skin and mucous membranes. They are usually employed as
vehicles for other dermatologic agents.

Prominent preparations include:
aluminum paste
benzoin tincture, compound
calamine lotion
collodion
collodion, flexible
dimethicone (Silicote®)
glycerol (glycerin)
hydrophilic ointment
lanolin (hydrous wool fat)
lanolin, anhydrous
methoxsalen (Oxsoralen®)
oatmeal, colloidal (Aveeno®)
olive oil
oxybenzone/dioxybenzone (Solbar®)
para-aminobenzoic acid ointment (Pabanol®, PreSun®)
petrolatum (petroleum jelly)
rose water ointment
starch
talc (talcum)
titanium dioxide preparations (A-Fil®, Surfadil®)
urea (Aquacare®, Carmol®)
zinc gelatin (Unna's boot)
zinc oxide
zinc oxide/salicylic acid (Lassar's paste)

Enzymes

Enzymes are the organic catalysts involved in all biochemical reactions. Those used in medicine include hyaluronidase, chymotrypsin, anti-inflammatory enzymes (see), debridement enzymes (see), and digestive enzymes, also known as digestants (see). Hyaluronidase (Alidase®, Hyazyme®, Wydase®) is a mucolytic enzyme that digests hyaluronic acid ("intercellular cement") and thereby facilitates absorption and distribution of infusions, local anesthetics, and drugs. (It is especially useful in hypodermoclysis.) Ophthalmic chymotrypsin (Alpha Chymar®) is used in cataract operations to loosen the suspensory ligaments attached to the lens.

Estrogens

Estrogens are female sex hormones; natural estrogens are steroids, while synthetic estrogens include both steroid and nonsteroid forms. Biologically, estrogens are responsible for the development of the sex organs at puberty and for secondary sex characteristics. Therapeutic indications, which are varied and numerous, include hypogonadism, menopause, postmenopausal osteoporosis, senile vaginitis, functional uterine bleeding, postpartum breast engorgement, prostatic carcinoma, and postmenopausal breast cancer. Estrogens combined with progestogens are used as oral contraceptives (see).

Prominent estrogens (other than those used as oral contraceptives) include:

> chlorotrianisene (Tace®)
> diethylstilbestrol (DES, stilbestrol)
> diethylstilbestrol diphosphate (Stilphostrol®)
> diethylstilbestrol/methyltestosterone (Tylosterone®)
> estradiol (Progynon®)
> estradiol benzoate
> estradiol cypionate (Depo®-Estradiol)
> estradiol valerate/testosterone enanthate (Deladumone®)
> estrogens, conjugated (Femest®, Premarin®)
> estrogens, esterified (Amnestrogen®, Evex®, Femogen®, Menest®)
> estrone/estradiol/estriol (Hormonin®)
> ethinyl estradiol (Estinyl®, Feminone®)
> piperazine estrone sulfate (Ogen®)

Expectorants

See ANTITUSSIVES AND EXPECTORANTS.

Fluoride preparations

Fluoride preparations contain sodium fluoride alone or combined with vitamins and minerals. Fluoride reacts with calcium and other minerals to form the apatite crystals of bone and teeth; it is recommended as a prophylaxis against dental caries in areas where the fluoride content of the drinking-water supply is known to be 0.7 parts per million or less. (Fluoride preparations should not be used when the water supply contains more than this level of fluoride.)

Prominent single-component products containing sodium fluoride are Fluoritab®, Luride®, and Pediaflor®.

Food formulations

Food formulations in clinical use include a variety of commercial preparations that may be generally categorized as dietetic, reducing, elemental, or supplemental. Elemental or molecular diets are preparations (e.g., Vivonex®) formulated out of known chemical nutrients; these are used when there is need for defined and balanced nutrition. Supplemental preparations (which may or may not be elemental) provide nutritional support orally or by nasogastric tube in patients with a wide range of medical, surgical, and psychological problems characterized by inadequate nutrition. Each 360 ml portion of a representative supplemental formulation (Sustacal®) provides 21.7 g protein (6.1% weight/volume), 8.3 g fat (2.3%), 46.9 g carbohydrate, and 360 Cal; supplies 33 to 35% of the RDA of vitamins and minerals; and contains 76% water and 1.1% ash.

Prominent supplemental preparations include:
Amin-Aid®
Citrogen®
Compleat®-B
Ensure®
Sustacal®
Sustagen®
Vivonex®

Fungicides

See ANTI-INFECTIVES, LOCAL.

Germicides

See ANTI-INFECTIVES, LOCAL.

Glucocorticoids

See CORTICOSTEROIDS.

Gonadotropics

Gonadotropics include natural gonadotropins (secreted by the anterior pituitary and, during pregnancy, by the placenta) and agents, such as clomiphene, which provoke their release. Gonadotropins stimulate the production of gametes (in both sexes) and the secretion of estrogens and progestogens in the female and androgens in the male. Clinically, they are used in the male to treat hypogenitalism and cryptorchidism, and in the female to treat secondary anovulatory infertility, hypogenitalism, and menstrual disorders.

Prominent gonadotropics include:
　　clomiphene citrate (Clomid®)
　　gonadotropin, chorionic (A.P.L.®, Follutein®)
　　menotropins (Pergonal®)

Heavy metal antagonists

Heavy metal antagonists are systemic antidotes used in poisoning due to arsenic, gold, iron, lead, mercury, and certain other metals. Their basic mechanism of action (chelation) involves the formation of a nontoxic chemical complex (chelate) with the poison.

Prominent heavy metal antagonists include:
　　calcium disodium edetate (Calcium Disodium Versenate™)
　　deferoxamine mesylate (Desferal®)
　　dimercaprol (BAL)
　　penicillamine (Cuprimine®)

Hematinics

Hematinics are agents used in the treatment of anemia. The fundamental agents include iron, folic acid, cyanocobalamin (vitamin B_{12}), intrinsic factor, vitamin C, liver extracts, and hydrochloric acid; these are employed alone or (more commonly) in combination.

Prominent hematinics include:
　　cyanocobalamin (vitamin B_{12}) (Redisol®, Rubramin PC®)
　　ferrous fumarate (Feostat®)
　　ferrous fumarate/dioctyl sodium sulfosuccinate
　　　(Ferro-Sequels®)
　　ferrous gluconate (Fergon®)
　　ferrous gluconate/ascorbic acid (Fergon® c̄ C)
　　ferrous gluconate/ascorbic acid/cyanocobalamin/intrinsic factor (Fergon® Plus)

ferrous sulfate (Feosol®, Fer-In-Sol®, Fero-Gradumet®)
ferrous sulfate/ascorbic acid (Fero-Grad-500®)
ferrous sulfate/vitamin B complex/ascorbic acid (Iberet®,
    Mol-Iron® Panhemic™ Chronosule®)
folic acid (Folvite®)
folic acid/ferrous sulfate (Folvron®)
folic acid/ferrous sulfate/ascorbic acid (Fero-Folic-500®)
glutamic acid hydrochloride (Acidulin®)
hydrochloric acid 10%
hydroxocobalamin (alphaREDISOL®, Neo-Betalin® 12)
intrinsic factor/cyanocobalamin/ferrous fumarate/ascorbic acid
    (Trinsicon®)
iron dextran injection (Imferon®)
leucovorin calcium (citrovorum factor)

Hemostatics

Hemostatics are agents that hasten the coagulation of blood or arrest
bleeding. Some act by mechanical means, while others act by directly
or indirectly affecting some step or steps in the actual biochemical
process.

Prominent hemostatics include:
aminocaproic acid (Amicar®)
antihemophilic factor (human) VIII (Humafac®, Koāte®,
    Profilate®)
antihemophilic factor (human) IX (Konȳne®)
cellulose, oxidized regenerated (Surgicel™ Absorbable
    Hemostat)
epinephrine (Adrenalin®)
estrogens, conjugated, for injection (Premarin®)
fibrinogen, human (Parenogen®)
gelatin film, absorbable (Gelfilm®)
gelatin sponge, absorbable (Gelfoam®)
microfibrillar collagen hemostat (Avitene®)
phytonadione (vitamin K_1) (AquaMEPHYTON®,
    Konakion®, Mephyton®)
protamine sulfate
thrombin, topical

Hormones

Hormones are chemical regulators produced by endocrine glands.
Some pass through the membrane of the target cell and directly
influence the biochemical processes within, while others attach
themselves to specialized receptor sites (on the surface of the cell)
and thereby activate the enzyme adenylate cyclase. In turn, adenylate cyclase converts adenosine triphosphate (ATP) into cyclic
adenosine monophosphate (cyclic AMP), which relays the signal

to the interior of the cell. Hormones are employed as replacement therapy in hypofunctional states (e.g., thyroid hormones in hypothyroidism) or in nonendocrine situations that are ameliorated by a particular hormone (e.g., corticosteroids in rheumatoid arthritis). In the latter use, classic side effects relate to hyperfunctional states; for example, corticosteroids may cause hyperadrenocortism. Hormonal preparations employed in medicine include the natural or synthetic products associated with the pituitary gland (see PITUITARY HORMONES, p. 59), thyroid (see THYROID PREPARATIONS, p. 65), pancreas (see **Insulin**, p. 294), adrenal glands (see CORTICOSTEROIDS, p. 37), ovaries (see ESTROGENS, p. 50, and PROGESTOGENS, p. 60), and testes (see ANDROGENS, p. 6).

Hydrocholeretics

See CHOLERETICS.

Hyperglycemics

Hyperglycemics are used to correct the acute hypoglycemia that may occur with insulin therapy. They include parenteral sugar solutions and the pancreatic hormone glucagon hydrochloride. Glucagon acts by stimulating the conversion of hepatic glycogen to glucose.

Hypoglycemics

See ANTIDIABETICS.

Hypnotics

See SEDATIVE-HYPNOTICS.

Immunosuppressives

Immunosuppressives are agents that induce immunosuppression. Standard preparations include corticosteroids (see), antilymphocytic serum (ALS), azathioprine (Imuran®), and $Rh_o(D)$ immune human globulin (Gamulin® Rh, RhoGAM®). Azathioprine is used as an adjunct for the prevention of rejection in renal homotransplantation; $Rh_o(D)$ immune human globulin is used in the prevention of $Rh_o(D)$ hemolytic disease of the newborn and Rh transfusion accidents.

Infant formulas

Infant formulas are of two types—those nearly identical to human milk, and those designed for special feeding needs (including formulas designed to be low in electrolytes, without cows' milk protein, or without lactose). Prominent human milk substitutes include Enfamil®, Similac®, and SMA® (all available with and without additional iron);

prominent special formulas include Probana®, Nursoy®, and Similac® PM 60/40. A representative formulation (SMA®) supplies 7.2% carbohydrate, 3.6% fat, 1.5% protein, 0.25% ash, and 68 Cal per 100 ml.

Irrigating solutions

Irrigating solutions are used to clean, soothe, deodorize, or medicate wounds, body orifices, or body cavities and to promote healing and harden suppuration. They *are not* to be injected.

Commonly used preparations include:
acetic acid 0.25%
glycine 1.5%
mannitol 5%
Ringer's solution
silver nitrate 0.5%
sodium chloride (0.45% and 0.9%) for irrigation
sorbitol 3.3%
sterile water
Suby's solution G

Keratolytics

Keratolytics are preparations that soften and loosen the outer horny layer of the skin. They are used to treat skin conditions marked by excessive keratinization (e.g., seborrheic dermatitis, corns, calluses, acne, and psoriasis) and are also used in conjunction with other dermatologic agents to enhance penetration.

Prominent preparations include:
anthralin (Anthra-Derm®, Lasan® Unguent)
benzoyl peroxide (present in Benoxyl® Lotion, Desquam-X®, Loroxide®, Persadox®, Persa-Gel®, Vanoxide®)
cantharidin (Cantharone®)
fluorouracil (Efudex®, Fluoroplex®)
podophyllum resin podophyllin
resorcinol
resorcinol/colloidal sulfur (Acne-Dome®)
salicylic acid (present in Fostex®, Keralyt®)
selenium sulfide (Exsel®, Selsun®)
silver nitrate
sulfur, colloidal (present in Bensulfoid®, Collosul®)
sulfurated lime solution (Vleminckx's solution)
trichloroacetic acid
tritinoin (RETIN-A®)
urea preparations (Aquacare®, Carmol®)

Keratoplastics

Keratoplastics are agents used to stimulate cell growth and promote healing. Indications include eczema, psoriasis, atopic dermatitis, and lichen simplex chronicus.

Prominent preparations include:
    coal tar (Cor-Tar-Quin®, Estar®, L.C.D.™)
    ichthammol (Ichthyol®)

Laxatives

See CATHARTICS.

Lubricants

See EMOLLIENT-PROTECTANTS.

Mineralocorticoids

See CORTICOSTEROIDS.

Miotics

Miotics are cholinergic drugs instilled in the eye to produce miosis and thereby relieve intraocular pressure in patients with glaucoma. They are also used to correct certain forms of strabismus and to counteract mydriasis.

Prominent miotics include:
    acetylcholine chloride (Miochol®)
    carbachol (Isopto® Carbachol)
    demecarium bromide (Humorsol®)
    echothiophate iodide (Phospholine® Iodide)
    isoflurophate (Floropryl®)
    physostigmine salicylate (eserine)
    pilocarpine hydrochloride (Isopto® Carpine, Pilocar®)

Mouthwashes

Mouthwashes are used to clean and soothe the mouth; they provide some antiseptic action. Those containing phenol and phenolates also provide a degree of local anesthesia.

Prominent mouthwashes include:
    alkaline aromatic solution
    borate/phenol/phenolate (Chloraseptic®)
    carbamide peroxide 10% (Gly-Oxide®)
    cetylpyridinium chloride (Cēpacol®)

hydrogen peroxide
methylbenzethonium chloride (Dalidyne®)
sodium borate compound
sodium perborate

Mucolytics

Mucolytic agents reduce the thickness of purulent and nonpurulent respiratory secretions and thereby facilitate their removal by coughing, postural drainage, or suction. They are useful in the treatment of chronic respiratory disorders, in patients who have had chest operations, and as adjuncts in bronchoscopy and tracheostomy.

Prominent agents include:
acetylcysteine (Mucomyst®, Respaire®)
desoxyribonuclease (Dornavac®)
tyloxapol (Alevaire®)

Mydriatics

Mydriatics are anticholinergic and adrenergic agents instilled in the eye to produce mydriasis and/or cycloplegia. These effects are advantageous in eye examinations (refraction) and in the management of inflammatory conditions.

Prominent mydriatics include:
atropine sulfate (Isopto® Atropine)
cyclopentolate hydrochloride (Cyclogyl®)
epinephrine (Adrenalin®)
homatropine hydrobromide
hydroxyamphetamine hydrobromide (Paredrine®)
phenylephrine hydrochloride (Neo-Synephrine®)
scopolamine hydrobromide
tropicamide (Mydriacyl®)

Narcoleptics

See CEREBRAL STIMULANTS.

Narcotic antagonists

See RESPIRATORY STIMULANTS.

Narcotics

See ANALGESICS.

Nasal decongestants

Nasal decongestants are adrenergic vasoconstrictors employed to shrink engorged mucous membranes of the nose. They are used both topically and systemically, often in combination with antihistamines, analgesics, and other "cold remedy" agents.

Prominent preparations include:
ephedrine sulfate (I-sedrin®)
naphazoline hydrochloride (Privine®)
oxymetazoline hydrochloride (Afrin®)
phenylephrine hydrochloride (Neo-Synephrine®)
phenylpropanolamine hydrochloride
phenylpropanolamine hydrochloride/chlorpheniramine maleate (Novahistine®, Triaminicin®)
propylhexedrine (Benzedrex®)
pseudoephedrine hydrochloride (Novafed®, Sudafed®)
pseudoephedrine hydrochloride/triprolidine hydrochloride (Actifed®)
tetrahydrozoline hydrochloride (Tyzine®)
xylometazoline hydrochloride (Otrivin®)

Oxytocics

Oxytocics are agents that hasten the process of childbirth by inducing contraction of the uterine muscle. They also prevent and control postpartum hemorrhage by hastening involution. Oxytocic hormones (oxytocin preparations) can be used to stimulate milk production in nursing mothers.

Prominent oxytocics include:
ergonovine maleate (Ergotrate®)
methylergonovine maleate (Methergine®)
oxytocin (Pitocin®, Syntocinon®, Syntocinon® Nasal Spray)
oxytocin citrate (Pitocin® Citrate, Buccal)

Parasympatholytics

See ANTICHOLINERGICS.

Parasympathomimetics

See CHOLINERGICS.

Parasiticides

See ANTI-INFECTIVES, LOCAL.

Parenteral alimentation

Parenteral alimentation involves the intravenous administration of electrolytes (see), vitamins (see), sugars, and amino acids.

Standard sugar and amino acid preparations include:*
    amino acid injection 8.5% (FreAmine® II, Travasol®)
    dextrose injections 5%, and 10%
    dextrose 5%/alcohol 5%
    dextrose 5% in lactated Ringer's injection (Hartmann's solution)
    dextrose 5% in Ringer's injection
    dextrose/sodium chloride injections

dextrose	sodium chloride
2.5%	0.45%
5%	0.2%
5%	0.33%
5%	0.45%
5%	0.9%
10%	0.9%

    fructose 5% and 10% (Levugen®, Travert®)
    invert sugar injections 5%, 10%, and 20%
    parenteral hyperalimentation kits (amino acids–dextrose)
      (Aminosol® Kit, FreAmine® Kit, Polynute® Kit)
    protein hydrolysate injection 5% and 10% (Amigen®,
    Aminosol®)

Pediculicides

See ANTI-INFECTIVES, LOCAL.

Pituitary hormones

The pituitary hormones used in medicine include the adrenocorticotropic hormone (corticotropin, ACTH), oxytocin, and vasopressin. The uses of corticotropin are similar to those of the corticosteroids (see). Vasopressin is used in the management of diabetes insipidus, and oxytocin is used in obstetrics to initiate labor and control postpartum hemorrhage.

Prominent preparations include:
    corticotropin injection (ACTH) (Acthar®)
    corticotropin injection, repository (H.P. Acthar®-Gel)
    lypressin (Diapid®)
    oxytocin (Pitocin®, Syntocinon®, Syntocinon® Nasal Spray)
    oxytocin citrate (Pitocin® Citrate, Buccal)
    vasopressin (Pitressin®)
    vasopressin tannate (Pitressin® Tannate)

*One gram dextrose (glucose) or fructose (levulose) supplies 4 Cal; thus, 500 ml of 10% dextrose (50 g) yields 200 Cal.

Plasma extenders (expanders)

See ELECTROLYTE SOLUTIONS AND WATER-BALANCE AGENTS.

Progestogens

Progestogens include progesterone (the natural hormone secreted by the corpus luteum) and its derivatives and synthetic congeners. Biologically, progesterone functions in the preparation and maintenance of the endometrium; supplements the action of estrogen on the myometrium and mammary glands; and, during pregnancy, decreases uterine irritability and suppresses ovulation. Pharmacologically, progestogens are used to treat functional uterine bleeding, endometriosis, amenorrhea, threatened and habitual abortion, and certain forms of cancer; in conjunction with estrogens, they are widely used as oral contraceptives (see).

Prominent progestogens (other than those used for contraception) include:

dydrogesterone (Duphaston®, Gynorest®)
hydroxyprogesterone caproate (Delalutin®)
medroxyprogesterone acetate (Amen®, Depo-Provera®, Provera®)
norethindrone (Norlutin®)
norethindrone acetate (Norlutate®)
progesterone (Corlutin®, Lipo-Lutin®, Proluton®)

Protein hydrolysates

See PARENTERAL ALIMENTATION.

Psychotropics

Psychotropics are drugs that affect the mental state; they include tranquilizers, antidepressants, and antimaniacals. Their mechanism of action is largely unknown, but there is evidence pointing to the involvement of CNS levels of biogenic amines (namely, epinephrine, norepinephrine, and serotonin); the tranquilizers tend to reduce these levels, and the antidepressants tend to increase these levels.

Tranquilizers

Tranquilizers are categorized as major (antipsychotics) and minor; antipsychotics are used, as indicated, in the treatment of schizophrenia, and minor tranquilizers are used in the treatment of anxiety and tension. (The antipsychotics are often referred to on a basis of molecular structure—namely, phenothiazines, butyrophenones, and thioxanthenes.)

Prominent antipsychotics include:

        acetophenazine maleate (Tindal®)

        butaperazine (Repoise®)

        chlorpromazine hydrochloride (Thorazine®)

        fluphenazine (Permitil®, Prolixin®)

        haloperidol (Haldol®)

        loxapine succinate (Daxolin®, Loxitane®)

        mesoridazine (Serentil®)

        molindone hydrochloride (Moban®)

        perphenazine (Trilafon®)

        perphenazine/amitriptyline hydrochloride (Etrafon®, Triavil®)

        piperacetazine (Quide®)

        prochlorperazine (Compazine®)

        promazine hydrochloride (Sparine®)

        thioridazine hydrochloride (Mellaril®)

        thiothixene hydrochloride (Navane®)

        trifluoperazine hydrochloride (Stelazine®)

        triflupromazine (Vesprin®)

Prominent minor tranquilizers include:

    chlordiazepoxide hydrochloride (Librium®)

    chlordiazepoxide hydrochloride/amitriptyline (Limbitrol®)

    clorazepate dipotassium (Tranxene®)

    clorazepate monopotassium (Azene™)

    diazepam (Valium®)

    droperidol (Inapsine®)

    hydroxyzine (Atarax®, Vistaril®)

    lorazepam (Ativan®)

    meprobamate (Equanil®, Miltown®)

    oxazepam (Serax®)

    prazepam (Verstran®)

Antidepressants

Antidepressants are used in the treatment of depressive states, including endogenous psychotic depression and reactive depression. These agents include tricyclic compounds (the term is derived from the fact that the molecule contains 3 cyclical groups) and monoamine oxidase (MAO) inhibitors. MAO inhibitors have serious side effects and are usually reserved for patients who do not respond to other drugs or to electroshock therapy.

Prominent tricyclic antidepressants include:

    amitriptyline hydrochloride (Elavil®, Endep®)

    desipramine hydrochloride (Norpramin®, Pertofrane®)

    doxepin hydrochloride (Adapin®, Sinequan®)

imipramine hydrochloride (Imavate®, Janimine®,
   Presamine®, Tofranil®)
nortriptyline hydrochloride (Aventyl®)
protriptyline hydrochloride (Vivactil®)

Prominent MAO inhibitors include:
   isocarboxazid (Marplan®)
   phenelzine sulfate (Nardil®)
   tranylcypromine (Parnate®)

Antimaniacals

Antimaniacals are agents used in the treatment and prophylaxis of manic and hypomanic phases of manic-depressive illnesses. The principal medicinal of this class is lithium carbonate (Eskalith®, Lithane®, Lithonate®, Lithotabs™).

Respiratory stimulants

Respiratory stimulants are used to counteract respiratory depression resulting from anesthesia and poisoning (barbiturate, narcotic, etc.). Some of these agents act upon the respiratory center (either directly or indirectly), while others compete with or antagonize narcotics.

Prominent respiratory stimulants include:
   ammonia spirit, aromatic
   caffeine/sodium benzoate
   doxapram hydrochloride (Dopram®)
   levallorphan tartrate (Lorfan®)
   nalorphine hydrochloride (Nalline®)
   naloxone hydrochloride (Narcan®)
   nikethamide (Coramine®)
   pentylenetetrazol (Metrazol®)

Rubefacients

Rubefacients are topical irritants that effect reactive hyperemia and thereby promote local circulation. Additionally, they serve as counterirritants (see).

Prominent rubefacients include:
   camphor
   menthol
   methyl nicotinate
   methyl salicylate

Scabicides

See ANTI-INFECTIVES, LOCAL.

Sclerosing agents

Sclerosing agents irritate the tunica intima of the blood vessels, thereby causing concretions and subsequent obliteration. They are used for injection therapy of varicose veins and internal hemorrhoids.

Prominent sclerosing agents include:
morrhuate sodium
sodium tetradecyl sulfate (Sotradecol®)

Sedative-hypnotics

Sedatives and hypnotics are agents that, respectively, allay anxiety and induce sleep; often, the same drug may achieve both effects at different dosages. These agents are generally categorized as barbiturates or nonbarbiturates, a barbiturate being defined as a derivative of barbituric acid. Barbiturates are classified according to their duration of action as ultrashort (IV anesthetics), short, intermediate, and long. (Many of the drugs classed as tranquilizers, here listed under psychotropics [see], are used for some of the same effects as conventional sedatives.)

Prominent barbiturates include:
amobarbital (Amytal®)
aprobarbital (Alurate®)
barbital/butalbital/phenobarbital dihydroergotamine/
scopolamine (Plexonal®)
butabarbital sodium (Buticaps®, Butisol®)
mephobarbital (Mebaral®)
methohexital sodium (Brevital®)
pentobarbital (Nembutal®)
phenobarbital (Luminal®)
secobarbital sodium (Seconal®)
secobarbital sodium/amobarbital sodium (Tuinal®)
talbutal (Lotusate®)
thiopental sodium (Pentothal®)
thiamylal sodium (Surital®)

Prominent nonbarbiturate hypnotics and sedatives include:
chloral hydrate (Aquachloral®, Felsules®, Noctec®,
Somnos®)
ethchlorvynol (Placidyl®)
ethinamate (Valmid®)
flurazepam hydrochloride (Dalmane®)
glutethimide (Doriden®)
methaqualone (Parest®, Quāālude®, Sopor®)
methyprylon (Noludar®)

paraldehyde
promethazine hydrochloride (Phenergan®)
triclofos (Triclos®)

Skeletal muscle relaxants

Skeletal muscle relaxants produce their effect either peripherally (at or beyond the myoneural junction) or by their action on the CNS. Peripheral agents cause the more pronounced response and, with certain exceptions, are used primarily to effect muscular relaxation during surgery; "central relaxants" are used in the management of musculoskeletal and neuromuscular conditions associated with muscle pain and spasticity.

Prominent skeletal muscle relaxants include:
baclofen (Lioresal®)
carisoprodol (Rela®, Soma®)
chlorphenesin carbamate (Maolate®)
chlorzoxazone (Paraflex®)
cyclobenzaprine hydrochloride (Flexeril™)
dantrolene sodium (Dantrium®)
diazepam (Valium®)
metaxalone (Skelaxin®)
methocarbamol (Robaxin®)
methocarbamol/aspirin (Robaxisal®)
metocurine iodide (Metubine®)
orphenadrine citrate (Norflex®)
orphenadrine citrate/APC (Norgesic®)
orphenadrine hydrochloride (Disipal®)
pancuronium bromide (Pavulon®)
succinylcholine chloride (Anectine®, Quelicin®, Sucostrin®)
tubocurarine chloride

Spermicides

See CONTRACEPTIVES, TOPICAL.

Sulfonamides

Sulfonamides are anti-infective agents derived from or related to the parent compound sulfanilamide (the first "sulfa drug"). These agents act via competitive inhibition; specifically, they compete with para-aminobenzoic acid (PABA). Organisms that require PABA to synthesize folic acid (a B-complex vitamin essential to growth) are thus inhibited by these drugs. Infections that yield to systemic sulfonamides include chancroid, trachoma, inclusion conjunctivitis, meningococcal meningitis, toxoplasmosis, nocardiosis, and most urinary tract infections. Some sulfonamides are used topically (e.g., sulfacetamide and silver sulfadiazine); nonabsorbable agents are employed for intestinal disinfection before and after bowel surgery.

Prominent sulfonamides include:
mafenide acetate cream (Sulfamylon®)
phthalylsulfathiazole (Sulfathalidine®)
silver sulfadiazine (Silvadene®)
sulfacetamide sodium (Sebizon®, Sulamyd®)
sulfachloropyridazine (Sonilyn®)
sulfacytine (Renoquid®)
sulfadiazine
sulfameter (Sulla®)
sulfamethizole (Thiosulfil®)
sulfamethizole/sulfadiazine/phenazopyridine hydrochloride
(Suladyne®)
sulfamethoxazole (Gantanol®)
sulfamethoxazole/phenazopyridine hydrochloride (Azo
Gantanol®)
sulfamethoxypyridazine (Midicel®)
sulfasalazine (Azulfidine®)
sulfisoxazole (Gantrisin®, Soxomide®)
sulfisoxazole/phenazopyridine (Azo Gantrisin®)
trimethoprim/sulfamethoxazole* (Bactrim™, Septra®)
trisulfapyrimidines (Terfonyl®)

Sympatholytics

See ANTIADRENERGICS.

Sympathomimetics

See ADRENERGICS.

Thyroid preparations

Thyroid preparations include thyroid extracts ("thyroid") and pure thyroid hormones; they are used in the treatment of hypothyroidism and in the management of certain conditions (such as arthritis, rickets, skin disorders, and menstrual disturbances) often associated with low metabolic levels of thyroid.

Standard thyroid preparations include:
levothyroxine sodium (Letter®, Synthroid®)
liothyronine sodium (Cytomel®)

*Drug of choice in treatment of *Pneumocystis carinii* infections.

liotrix* (Euthroid®, Thyrolar®)
thyroglobulin (Proloid®)
thyroid

Toxoids

See BIOLOGICALS.

Tranquilizers

See PSYCHOTROPICS.

Trichomonacides

See ANTIPROTOZOALS.

Uricosurics

Uricosurics are agents that promote the excretion of uric acid; they are used in the management of chronic gout.

Prominent uricosurics include:
probenecid (Benemid®)
probenecid/colchicine (ColBENEMID®)
sulfinpyrazone (Anturane®)

Urinary antiseptics

Urinary antiseptics are agents used in the treatment of urinary tract infections; these agents include antibiotics, sulfonamides, and miscellaneous anti-infectives. They are commonly combined with analgesics and antispasmodics.

Prominent urinary antiseptics include:
methenamine hippurate (Hiprex®, Urex®)
methenamine mandelate (Mandelamine®)
methenamine mandelate/phenazopyridine hydrochloride
   (Azo-Mandelamine®)
methenamine mandelate/phenazopyridine hydrochloride/
   belladonna alkaloids/phenobarbital (Donnasep®)
methylene blue (Urolene® Blue, M-B Tabs)
nalidixic acid (NegGram®)
nitrofurantoin (Cyantin®, Furadantin®, Macrodantin®)
oxolinic acid (Utibid®)
oxytetracycline hydrochloride/sulfamethizole/phenazopyridine
   hydrochloride (Urobiotic®)
sulfamethoxazole (Gantanol®)

*Liotrix contains levothyroxine sodium (T_4) and liothyronine sodium (T_3) in a ratio of 4 : 1 by weight.

sulfamethoxazole/phenazopyridine hydrochloride (Azo
Gantanol®)
sulfisoxazole (Gantrisin®, Soxomide®)
sulfisoxazole/phenazopyridine hydrochloride (Azo Gantrisin®)
tetracycline phosphate complex/sulfamethizole/phenazopyri-
dine hydrochloride (Azotrex®)
trimethoprim/sulfamethoxazole (Bactrim™, Septra®)

Vaccines

See BIOLOGICALS.

Vasodilators, coronary

See CARDIACS.

Vasodilators, peripheral

Peripheral vasodilators relax vascular smooth muscle (directly or
indirectly via alpha-adrenergic stimulation or beta blockade) and
thus increase blood flow in the extremities and brain. They are indicated for adjunctive therapy in arteriosclerosis, arteriosclerosis
obliterans, intermittent claudication, thrombophlebitis, Buerger's
disease, Raynaud's phenomenon, gangrene, endarteritis, frostbite,
varicose ulcers, chilblain, and scleroderma. Certain vasodilators
are possibly effective in selected cases of ischemic cerebral vascular
disease.

Prominent peripheral vasodilators include:
cyclandelate (Cyclospasmol®)
ethaverine hydrochloride (Cebral®, Eta-Lent®, Ethaquin®,
Isovex-100®)
isoxsuprine hydrochloride (Vasodilan®)
niacin (nicotinic acid) (Niac®, Nicotinex®)
nicotinyl alcohol (Roniacol®)
nylidrin hydrochloride (Arlidin®)
papaverine hydrochloride (Cerespan®, Pavabid®, Pavakey®,
Vasospan®)
phenoxybenzamine hydrochloride (Dibenzyline®)
tolazoline hydrochloride (Priscoline®)

Vasoconstrictors

See ADRENERGICS.

Vitamins

Vitamins are essential nutrients that the balanced diet supplies in
appropriate amounts. Medically, vitamins are used to bolster the
constitution (in debilitation and illness) and to treat deficiencies

(avitaminoses). By convention, they are classified as fat-soluble or water-soluble.

Standard vitamin preparations include the following:
- fat-soluble vitamins:
  - ergocalciferol (vitamin D_2) (Calciferol™, Drisdol®)
  - menadiol sodium diphosphate (vitamin K) (Synkayvite®)
  - phytonadione (vitamin K_1) (AquaMEPHYTON®, Konakion®, Mephyton®)
  - vitamin A (Aquasol® A, Vi-Dom-A®)
  - vitamin E (Aquasol® E, Tokols®)
- water-soluble vitamins:
  - ascorbic acid (vitamin C)
  - vitamin B complex:
    - biotin
    - cyanocobalamin injection (vitamin B_{12}) (Redisol®, Rubramin PC®)
    - dexpanthenol* (Ilopan®)
    - folic acid (Folvite®)
    - hydroxocobalamin (alphaREDISOL®, Neo-Betalin® 12)
    - leucovorin calcium (citrovorum factor)
    - niacin (nicotinic acid)
    - niacinamide (nicotinamide)
    - pantothenic acid†
    - pyridoxine hydrochloride (vitamin B_6) (Hexa-Betalin®)
    - riboflavin (vitamin B_2, vitamin G)
    - thiamine hydrochloride or mononitrate (vitamin B_1)

Vitamins, multiple

There are hundreds of multivitamin preparations, but basically they differ only in regard to their spectrum (i.e., which vitamins are included) and strength. These preparations may also contain iron and other minerals. At the pharmaceutical level, they vary in formulation and in the particular derivatives employed (e.g., one preparation may use dexpanthenol while another contains calcium pentothenate). Generally, an oral preparation (capsules, tablets, liquid, or drops) is characterized as *supplemental* or *therapeutic,* depending on its strength. Parenteral preparations are used in the treatment of patients before and after surgery, and in patients with increased metabolic needs resulting from fever, severe burns, hyperthyroidism, gastrointestinal disorders, wasting diseases, or alcoholism.

*Converted (in the body) to pantothenic acid.
†Usually used as calcium and sodium salts.

Prominent oral vitamin preparations include the following (with the amount of each ingredient per capsule or tablet, except where noted):

Adabee®

vitamin A	10,000	IU
ascorbic acid	250	mg
niacinamide	50	mg
pyridoxine hydrochloride	5	mg
riboflavin	10	mg
thiamine mononitrate	15	mg

Adabee® with Minerals

The same as Adabee® Tablets plus:

calcium (as calcium phosphate)	103	mg
iron (as ferrous sulfate)	15	mg
phosphorus (as calcium phosphate)	80	mg

Allbee-T® Tablets

ascorbic acid	500	mg
calcium pantothenate	25	mg
cyanocobalamin	5	μg
niacinamide	100	mg
pyridoxine hydrochloride	10	mg
thiamine mononitrate	15	mg
desiccated liver	150	mg

Berocca® Tablets

ascorbic acid	500	mg
calcium pantothenate	20	mg
cyanocobalamin	5	μg
folic acid	500	μg
niacinamide	100	mg
pyridoxine hydrochloride	5	mg
riboflavin	15	mg
thiamine mononitrate	15	mg

Dayalets® Tablets

vitamin A	5,000	IU
vitamin D	400	IU
vitamin E	30	IU
ascorbic acid	60	mg
cyanocobalamin	6	μg
folic acid	400	μg
niacinamide	20	mg
pyridoxine hydrochloride	2	mg
riboflavin	1.7	mg
thiamine hydrochloride	1.5	mg

Dayalets® plus Iron
The same as Dayalets® Tablets plus 18 mg of iron (as ferrous sulfate)

Decavitamin capsules and tablets

vitamin A	4,000	IU
vitamin D	400	IU
ascorbic acid	70	mg
calcium pantothenate	10	mg
cyanocobalamin	1	μg
folic acid	50	μg
niacinamide	20	mg
pyridoxine hydrochloride	2	mg
riboflavin	2	mg
thiamine hydrochloride	2	mg

Lederplex® Capsules

calcium pantothenate	3	mg
choline	20	mg
cyanocobalamin	1	μg
inositol	10	mg
niacinamide	10	mg
pyridoxine hydrochloride	200	μg
riboflavin	2	mg
thiamine mononitrate	2	mg

Multicebrin® Tablets

vitamin A	10,000	IU
vitamin D	400	IU
vitamin E	6.6	IU
ascorbic acid	75	mg
cyanocobalamin	3	μg
niacinamide	25	mg
pantothenic acid	5	mg
pyridoxine hydrochloride	1.2	mg
riboflavin	3	mg
thiamine hydrochloride	3	mg

Stresscaps®

ascorbic acid	300	mg
calcium pantothenate	20	mg
cyanocobalamin	4	μg
niacinamide	100	mg
pyridoxine hydrochloride	2	mg
riboflavin	10	mg
thiamine mononitrate	10	mg

Theragran-M® Tablets

vitamin A	10,000	IU
vitamin D	400	IU
vitamin E	15	IU
ascorbic acid	200	mg
calcium pantothenate	20	mg
cyanocobalamin	5	μg
niacinamide	100	mg
pyridoxine hydrochloride	5	mg
riboflavin	10	mg
thiamine mononitrate	10	mg
copper (as copper sulfate)	2	mg
iodine (as potassium iodide)	150	μg
iron (as ferrous carbonate)	12	mg
magnesium (as magnesium carbonate)	65	mg
manganese (as manganese sulfate)	1	mg
zinc (as zinc sulfate)	1.5	mg

Vi-Daylin® ADC Drops (quantities are per milliliter)

vitamin A	1,500	IU
vitamin D	400	IU
ascorbic acid	60	mg

Vigran® Capsules

vitamin A	5,000	IU
vitamin D	400	IU
vitamin E	30	IU
ascorbic acid	60	mg
cyanocobalamin	6	μg
folic acid	400	μg
niacin	20	mg
pyridoxine hydrochloride	2	mg
riboflavin	1.7	mg
thiamine hydrochloride	1.5	mg

Vi-Penta® F Multivitamin Drops (quantities are per 0.6 ml)

vitamin A palmitate	5,000	IU
vitamin E	2	IU
ascorbic acid	50	mg
d-biotin	30	μg
ergocalciferol	10	μg
niacinamide	10	mg
dexpanthenol	10	mg
pyridoxine hydrochloride	1	mg
riboflavin	1	mg
thiamine hydrochloride	1	mg
fluoride (as sodium fluoride)	500	μg

Prominent parenteral vitamin preparations include the following (with the amount of each ingredient per milliliter):

Berocca®-C

ascorbic acid	50	mg
d-biotin	100	μg
dexpanthenol	10	mg
niacinamide	40	mg
pyridoxine hydrochloride	10	mg
riboflavin	5	mg
thiamine hydrochloride	5	mg

Berocca®-C 500

The same as Berocca®-C
plus 200 mg of ascorbic
acid

Betalin® Complex

cyanocobalamin	2.5	μg
niacinamide	75	mg
pantothenic acid	2.5	mg
pyridoxine hydrochloride	5	mg
riboflavin	2	mg
thiamine hydrochloride	5	mg

Betalin® Complex F.C.

ascorbic acid	75	mg
niacinamide	50	mg
pantothenic acid	2.5	mg
pyridoxine hydrochloride	5	mg
riboflavin	3	mg
thiamine hydrochloride	12.5	mg

Folbesyn®

ascorbic acid	150	mg
cyanocobalamin	7.5	μg
folic acid	500	μg
niacinamide	37.5	mg
pyridoxine hydrochloride	7.5	mg
riboflavin	5	mg
sodium pantothenate	5	mg
thiamine hydrochloride	5	mg

M.V.I.®

vitamin A	1,000	IU
vitamin D	100	IU
vitamin E	0.5	IU
ascorbic acid	50	mg
dexpanthenol	2.5	mg
niacinamide	10	mg
pyridoxine hydrochloride	1.5	mg
riboflavin	1	mg
thiamine hydrochloride	5	mg

Solu-B-Forte® (S-B-F®)

ascorbic acid	100	mg
niacinamide	125	mg
pyridoxine hydrochloride	5	mg
riboflavin	5	mg
sodium pantothenate	50	mg
thiamine hydrochloride	25	mg

Section 2
Standard and
Commonly Used
Drugs

SPECIAL NOTES

Brand Names (Trademarks)
The listing of two or more brand names following a generic designation implies nothing beyond the fact that the same drug or active ingredient is involved. As indicated under "Composition and Supply," brands may vary in regard to pharmaceutic form, dosage, route of administration, or all three. Even when two brands are "identical" (e.g., 5 mg tablets of drug X), there is the matter of bioavailability (see Glossary). For convenience, drug mixtures are indicated by slashes; e.g., aspirin/phenacetin/caffeine (Empirin® Compound).

Dosage
Pediatric. Unless otherwise indicated, the dosages cited in the monographs are for adults; dosages for infants and children can be calculated by using the rules given in Appendix 8. It must be stressed, however, that such calculations are approximate values and that infants and young children are highly sensitive to certain drugs (e.g., opiates) and are relatively resistant to others (e.g., belladonna). As pointed out by many authorities, untoward reactions in children arise from problems in growth and development rather than size.

Weight and measures. Dosages (and other values) follow the modernized metric system as stated by the U.S. Bureau of Standards (Appendix 7). For example, the official symbol for gram is g (lowercase g, no period), and decimal expressions less than 1.0 are not used; thus, 0.3 g becomes 300 mg, and 0.3 mg becomes 300 μg. Since the microliter (μl) unit is not widely used in clinical situations, the ml equivalent is given first, followed by the μl. Also "per kg" implies "per kilogram *of body weight.*"

Cross-References
Drugs are described in detail only under the generic listing in this section. A cross-reference in all CAPITAL LETTERS indicates that you should look at the information under the designation in Section 1. A cross-reference in **boldface type** refers to a monograph in Section 2. The expression "See under" relates to drug combinations. For example, the entry "Butazolidin® Alka, see under Phenylbutazone" refers to a drug combination found under "Composition and Supply" in the monograph "Phenylbutazone (Butazolidin®)."

Cautions
In the interest of conciseness and to underscore crucial highlights, "Cautions" (as used here) encompasses "Contraindications," "Warnings," "Precautions," "Drug interactions," and "Incompatibilities." In some instances it was possible to present everything cited by the manufacturer or reference source, while in others material was either condensed or abbreviated, as indicated.

Legal Status

Schedule. A schedule number is given for "controlled drugs" (see Appendix 2).

Prescription. The drug in question can only be dispensed by a pharmacist under order by a physician, dentist, or authorized agent.

Nonprescription. The drug described is sold "over the counter" (OTC); that is, it is not required by law to be sold by prescription only.

DRUG DESCRIPTIONS

Aarane®

See **Cromolyn sodium.**

Abbokinase® (urokinase)

See ANTICOAGULANTS.

Acenocoumarol (Sintrom®)

See ANTICOAGULANTS.

Acetaminophen (Datril®, Nebs®, Tempra®, Tylenol®, Valadol®)

Action and Use
Nonaddictive analgesic and antipyretic.

Dosage and Administration
325 to 1,000 mg every 4 hours up to 4 g daily, orally. Acetaminophen may also be administered rectally.

Cautions
If arthritic or rheumatic pain persists for longer than 10 days or is accompanied by redness or swelling, consult the physician immediately. Prolonged use of large doses is reported to enhance slightly the effect of coumarin anticoagulants.

Adverse Reactions
Side effects are uncommon and nonspecific. Overdosage may cause hepatotoxicity.

Composition and Supply
Capsules   500 mg
Drops   60 mg/0.6 ml
Elixir, syrup   120 mg/5 ml
Elixir with codeine (Tylenol® with Codeine Elixir)   120 mg/5 ml with codeine 12 mg/5 ml
Suppositories   300 mg and 600 mg
Tablets   325 mg and 500 mg
Tablets, chewable   120 mg
Tablets   300 mg with codeine 30 mg (Empracet® with Codeine No. 3)
Tablets   300 mg with codeine (Tylenol® with Codeine): 7.5 mg codeine (No. 1), 15 mg codeine (No. 2), 30 mg codeine (No. 3), 60 mg codeine (No. 4)

Note: the preparations that contain codeine may be habit-forming (see **Codeine phosphate**).

Legal Status
Nonprescription (except for codeine preparations)
Schedule III (codeine preparations)

Acetaminophen/allobarbital (Dialog®)

See ANALGESICS, nonnarcotic.

Acetazolamide (Diamox®)

Action and Use
Carbonic anhydrase inhibitor (and diuretic) used for the adjunctive treatment of chronic open-angle glaucoma, secondary glaucoma, and (preoperatively) acute angle-closure glaucoma. It is also used to treat edema due to congestive heart failure and certain convulsive disorders (e.g., petit mal epilepsy).

Dosage and Administration
Chronic open-angle glaucoma: 250 mg to 1 g every 24 hours in divided doses, orally.
Secondary glaucoma and preoperative acute angle-closure (narrow-angle) glaucoma: 250 mg every 4 hours, orally; 500 mg, IV.
Epilepsy: 8 to 30 mg per kg daily in divided doses, orally.
Diuresis in congestive heart failure: 250 to 375 mg once daily, orally.

Cautions
Contraindicated when sodium and/or potassium blood serum levels are depressed and in patients with marked kidney or liver dysfunction or hyperchloremic acidosis. It is strongly recommended that the injection be used within 24 hours of reconstitution.

Adverse Reactions
Reported side effects include paresthesias (especially tingling of the fingers and toes), anorexia, polyuria, drowsiness, confusion, transient myopia, urticaria, hematuria, glycosuria, flaccid paralysis, agranulocytosis, and convulsions. Acidosis may occur during long-term treatment.

Composition and Supply
Capsules, sustained-release (Diamox® Sequels®)   500 mg (*Note:* the usual dose is 1 capsule in the morning and 1 capsule in the evening.)
Injection (sodium salt)   500 mg vials
Tablets   125 mg and 250 mg

Legal Status
Prescription

Acetic acid preparations (VōSol® Otic Solution)

See ANTI-INFECTIVES, LOCAL, miscellaneous antiseptic-disinfectants.

Acetic acid/aluminum acetate (Otic Domeboro® Solution)

See ANTI-INFECTIVES, LOCAL, miscellaneous antiseptic-disinfectants.

Acetohexamide (Dymelor®)

Action and Use
Oral hypoglycemic.

Dosage and Administration
250 mg to 1.5 g, orally.

Cautions
Contraindicated in patients with hepatic, renal, or thyroid impairment, and in those with diabetes mellitus controlled with diet. For further cautions, see **Chlorpropamide.**

Adverse Reactions
See **Chlorpropamide.**

Composition and Supply
Tablets   250 mg and 500 mg

Legal Status
Prescription

Acetophenazine maleate (Tindal®)

See PSYCHOTROPICS, antipsychotics.

Acetylcholine chloride (Miochol®)

Action and Use
Short-acting miotic used during eye surgery involving anterior chamber, cataract, or peripheral iridectomy, and in certain other procedures.

Dosage and Administration
0.5 ml (500 μl) to 2.0 ml, by instillation.

Cautions
See **Carbachol.**

Adverse Reactions
See **Carbachol.**

Composition and Supply
Solution, ophthalmic   1%

Legal Status
Prescription

Acetylcysteine (Mucomyst®, Respaire®)

Action and Use
Mucolytic agent used in bronchopulmonary disorders.

Dosage and Administration
3 to 5 ml of 20% solution or 6 to 10 ml of 10% solution 3 to 4 times a day; applied directly, by nebulization, or by intratracheal instillation.

Cautions
Use with caution in asthmatic patients because bronchospasm might occur. Liquefied secretions may occlude the airway passages. Antimicrobials should not be administered in the same solution. The solutions harden rubber and become discolored on contact with certain metals; the equipment used with this drug should be made of glass, plastic, or stainless steel. If the vacuum seal is broken, refrigerate the solution to retard oxidation, and use it within 48 hours.

Adverse Reactions
Stomatitis, nausea, and rhinorrhea may occur. Other side effects include bronchospasm (especially in patients with bronchial asthma), hemoptysis, and vomiting.

Composition and Supply
Solution   10% and 20% in 10 ml and 30 ml vials

Note: solution may develop a purple tinge, which is not harmful.

Legal Status
Prescription

Acetyldigitoxin (Acylanid®)

See **CARDIACS,** cardiac glycosides.

Acetylsalicylic acid

See **Aspirin.**

Achromycin®

See **Tetracycline hydrochloride.**

Achromycin® V

See **Tetracycline hydrochloride.**

Achrostatin® V

See **Tetracycline hydrochloride.**

Acidulin®

See **Glutamic acid hydrochloride.**

Acne-Dome® (resorcinal colloidal sulfur)

See KERATOLYTICS.

Acrisorcin (Akrinol®)

See ANTI-INFECTIVES, LOCAL, fungicides.

ACTH

See **Corticotropin.**

Acthar®

See **Corticotropin.**

Actidil® (triprolidine hydrochloride)

See ANTIHISTAMINES.

Actifed®

See under **Pseudoephedrine hydrochloride.**

Actifed-C® Expectorant

See COUGH-COLD PREPARATIONS, cough preparations.

Actifed® Syrup

See under **Pseudoephedrine hydrochloride.**

Actinomycin D

See **Dactinomycin.**

Acylanid® (acetyldigitoxin)

See CARDIACS, cardiac glycosides.

Adabee®

See VITAMINS, MULTIPLE, oral.

Adabee® with Minerals

See VITAMINS, MULTIPLE, oral.

Adapin®

See **Doxepin hydrochloride.**

Adiphenine hydrochloride (Trasentine®)

See ANTICHOLINERGICS.

Adrenalin®

See **Epinephrine.**

Adriamycin® (doxorubicin hydrochloride)

See ANTINEOPLASTICS, antibiotics.

Aerolate® (theophylline)

See ANTIASTHMATICS, xanthine preparations.

Aerosporin®

See **Polymyxin B sulfate.**

A-Fil® (titanium dioxide preparation)

See EMOLLIENT-PROTECTANTS.

Afrin®

See **Oxymetazoline hydrochloride.**

Agoral®

See under **Mineral oil.**

Akineton®

See **Biperiden hydrochloride.**

Akrinol® (acrisorcin)

See ANTI-INFECTIVES, LOCAL, fungicides.

Albumin, normal human serum (Albuspan®)

See ELECTROLYTE SOLUTIONS AND WATER-BALANCE AGENTS, plasma extenders.

Albuspan® (albumin, normal human serum)

See ELECTROLYTE SOLUTIONS AND WATER-BALANCE AGENTS, plasma extenders.

Alcaine®

See **Proparacaine hydrochloride.**

Alcohol

See ANTI-INFECTIVES, LOCAL.

Alcopara®

See **Bephenium hydroxynaphthoate.**

Aldactazide®

See under **Spironolactone.**

Aldactone®

See **Spironolactone.**

Aldinamide®

See **Pyrazinamide.**

Aldomet®

See **Methyldopa.**

Aldoril®

See under **Methyldopa.**

Alevaire® (tyloxapol)

See MUCOLYTICS.

Alglyn® (dihydroxyaluminum aminoacetate)

See ANTACIDS.

Alidase®

See **Hyaluronidase.**

Alkaline aromatic solution

See MOUTHWASHES.

Alka-Seltzer® Effervescent Pain Reliever and Antacid (sodium bicarbonate/citric acid/aspirin)

See ANALGESICS, nonnarcotic; ANTACIDS.

Alkeran®

See **Melphalan.**

Allbee-T® Tablets

See VITAMINS, MULTIPLE, oral.

Allergenic extracts

See BIOLOGICALS; DIAGNOSTICS, allergy (skin tests).

Allopurinol (Zyloprim®)

Action and Use
Allopurinol inhibits the formation of uric acid; it is indicated in gout, uric acid nephropathy, and recurrent uric acid stone formation. It is also used to prevent urate deposition, renal calculi, or uric acid nephropathy in patients receiving antineoplastics (which cause increased serum uric acid levels).

Dosage and Administration
100 to 800 mg maximum daily in divided doses, orally.

Cautions
The patient should be encouraged to maintain a fluid intake sufficient to produce at least 2 liters of neutral to alkaline urine per day. Liver function tests may be altered. Kidney or liver damage may occur; patients with impaired renal and/or hepatic function should be closely followed. The effects of coumarin anticoagulants may be prolonged. Contraindicated in children and nursing mothers. Avoid concomitant use of iron salts.

Adverse Reactions
The most common side effects include skin eruptions and drowsiness. Occasional side effects include headache, nausea, vomiting, vertigo, and diarrhea. Rare side effects include alopecia, fever, chills, blood dyscrasias, arthralgia, rash, and pruritus.

Composition and Supply
Tablets   100 mg and 300 mg

Legal Status
Prescription

Alpen®

See **Ampicillin.**

Alpha Chymar® (chymotrypsin, ophthalmic)

See ENZYMES.

Alphaprodine hydrochloride (Nisentil®)

Action and Use
Rapid-acting narcotic analgesic with a short duration of action.

Dosage and Administration
20 to 40 mg, IV or SC repeated every 2 hours as needed.

Cautions
A narcotic, which can lead to physical dependence. Should not be injected intramuscularly. The depressant effects of barbiturates, MAO inhibitors, general anesthetics, alcohol, and some phenothiazines are potentiated. Use with caution in patients with increased intracranial pressure, hepatic insufficiency, severe CNS depression, myxedema, acute alcoholism, delirium tremens, convulsive disorders, and Addison's disease, and in women in the first trimester of pregnancy. Intravenous administration should be done with caution to avoid respiratory depression, especially in patients with pulmonary disease and in elderly persons. Alphaprodine hydrochloride crosses the placental barrier, especially if it is given in conjunction with a barbiturate; and it can depress respirations in the fetus unless it is given long enough before the time of delivery.

Adverse Reactions
Side effects include euphoria, mild sedation, slight dizziness, itching, and diaphoresis. Toxic effects include respiratory depression, coma, hypotension, and pinpoint pupils.

Composition and Supply
Injection   40 mg/ml and 60 mg/ml, in 1 ml ampuls; 60 mg/ml in 10 ml vials

Legal Status
Schedule II

AlphaREDISOL® (hydroxocobalamin)

See HEMATINICS; VITAMINS, water-soluble.

Aludrox®

See **Magnesium hydrochloride/aluminum hydroxide.**

Aluminum acetate, modified (Bluboro® Powder, Domeboro® Powder)

See ASTRINGENTS.

Aluminum acetate solution (Burow's solution)
Aluminum subacetate solution

Action and Use
Astringent, antiseptic, and antipruritic.

Dosage and Administration
Acetate: dilute with 10 to 40 parts water before application (as wet dressing).
Subacetate: dilute with 20 to 40 parts water.

Caution
Avoid contact with the eyes. Evaporation should be prevented by covering the area with plastic or other impervious materials. If applied with a dressing, do not allow the dressing to dry.

Adverse Reactions
Relatively nonirritating.

Composition and Supply
Solution (acetate)   aluminum oxide 1.2 to 1.5 g/100 ml with acetic acid 4.2 to 5.1 g/100 ml
Solution (subacetate)   aluminum oxide 2.3 to 2.6 g/100 ml with acetic acid 5.4 to 6.1 g/100 ml

Legal Status
Nonprescription

Aluminum carbonate gel (Basaljel®)

See ANTACIDS.

Aluminum chloride (Drysol™)

See ASTRINGENTS.

Aluminum glycinate/magnesium carbonate (Di-Alminate®)

See ANTACIDS.

Aluminum hydroxide gel (Amphojel®)

Action and Use
Antacid.

Dosage and Administration
Suspension, 5 to 30 ml every 2 to 4 hours; 2 tablets (300 mg) or 1 tablet (600 mg), well chewed and taken with water, 5 or 6 times a day.

Cautions
Prolonged use may interfere seriously with phosphate absorption. Should not be used with any form of tetracycline.

Adverse Reactions
May cause constipation.

Composition and Supply
Suspension   320 mg/5 ml
Tablets   300 mg and 600 mg

Legal Status
Nonprescription

Aluminum hydroxide/magnesium hydroxide (Maalox®)

See **Magnesium hydroxide/aluminum hydroxide.**

Aluminum hydroxide/magnesium hydroxide/ simethicone (Mylanta®)

See **Magnesium hydroxide/aluminum hydroxide/simethicone.**

Aluminum hydroxide/magnesium trisilicate (Gelusil®)

Action and Use
Antacid.

Dosage and Administration
Suspension: 5 to 30 ml between meals and at bedtime.
Tablets: 2 to 6 tablets, chewed, with water, between meals and at bedtime.

Cautions
Should not be taken with any form of tetracycline. Tablets should be well chewed.

Adverse Reactions
None of significance if not taken with any form of tetracycline.

Composition and Supply
Suspension
Tablets
Tablets and suspension with magnesium hydroxide (Gelusil-M®)

Legal Status
Nonprescription

Aluminum paste

Action and Use
Protectant.

Dosage and Administration
Apply to skin.

Cautions
None.

Adverse Reactions
None.

Composition and Supply
Paste   10%

Legal Status
Nonprescription

Aluminum phosphate (Phosphaljel®)

See ANTACIDS.

Alupent®

See **Metaproterenol sulfate.**

Alurate® (aprobarbital)

See SEDATIVE-HYPNOTICS, barbiturates.

Alzinox® (dihydroxyaluminum aminoacetate)

See ANTACIDS.

Amantadine hydrochloride (Symmetrel®)

Action and Use
Antiviral used in the treatment of idiopathic Parkinson's disease, postencephalitic parkinsonism, and symptomatic parkinsonism, and in the prevention of influenza (type A).

Dosage and Administration
100 mg twice daily, orally; the maximum dose is 400 mg per day.

Cautions
Contraindicated in nursing mothers. Epilepsy may be aggravated. Use with caution in patients with congestive heart failure or liver disease, and in those concurrently being treated with CNS stimulants. The drug should not be discontinued abruptly when used in patients with Parkinson's disease. The dosage needs careful adjustment in patients with congestive heart failure, kidney disease, edema, or orthostatic hypotension.

Adverse Reactions
Occasional side effects include confusion, irritability, lethargy, drowsiness, slurred speech, nervousness, insomnia, dizziness, ataxia, giddiness, depression, convulsions, congestive heart failure, orthostatic hypotension (the patient should exert caution on rising), urinary retention, and mental symptoms in patients with a history of psychiatric disorders. Other reported side effects include hallucinations, nightmares, blurred vision, dry mouth, nausea, vomiting, anorexia, constipation, tremors, skin rash, leukopenia, peripheral edema, dermatitis.

Composition and Supply
Capsules   100 mg
Syrup   50 mg/5 ml

Legal Status
Prescription

Ambenonium chloride (Mytelase®)

Action and Use
Cholinergic used chiefly in the symptomatic treatment of myasthenia gravis.

Dosage and Administration
5 to 25 mg 3 or 4 times a day, orally (usual range).

Cautions
Atropine and other anticholinergic drugs should not be administered along with ambenonium chloride. Administer with caution to patients with bronchial asthma or mechanical obstruction of the intestine or urinary tract.

Adverse Reactions
Similar to but less pronounced than adverse reactions to neostigmine.

Composition and Supply
Tablets   10 mg

Legal Status
Prescription

Ambenyl® Expectorant

See COUGH-COLD PREPARATIONS, cough preparations.

Ambilhar® (niridazole)

See ANTHELMINTICS, schistosomiasis.

Ambodryl® (bromodiphenhydramine)

See ANTIHISTAMINES.

Amcill®

See **Ampicillin.**

Amen®

See **Medroxyprogesterone acetate.**

Amenestrogen®

See **Estrogens, esterified.**

Americaine® (benzocaine)

See ANESTHETICS, LOCAL; ANTIPRURITICS, topical preparations.

Amicar®

See **Aminocaproic acid.**

Amigen® (protein hydrolysate injection 5% and 10%)

See PARENTERAL ALIMENTATION.

Amikacin sulfate (Amikin™)

Action and Use
Semisynthetic aminoglycoside antibiotic (derived from kanamycin) effective in the treatment of serious gram-negative infections, particularly those due to gentamicin-resistant organisms.

Dosage and Administration
15 mg/kg per day divided into 2 or 3 equal doses at equally divided intervals, IM or IV for 7 to 10 days; beyond this, re-evaluation should be considered.

Cautions
Ototoxic and nephrotoxic. Avoid concurrent or sequential use of antibiotics that are topically or systemically neurotoxic or nephrotoxic.

Adverse Reactions
In addition to ototoxic and nephrotoxic effects, other reactions include skin rash, drug fever, headache, paresthesia, tremor, nausea and vomiting, arthralgia, hypotension, anemia, and eosinophilia.

Composition and Supply
Injection   100 mg and 500 mg in 2 ml vials and 1 g in 4 ml vials

Legal Status
Prescription

Amikin™

See **Amikacin sulfate.**

Amin-Aid®

See FOOD FORMULATIONS.

Amino acid injection (FreAmine® II, Travasol®)

See PARENTERAL ALIMENTATION.

Aminocaproic acid (Amicar®)

Action and Use
Systemic hemostatic agent useful in the treatment of excessive bleeding resulting from systemic hyperfibrinolysis and urinary fibrinolysis.

Dosage and Administration
4 to 5 g during the first hour, followed by 1 to 1.25 g hourly, orally or by IV infusion; the maximum dose is 30 g daily.

Cautions
Should not be used without a definite diagnosis of hyperfibrinolysis. Use with caution in patients with cardiac, renal, or hepatic disease. Intravenous injection should be slow, and medication should be diluted. Contraindicated in patients with intravascular coagulation and in pregnant women.

Adverse Reactions

Occasional side effects include nausea, cramps, diarrhea, dizziness, tinnitus, malaise, conjunctival suffusion, nasal stuffiness, headache, and skin rash. Rapid intravenous administration may produce hypotension, bradycardia and/or arrhythmias, and thrombophlebitis.

Composition and Supply

Injection   250 mg/ml, in 20 ml vials
Syrup   1.25 g/5 ml
Tablets   500 mg

Legal Status

Prescription

Aminodur® Dura-Tabs®

See under **Aminophylline.**

Aminophylline (theophylline ethylenediamine)

Action and Use

Bronchodilator.

Dosage and Administration

100 to 200 mg 3 to 4 times a day, orally; 500 mg at bedtime, rectally; 250 to 500 mg, IM or slowly IV.

Cautions

Contraindicated when the patient's blood pressure is low. Intravenous solutions must be diluted and warmed to body temperature, and should be injected slowly. Cardiac arrest or ventricular fibrillation may result.

Adverse Reactions

Intramuscular administration may produce pain at the injection site. Intravenous preparation may produce flushing, headache, palpitations, dizziness, nausea, hypotension, and precordial pain. Repeated use of rectal preparation can cause anorectal irritation.

Composition and Supply

Elixir   105 mg/15 ml (Somophyllin®)
Injection   25 mg/ml, in 10 ml and 20 ml ampuls
Solution, rectal   300 mg/5 ml (Somophyllin®)
Suppositories   250 mg and 500 mg
Tablets   100 mg and 200 mg
Tablets, prolonged-release   300 mg (Aminodur® Dura-Tabs®)

Legal Status
Prescription

Aminophylline/guaifenesin/ephedrine/phenobarbital
(Mudrane®-GG)

See ANTIASTHMATICS, xanthine preparations.

Aminosalicylic acid (*p*-aminosalicylic acid [PAS]) (Pamisyl®, Rezipas®)

Action and Use
Antituberculotic.

Dosage and Administration
10 to 15 g daily in divided doses, orally.

Cautions
Aminosalicylic acid can cause hypersensitivity, hepatic damage, goiter, hypothyroidism, and gastrointestinal disturbances. Use with caution in patients with peptic ulcer; contraindicated in those with kidney disease. The patient should avoid other salicylates (because salicylate poisoning might result).

Adverse Reactions
Allergic reactions may occur from the second to eighth week; these reactions include skin eruptions, fever, malaise, sore throat, and painful joints. Occasional side effects include hepatitis (with inhibition of prothrombin synthesis), renal failure (including negative potassium balance and acidosis), and blood dyscrasias (with leukopenia, agranulocytosis, eosinophilia, lymphocytosis, and thrombocytopenia). With extended therapy, clotting time may be prolonged. Rare side effects include radiculitis and meningitis, pancreatitis, exfoliation, encephalopathy, and pulmonary difficulties.

Composition and Supply
Resin 50%, in 4 g or 8 g packets
Tablets 500 mg
Tablets 500 mg with vitamin C (PAS-C)(Pascorbic)

Legal Status
Prescription

Aminosol® (protein hydrolysate injection 5% and 10%)

See PARENTERAL ALIMENTATION.

Aminosol® Kit (parenteral hyperalimentation kit [amino acids–dextrose])

See PARENTERAL ALIMENTATION.

Amitriptyline hydrochloride (Elavil®, Endep®)

Action and Use
Tricyclic antidepressant.

Dosage and Administration
75 to 300 mg daily, orally; 20 to 30 mg 4 times a day, IM.

Cautions
Contraindicated in patients with pyloric stenosis, urinary retention, prostatic hypertrophy, kidney disease, and angle-closure glaucoma. Do not give concomitantly with MAO inhibitors. Adrenergics, anticholinergics, and CNS depressants may be potentiated. Transient delirium may occur in patients receiving large doses of ethchlorvynol. Use cautiously in patients with impaired liver function.

Adverse Reactions
Frequently occurring symptoms include rash, impairment of mental and/or physical abilities with drowsiness, postural hypotension, faintness, dizziness, weakness (monitor blood pressure and caution the patient to rise slowly), insomnia, excitement, paresthesias, tremors, dry mouth, blurred vision, constipation, urinary retention, nausea, vomiting, anorexia, impotence, headache, and perspiration; these symptoms may be relieved or controlled by decreasing the dosage. Other possible side effects include tachycardia, palpitations, arrhythmia, myocardial infarction, heart block, cerebrovascular accident, accommodation disturbance, paralytic ileus, photosensitivity (patient should avoid sun rays), edema of face and tongue, bone marrow depression (periodic blood tests are recommended), stomatitis, black tongue, parotid swelling, peculiar taste, diarrhea, testicular swelling and gynecomastia, breast enlargement and galactorrhea, change in libido, hypoglycemia or hyperglycemia, fatigue, weight gain, frequent urination, mydriasis, alopecia, and jaundice (periodic liver function studies are recommended). Late symptoms may include confusion, disorientation, delusions, hallucinations, anxiety, restlessness, nightmares, ataxia, seizures, tinnitus, and mild extrapyramidal reactions. Abrupt discontinuance of the drug may produce nausea, headache, and malaise.

Composition and Supply
Injection   10 mg/ml
Tablets   10 mg, 25 mg, 50 mg, and 100 mg
Tablets   10 mg with perphenazine 2 mg (Triavil® 2-10)

Tablets   10 mg with perphenazine 4 mg (Triavil® 4-10)
Tablets   25 mg with perphenazine 2 mg (Triavil® 2-25)
Tablets   25 mg with perphenazine 4 mg (Triavil® 4-25)

Note: Triavil® is a tranquilizer-antidepressant combination for depression with moderate anxiety. The usual initial dosage is 1 Triavil® 2-25 or 1 Triavil® 4-25 3 or 4 times a day. Cautions and adverse reactions for perphenazine are similar to those for chlorpromazine hydrochloride.

Legal Status
Prescription

Ammonia spirit, aromatic

Action and Use
Reflex respiratory stimulant used to treat syncope or threatened fainting.

Dosage and Administration
Ampuls are crushed and the vapor inhaled; or 2 to 4 ml is well diluted with water and taken orally.

Cautions
High concentrations of inhaled vapor are injurious to the lungs, and may result in pulmonary edema.

Adverse Reactions
No important side effects when used as directed.

Composition and Supply
Ampuls (or pearls) (Vaporole®)
Bottles   2 oz

Legal status
Nonprescription

Ammonium chloride

Action and Use
Acidifying agent and expectorant.

Dosage and Administration
Acidifying agent: 4 to 12 g in divided doses, orally.
To combat alkalosis: as indicated, IV.
Expectorant: 250 to 500 mg every 2 to 4 hours, with water.

Cautions
Large doses may lead to metabolic acidosis. Contraindicated in patients with renal impairment. Ammonium chloride may cause hypokalemia.

Adverse Reactions
Gastrointestinal irritation may occur.

Composition and Supply
Injection   160 mg (3 mEq) in 30 ml
Tablets   300 mg and 500 mg
Tablets, enteric-coated   300 mg and 500 mg

Legal Status
Prescription

Amnestrogen®

See **Estrogens, esterified.**

Amobarbital (Amytal®)

Action and Use
Short-acting barbiturate (sedative-hypnotic).

Dosage and Administration
15 to 480 mg orally (usual hypnotic dose 100 to 200 mg); 65 to 200 mg (maximum dose 500 mg), IM, IV.

Cautions
Habit-forming. May cause respiratory depression and hypotension if injected rapidly. Should not be combined with alcohol or other CNS depressants or given to patients with uncontrolled pain. Use with caution in patients with hypertension, hypotension, pulmonary or cardiovascular disease, narrow-angle glaucoma, or epilepsy. Contraindicated in patients with severe liver or kidney disease and in those with a history of porphyria. Superficial intramuscular or subcutaneous injection may be painful and may produce a sterile abscess or tissue slough.

Adverse Reactions
Common side effects include hangover, listlessness, nausea, vomiting, emotional disturbances, rash, pruritus, asthmatic attack, restlessness, delirium, and nightmares. Acute overdose may cause deep sleep, coma, respiratory depression, and miosis.

Composition and Supply
Capsules   65 mg and 200 mg
Injection (as sodium salt)   65 mg, 125 mg, and 500 mg ampuls;
   1 g vials
Tablets   15 mg, 30 mg, 50 mg, and 100 mg

Legal Status
Schedule II

Amodiaquine hydrochloride (Camoquin®)

Action and Use
Antimalarial.

Dosage and Administration
For malaria suppression: 400 to 600 mg per week, orally.
For malaria treatment: 600 mg to 1 g, orally, initially; followed by 400 mg a day for 2 days, orally.

Cautions
See **Chloroquine.**

Adverse Reactions
Similar to adverse reactions to chloroquine (see).

Composition and Supply
Tablets   200 mg

Legal Status
Prescription

Amoxicillin (Amoxil®, Larotid®)

Action and Use
Broad-spectrum antibiotic.

Dosage and Administration
250 to 500 mg every 8 hours, orally.

Cautions
Penicillin cross-sensitivity. Use with caution in patients who are allergic to penicillin or have a history of allergic reactions. See **Penicillin G potassium** for further cautions.

Adverse Reactions
See **Penicillin G potassium.**

Composition and Supply
Capsules   250 mg and 500 mg
Suspension   125 mg/5 ml and 250 mg/5 ml

Legal Status
Prescription

Amoxil®

See **Amoxicillin.**

Amphetamine sulfate (Benzedrine®)

See CEREBRAL STIMULANTS.

Amphojel®

See **Aluminum hydroxide gel.**

Amphotericin B (Fungizone®)

Action and Use
Systemic antifungal antibiotic; also used topically in candidiasis.

Dosage and Administration
Injection: initially 250 μg per kg daily, by slow IV infusion, increased to 1 to 1.5 mg per kg on alternate days.
Topical application: apply 2 to 4 times a day.

Cautions
Under no circumstances should the dose exceed 1.5 mg/kg per day. Use only in life-threatening situations and only under close medical supervision. Toxic effects are frequent and serious. Monitor kidney function. Acidic solutions, solutions of electrolytes, or solutions with preservatives should not be used in mixing the powder because they produce precipitation. Discard solutions with a precipitate.

Adverse Reactions
Hypersensitivity reactions include anaphylaxis, thrombocytopenia, flushing, generalized pain, and convulsions. Liver dysfunction may be aggravated. Phlebitis and thrombophlebitis may occur at the injection site. Intrathecal injection may produce pain along the distribution of lumbar nerves, headache, paresthesias, nerve palsies, difficult micturition, vision impairment, and meningitis.

Composition and Supply
Cream, lotion, and ointment   3%
Injection   50 mg vials.

Legal Status
Prescription

Ampicillin (Alpen®, Amcill®, Omnipen®, Omnipen®-N, Penbritin®, Penbritin®-S, Pensin®, Polycillin®, Polycillin® N, Principen®, Totacillin®, Totacillin®-N)

Action and Use
Broad-spectrum antibiotic.

Dosage and Administration
250 to 500 mg every 6 hours, up to 200 mg/kg per day, orally, IM, or IV.

Cautions
Use with caution in patients who are allergic to penicillin or have a history of allergic reactions. Use with caution in patients with renal failure. See **Penicillin G potassium** for further cautions.

Adverse Reactions
See **Penicillin G potassium.**

Composition and Supply
Capsules (as trihydrate)   250 mg and 500 mg
Injection (as sodium salt)   125 mg, 250 mg, 500 mg, 1 g, 2 g, and 4 g
Suspension (as trihydrate)   125 mg/5 ml, 250 mg/5 ml, and 500 mg/5 ml

Legal Status
Prescription

Amyl nitrite

Action and Use
Coronary vasodilator used in angina pectoris and as an antidote (along with sodium nitrite) in cyanide poisoning.

Dosage and Administration
The ampuls are crushed in a handkerchief, and the vapors are inhaled at once.

Cautions
The patient should be seated. Intense and rapid lowering of blood pressure may occur.

Adverse Reactions
Throbbing headache, flushing, or nausea and vomiting may result. (*Note:* amyl nitrite is very flammable.)

101

Composition and Supply
Ampuls (or perles), covered with silk   0.2 ml (200 µl) and 0.3 ml (300 µl)

Legal Status
Prescription

Amytal®

See **Amobarbital.**

Anacin® (aspirin/caffeine)

See ANALGESICS, nonnarcotic.

Anadrol®-50 (oxymetholone)

See ANDROGENS.

Ananase®

See **Bromelains.**

Ancef® (cefazolin)

See ANTIBIOTICS, cephalosporins.

Ancobon® (flucytosine)

See ANTIFUNGALS.

Android®

See **Methyltestosterone.**

Anectine®

See **Succinylcholine chloride.**

Anileridine (Leritine®)

Action and Use
Narcotic analgesic.

Dosage and Administration
25 to 50 mg every 4 to 6 hours (not to exceed 200 mg), orally, SC, or IM.

Cautions
The injection has a wide range of incompatibilities with other drugs. Anileridine enhances MAO inhibitors; phenothiazines tend to increase its sedative effects. It is addicting.

Adverse Reactions
Side effects include drowsiness, euphoria, nausea, vomiting, dizziness, and palpitations. Hypotension and syncope may occur in ambulatory patients. Morphine-like effects include miosis, constipation, diaphoresis, decreased body temperature, urine retention, frequency of urination, and ureteral and/or biliary spasm. Toxic effects include respiratory and circulatory depression.

Composition and Supply
Injection (phosphate)   25 mg/ml
Tablets (hydrochloride)   25 mg

Legal Status
Schedule II

Anisindione (Miradon®)

See ANTICOAGULANTS.

Anspor® (cephradine)

See ANTIBIOTICS, cephalosporins.

Antabuse®

See **Disulfiram.**

Antepar®

See **Piperazine citrate.**

Anthra-Derm®

See **Anthralin.**

Anthralin (Anthra-Derm®, Lasan® Unguent)

Action and Use
Antipsoriatic.

Dosage and Administration
Apply in a thin layer to affected areas. The lowest concentration should be used first.

Cautions
Not to be used near eyes, face, scalp, genitalia, intertriginous skin areas or on inflamed areas. Contraindicated in renal dysfunction. Wash hands thoroughly after use.

Adverse Reactions
Skin is stained yellow. Warn patient that urine will turn red.

Composition and Supply
Ointment   0.1%, 0.25%, 0.5%, and 1% (Anthra-Derm®)
Ointment   0.4% (Lasan® Unguent)

Legal Status
Prescription

Antihemophilic factor (human) VIII (Humafac®, Koāte®, Profilate®)

See HEMOSTATICS.

Antihemophilic factor (human) IX (Konȳne®)

See HEMOSTATICS.

Antilirium®

See **Physostigmine salicylate.**

Antiminth® (pyrantel pamoate)

See ANTHELMINTICS, pinworm, roundworm.

Antimony potassium tartrate (tartar emetic)

Action and Use
Anthelmintic for use in schistosomiasis caused by *Schistosoma japonicum.*

Dosage and Administration
Given IV according to the manufacturer's directions.

Cautions
Contraindicated in hepatic, renal, or cardiac insufficiency. The patient should be hospitalized during treatment and should remain recumbent for 7 hours after administration.

Adverse Reactions
Common side effects include nausea, vomiting, and muscle and joint pains. If the injection is too rapid, a hacking cough, vomiting, and severe or even fatal reactions may result.

Composition and Supply
Injection   10 mg/ml

Legal Status
Prescription

Antipyrene/benzocaine/glycerin (Auralgen®)

See ANESTHETICS, local.

Antirabies serum

See BIOLOGICALS, immune serums–antitoxins.

Antivenin, *Latrodectus mactans*

Action and Use
Provides neutralizing antibodies (antitoxins) against the toxins of the black widow spider.

Dosage and Administration
Mild to moderate envenomation: inject the entire contents of a restored vial (2.5 ml), IM.
Severe cases: infuse entire vial mixed with 10 to 50 ml of saline solution, IV, over a 15 minute period.

Cautions
Test first for sensitivity to horse serum. Desensitization should be attempted only when antivenin is considered necessary to save the patient's life. Epinephrine must be available in case an untoward reaction occurs.

Adverse Reactions
Serum sickness (with fever, urticaria, or pruritus) may develop 5 to 13 days after administration of antivenin.

Composition and Supply
Combination package:
    6,000 unit vial
    Horse serum for sensitivity testing (1 ml)
    Sterile water (2.5 ml)

Note: supplied by Merck Sharp and Dohme, West Point, PA.

Legal Status
Prescription

Antivenin, *Micrurus fulvius*

Action and Use
Provides neutralizing antibodies (antitoxins) against the toxins of the North American coral snake.

Dosage and Administration
Follow manufacturer's directions carefully. The IV route is most effective, except in shock, when the antivenin may have to be given intraperitoneally.

Cautions
See **Antivenin,** *Latrodectus mactans.*

Adverse Reactions
Serum sickness (with fever, urticaria, or pruritus) may develop.

Composition and Supply
Combination package:
    Vial of lyophilized antivenin
    Vial of diluent (10 ml)

Note: available at Wyeth Laboratories, Philadelphia, PA, and at depots and hospitals within range of coral snakes.

Legal Status
Prescription

Antivenin, polyvalent crotaline

Action and Use
Provides neutralizing antibodies (antitoxins) against pit vipers, which include copperhead, water moccasin, pigmy rattler, timber rattler, eastern diamondback rattler, western diamondback rattler, prairie rattler, and Pacific rattler.

Dosage and Administration
See **Antivenin,** *Micrurus fulvius.*

Cautions
See **Antivenin,** *Latrodectus mactans.*

Adverse Reactions
See **Antivenin,** *Latrodectus mactans.*

Composition and Supply
Combination package:
    Vial of lyophilized antivenin
    10 ml water for injection in disposable syringe
    Applicator vial of tincture of iodine
    Horse serum for sensitivity testing

Note: available at Wyeth Laboratories, Philadelphia, PA, and at depots and hospitals within range of pit vipers.

Legal Status
Prescription

Antivert®

See **Meclizine hydrochloride.**

Antrypol® (suramin)

See ANTIPROTOZOALS, antitrypanosomals.

Anturane®

See **Sulfinpyrazone.**

APC

See **Aspirin/phenacetin/caffeine.**

A.P.L.®

See **Gonadotropin, chorionic.**

Aplisol®

See **Tuberculin, purified protein derivative (PPD).**

Apomorphine hydrochloride

Action and Use
Central-acting narcotic emetic.

Dosage and Administration
5 mg SC; *do not repeat.*

Cautions
Contraindicated in patients who have ingested petroleum products or corrosive or caustic substances, and in comatose or semicomatose individuals who may aspirate vomitus. Excessive doses may produce violent emesis, cardiac depression, or death.

Adverse Reactions
Therapeutic doses may produce CNS depression or, at times, tremors.

Composition and Supply
Hypodermic tablets   6 mg

Note: color changes with age; protect from light and keep in tightly closed bottles.

Legal Status
Schedule II

Apresazide™

See under **Hydralazine hydrochloride.**

Apresoline®

See **Hydralazine hydrochloride.**

Aprobarbital (Alurate®)

See SEDATIVE-HYPNOTICS, barbiturates.

Aquacare® (urea preparation)

See EMOLLIENT-PROTECTANTS; KERATOLYTICS.

Aquachloral®

See **Chloral hydrate.**

AquaMEPHYTON®

See **Phytonadione.**

Aquasol® A

See **Vitamin A.**

Aquasol® E (Vitamin E)

See VITAMINS, fat-soluble.

Aralen® hydrochloride

See **Chloroquine hydrochloride.**

Aralen® phosphate

See **Chloroquine phosphate.**

Aramine®

See **Metaraminol bitartrate.**

Arfonad® (trimethaphan camsylate)

See ANTIHYPERTENSIVES, nondiuretic.

Arginine glutamate

See ELECTROLYTE SOLUTIONS AND WATER-BALANCE AGENTS, ammonia detoxicants.

Arginine hydrochloride (R-Gene™ 10)

Action and Use
Ammonia detoxicant for use in patients with hepatic disease.

Dosage and Administration
20 g in 500 to 1,000 ml of 5% or 10% dextrose over 1 to 4 hours by IV infusion.

Cautions
Use with caution in patients with renal disease. Creatine and creatinine levels may be elevated.

Adverse Reactions
None when used as directed.

Composition and Supply
Injection   10%, 300 ml in 500 ml flask

Legal Status
Prescription

Aristocort®

See **Triamcinolone.**

Aristocort® A

See **Triamcinolone acetonide.**

Aristospan®

See **Triamcinolone hexacetonide.**

Arlidin®

See **Nylidrin hydrochloride.**

Aromatic cascara fluidextract

See under **Cascara sagrada.**

Arsthinol (Balarsen®)

See ANTIPROTOZOALS, antiamebials.

Artane®

See **Trihexyphenidyl hydrochloride.**

Ar-Tet®

See **Tetanus immune human globulin.**

Arthropan® (choline salicylate)

See ANALGESICS, nonnarcotic.

Ascodeen-30® (aspirin/codeine)

See ANALGESICS, narcotic.

Ascorbic acid (vitamin C)

Action and Use
Vitamin supplement.

Dosage and Administration
100 to 500 mg daily, orally; 100 to 500 mg daily, IM or IV.

Cautions
Possibility of kidney stones.

Adverse Reactions
None within usual dosage range; large doses may cause gastrointestinal upsets.

Composition and Supply
Injection   50 to 500 mg/ml, in 1 ml and 10 ml ampuls
Liquid   100 mg/ml
Tablets   25 mg, 50 mg, 100 mg, 250 mg, and 500 mg

Legal Status
Prescription (injection)
Nonprescription (liquid and tablets)

Asparaginase (Elspar®)

See ANTINEOPLASTICS, miscellaneous.

Aspirin (acetylsalicylic acid)

Action and Use
Analgesic and antipyretic.

Dosage and Administration
325 to 975 mg every 4 hours, orally; or 650 mg every 4 hours, rectally.

Cautions
Exacerbates peptic ulcer and erosive gastritis. Allergic reactions may occur. Enhances the activity of oral anticoagulants, probenecid, sul-

fonylureas, methotrexate, penicillin, and phenytoin sodium. Concurrent use of methotrexate and aspirin may produce toxic effects, including bone marrow depression, nausea, vomiting, and diarrhea. Aspirin may produce gastrointestinal bleeding when combined with alcohol. Use with caution in renal or hepatic insufficiency and in hypoprothrombinemia.

Adverse Reactions
Irritation of gastrointestinal mucosa may occur, especially with prolonged use. Prothrombin level is decreased and platelet survival time is prolonged. High doses may decrease hematocrit, hemoglobin, and plasma iron levels and may shorten erythrocyte survival time. Hemolysis may result in individuals with glucose-6-phosphate dehydrogenase deficiency. Skin eruptions and dyspnea may occur. An overdose may cause salicylism, tinnitus, dizziness, disturbances of hearing and vision, diaphoresis, nausea, vomiting, diarrhea, thirst, hyperventilation, hypotension, inconstant pulse, and skin eruptions. A massive dose may produce delirium, coma, depressed respirations, and alterations in acid-base balance.

Composition and Supply
Suppositories   325 mg and 650 mg
Tablets   325 mg
Tablets, buffered   325 mg with aluminum glycinate and magnesium
   carbonate (Bufferin®)
Tablets, enteric-coated   325 mg and 650 mg

Legal Status
Nonprescription

Aspirin/caffeine (Anacin®)

See ANALGESICS, nonnarcotic.

Aspirin/codeine (Ascodeen-30®)

See ANALGESICS, narcotic.

Aspirin compound

See **Aspirin/phenacetin/caffeine.**

Aspirin/phenacetin/caffeine (APC, aspirin compound) (Empirin® Compound)

Action and Use
Analgesic and antipyretic.

Dosage and Administration
1 or 2 tablets every 4 hours.

Cautions
See **Aspirin.**

Adverse Reactions
Side effects are uncommon, but overdosage is serious (see **Aspirin;** see also Phenacetin poisoning in Appendix 3).

Composition and Supply
Tablets   aspirin 200 to 250 mg, phenacetin 120 to 150 mg, caffeine 15 to 30 mg
Tablets   APC with codeine (Empirin® Compound with Codeine): 7.5 mg codeine (No. 1), 15 mg codeine (No. 2), 30 mg codeine (No. 3), and 60 mg codeine (No. 4)
Tablets, capsules   APC with 50 mg butalbital (Fiorinal®)
Capsules   Fiorinal® with Codeine: 7.5 mg codeine (No. 1), 15 mg codeine (No. 2), and 30 mg codeine (No. 3)

Note: dosage for the compounds containing butalbital or codeine is 1 or 2 tablets, repeated if necessary up to 6 per day or as directed by physician; may be habit-forming.

Legal Status
Nonprescription (APC)
Prescription (Fiorinal®)
Schedule III (Empirin® Compound with Codeine, Fiorinal® with Codeine)

Aspirin/salicylamide/acetaminophen/caffeine (Excedrin®)

See ANALGESICS, nonnarcotic.

Atabrine®

See **Quinacrine hydrochloride.**

Atarax®

See **Hydroxyzine.**

Ativan® (lorazepam)

See PSYCHOTROPICS, tranquilizers, minor.

Atromid-S®

See **Clofibrate.**

Atropine sulfate

Action and Use
Belladonna alkaloid anticholinergic. Useful as an antispasmodic, mydriatic, and cycloplegic; also used to increase the heart rate.

Dosage and Administration
Usual dose is 500 μg, orally, SC, or IV. 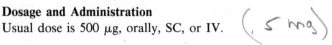 (, 5 mg)

Cautions
Blindness may result in patients with narrow-angle glaucoma. An overdose may lead to elevated temperature and delirium.

Adverse Reactions
Common side effects include dry mouth, mydriasis, blurred vision, and flushing. Occasional side effects include nausea, vomiting, giddiness, staggering, and stupor. Increased intraocular pressure, impotence, or circulatory failure may occur.

Composition and Supply
Injection   400 μg/ml, in 1 ml and 20 ml ampuls
Ophthalmic ointment   0.5% and 1%
Ophthalmic solution   0.5% and 1% (Isopto®-Atropine)
Tablets   300 μg, 400 μg, and 600 μg
Tablets, capsules, or elixir with hyoscyamine, hyoscine, and phenobarbital (Donnatal®): each tablet, capsule, or 5 ml of elixir contains atropine sulfate 19.4 μg, hyoscyamine sulfate 103.7 μg, hyoscine hydrobromide 6.5 μg, and phenobarbital 16.2 mg (*Note:* the dosage for Donnatal® is 1 or 2 tablets or capsules, or 5 to 10 ml of elixir, 3 or 4 times a day according to patient's condition and severity of symptoms; or 1 or 2 Donnatal® Extentabs® morning and night. 1 Donnatal® Extentab® equals 3 Donnatal® tablets. *Caution:* phenobarbital may be habit-forming [see **Phenobarbital**].)

Legal Status
Prescription

Attenuvax®

See **Measles virus vaccine, live attenuated.**

Auralgen® (antipyrene/benzocaine/glycerin)

See ANESTHETICS, local.

Aureomycin® (chlortetracycline hydrochloride)

See ANTIBIOTICS, tetracyclines.

Aureotope® (gold Au 198)

See ANTINEOPLASTICS, radioisotopes.

Aurothioglucose (Solganal®)

Action and Use
Gold salt useful in the treatment of rheumatoid arthritis.

Dosage and Administration
Usual IM schedule: first dose, 10 mg; second and third doses, 25 mg; fourth and subsequent doses, 50 mg. There should be a 1 week interval between doses up to 1 g. If patient improves with no toxic signs, then 25 to 50 mg is given at 3 to 4 week intervals.

Cautions
Contraindicated in patients with kidney disease, a history of infectious hepatitis, blood dyscrasias, urticaria, eczema, or colitis, in the aged, and in those who have recently been exposed to radiation. Periodic blood studies and urinalysis are recommended. At the first signs of a severe reaction, treat the patient with dimercaprol.

Adverse Reactions
The most common side effects are transient albuminuria, lesions of the mucous membranes, dermatitis, diarrhea, and abdominal cramps. There is a low incidence of serious reactions, including encephalitis, peripheral neuritis, hepatitis, blood dyscrasias (thrombocytopenia may develop many months after gold is administered), and kidney toxicity with albuminuria.

Composition and Supply
Injection   50 mg/ml, in 10 ml vials

Legal Status
Prescription

Aveeno®

See **Oatmeal, colloidal.**

Aventyl®

See **Nortriptyline hydrochloride.**

Avitene® (microfibrillar collagen hemostat)

See HEMOSTATICS.

114

Avlosulfon® (dapsone)

See ANTILEPROTICS.

Azathioprine (Imuran®)

Action and Use
Immunosuppressive used to help prevent rejection in renal homotransplantation.

Dosage and Administration
Dosage is individualized, based on clinical and hematologic response. The usual initial dose is about 3 to 5 mg/kg per day, orally or IV; the maintenance dose averages about 1 to 2 mg/kg per day.

Cautions
Azathioprine is highly toxic and must be used under close medical supervision; it may be teratogenic. Irreversible bone marrow depression may result. Complete blood counts, including platelets, should be performed periodically. Clotting time is prolonged.

Adverse Reactions
Similar to mercaptopurine (see), which is the active metabolite of azathioprine.

Composition and Supply
Injection (as sodium salt)   100 mg in 20 ml vials
Tablets   50 mg

Legal Status
Prescription

Azene™ (clorazepate monopotassium)

See PSYCHOTROPICS, tranquilizers, minor.

Azo Gantanol®

See under **Sulfamethoxazole.**

Azo Gantrisin®

See under **Sulfisoxazole.**

Azolid®

See **Phenylbutazone.**

Azolid®-A

See under **Phenylbutazone.**

Azo-Mandelamine® (methenamine mandelate/phenazopyridine hydrochloride)

See URINARY ANTISEPTICS.

Azotrex® (tetracycline phosphate complex/sulfamethizole/phenazopyridine hydrochloride)

See URINARY ANTISEPTICS.

Azulfidine®

See **Sulfasalazine.**

Bacid®

See under *Lactobacillus acidophilus/L. bulgaricus*

Baciquent®

See under **Bacitracin.**

Bacitracin

Action and Use
Antibiotic effective against a variety of gram-positive organisms and a few gram-negative organisms. It is often combined with other antibiotics (see **Polymyxin B sulfate).**

Dosage and Administration
Applied topically as solution or ointment. Parenteral (IM) use is restricted to infants with staphylococcal pneumonia and empyema caused by susceptible organisms.

Cautions
May cause renal failure with parenteral use. Renal function should be determined prior to therapy and daily during therapy. Fluid intake should be high enough to insure adequate excretion.

Adverse Reactions
Pain may occur at the site of intramuscular injection (rotate sites and inject deeply). In addition to nephrotoxicity, toxicity may include damage to eighth cranial nerve with parenteral use. Rarely, hypersensitivity occurs with topical use.

Composition and Supply
Ointment   500 units/g (Baciquent®)
Solution   50,000 unit sterile vials
Injection   10,000 unit and 50,000 unit vials

Legal Status
Nonprescription (topical preparations)
Prescription (injection)

Baclofen (Lioresal®)

See SKELETAL MUSCLE RELAXANTS.

Bactocill®

See **Oxacillin sodium.**

Bactrim™

See **Trimethoprim/sulfamethoxazole.**

Bactrim™ DS

See under **Trimethoprim/sulfamethoxazole.**

Baking soda

See **Sodium bicarbonate.**

BAL

See **Dimercaprol.**

Balarsen® (arsthinol)

See ANTIPROTOZOALS, antiamebials.

Banthīne® (methantheline bromide)

See ANTICHOLINERGICS.

Barbital/butalbital/phenobarbital/ dihydroergotamine/scopolamine (Plexonal®)

See SEDATIVE-HYPNOTICS, barbiturates.

Barium sulfate (Barosperse®, Barotrast®)

Action and Use
Radiopaque diagnostic agent used to visualize the alimentary tract.

Dosage and Administration
Varies according to area to be visualized: 200 to 300 g for barium meal; 650 to 750 g for barium enema.

Cautions
Barium sulfate should not be confused with the highly poisonous barium sulfide or barium sulfite. The patient should be informed that

the stool will be a light color after the examination. Large amounts orally may cause fecal impaction in patients with impaired evacuation.

Adverse Reactions
Relatively nontoxic; rarely, with barium enema, granulomas of the rectum and colon may occur.

Composition and Supply
Powder

Legal Status
Prescription

Barosperse®

See **Barium sulfate.**

Barotrast®

See **Barium sulfate.**

Basaljel® (aluminum carbonate gel)

See ANTACIDS.

BCG vaccine (tuberculosis vaccine)

Action and Use
Attenuated strain of *Mycobacterium bovis* (of bovine origin) used for active immunization against tuberculosis in persons at high risk.

Dosage and Administration
Intradermal injection of 0.1 ml (100 μl), diluted, to produce a wheal of 8 to 10 mm (may also be given by multiple-puncture technique).

Cautions
Contraindicated in tuberculin-positive individuals and in persons with congenital immunologic deficiencies.

Adverse Reactions
Local induration. Hypersensitivity may occur. The use of vaccine negates diagnostic value of tuberculin test.

Composition and Supply
Vaccine, freeze-dried (to be diluted)

Legal Status
Prescription

BCNU (carmustine)

See ANTINEOPLASTICS, miscellaneous.

Because® (nonylphenoxypolyoxyethylene ethanol)

See CONTRACEPTIVES, TOPICAL.

Beclomethasone dipropionate (Vanceril®)

Action and Use
Synthetic corticosteroid indicated only for patients who require chronic treatment with corticosteroids for control of bronchial asthma.

Dosage and Administration
3 to 16 inhalations daily, up to a maximum of 20 inhalations (1 mg).

Cautions
Deaths have occurred in asthmatic patients during and after transfer from systemic corticosteroids to beclomethasone. Contraindicated in the primary treatment of status asthmaticus and other episodes of asthma where intensive measures are required.

Adverse Reactions
Suppresses hypothalamic-pituitary-adrenal (HPA) function in adults when administered beyond recommended dosage. Dry mouth and hoarseness are possible side effects.

Composition and Supply
Inhaler   beclomethasone dipropionate 10 mg (200 inhalations)

Legal Status
Prescription

Belladenal® (belladonna alkaloids/phenobarbital)

See ANTICHOLINERGICS.

Belladonna alkaloids (Bellafoline®, Prydon®)

See ANTICHOLINERGICS.

Belladonna alkaloids/phenobarbital (Belladenal®)

See ANTICHOLINERGICS.

Belladonna alkaloids/phenobarbital/simethicone (Kinesed®)

See ANTICHOLINERGICS.

Belladonna tincture

Action and Use
Anticholinergic and spasmolytic.

Dosage and Administration
0.3 ml (300 μl) to 1 ml 3 times a day, orally.

Cautions
Contraindicated in patients with glaucoma, renal or hepatic disease, or obstructive uropathy. See **Atropine sulfate** for further cautions.

Adverse Reactions
Same as for atropine sulfate (see).

Composition and Supply
Tincture   alkaloids 30 mg/100 ml

Legal Status
Prescription

Bellafoline® (belladonna alkaloids)

See ANTICHOLINERGICS.

Benadryl®

See **Diphenhydramine hydrochloride.**

Bendectin® (doxylamine succinate/pyridoxine hydrochloride)

See ANTIEMETICS.

Bendopa®

See **Levodopa.**

Bendroflumethiazide (Naturetin®)

Action and Use
Diuretic and antihypertensive.

Dosage and Administration
2.5 to 20 mg daily, orally.

Cautions
See **Chlorothiazide.**

Adverse Reactions
See **Chlorothiazide.**

Composition and Supply
Tablets   2.5 mg and 5 mg

Legal Status
Prescription

Benemid®

See **Probenecid.**

Benisone®

See **Betamethasone.**

Benoxyl® (benzoyl peroxide)

See ANTI-INFECTIVES, LOCAL; KERATOLYTICS.

Bensulfoid® (sulfur, colloidal)

See KERATOLYTICS.

Bentyl®

See **Dicyclomine hydrochloride.**

Benylin® Cough Syrup

See COUGH-COLD PREPARATIONS, cough preparations.

Benzalkonium chloride (Zephiran®)

Actions and Use
Local anti-infective.

Dosage and Administration
Use as indicated for disinfection.

Cautions
Use only after all soap or detergent has been rinsed from the skin (to avoid inactivation). Concomitant use of antibiotics may sensitize the patient and may result in the production of resistant strains of bacteria.

Adverse Reactions
Irritates the skin if used in concentrations exceeding 1%. Irritation and chemical burns are possible if used on occlusive dressings or as rectal or vaginal packing.

Composition and Supply
Solution   1 : 750
Tincture   1 : 750

Legal Status
Nonprescription

Benzedrex® (propylhexedrine)

See ADRENERGICS; NASAL DECONGESTANTS.

Benzedrine® (amphetamine sulfate)

See CEREBRAL STIMULANTS.

Benzocaine (Americaine®)

See ANESTHETICS, local; ANTIPRURITICS, topical preparations.

Benzoic acid/salicylic acid ointment (Whitfield's ointment)

Action and Use
Antifungal agent used to treat tinea pedis (athlete's foot).

Dosage and Administration
Apply 2 or 3 times a day.

Cautions
Avoid contact with mucous membranes.

Adverse Reactions
Skin irritation may occur.

Composition and Supply
Ointment   benzoic acid 6%, salicylic acid 3%

Legal Status
Nonprescription

Benzoin tincture, compound

Action and Use
Protectant and mild antiseptic.

Dosage and Administration
Applied topically. Should be dry before applying dressing to prevent sticking.

Cautions
Flammable.

Adverse Reactions
Stings on open wounds.

Composition and Supply
Tincture, contains benzoin, aloe, storax, and tolu balsam

Legal Status
Nonprescription

Benzonatate (Tessalon®)

Action and Use
Nonnarcotic antitussive.

Dosage and Administration
100 to 600 mg daily, orally.

Cautions
Capsules or "perles" should be swallowed whole; the release of the drug in the mouth can produce local anesthesia of oral mucosa.

Adverse Reactions
Side effects include drowsiness, nausea, tightness in chest, dizziness, nasal congestion, headache, pruritus, skin eruptions, constipation, and a burning sensation in the eyes. Overdose may cause convulsions and consequent CNS depression.

Composition and Supply
Capsules ("perles")   50 mg and 100 mg

Legal Status
Nonprescription

Benzoyl peroxide (Benoxyl®, Persadox®, Persa-Gel®)

See ANTI-INFECTIVES, LOCAL, miscellaneous antiseptic-disinfectants; KERATOLYTICS.

Benzphetamine hydrochloride (Didrex™)

See CEREBRAL STIMULANTS, anorectics.

Benzquinamide hydrochloride (Emete-con®)

Action and Use
Antiemetic.

Dosage and Administration
50 mg IM. First dose may be repeated within 1 hour, with subsequent doses every 3 to 4 hours. 25 mg IV slowly.

Cautions
When reconstituted with saline, a precipitate forms. The IV route is restricted to patients without cardiovascular disease.

Adverse Reactions
Drowsiness is common. Occasional side effects include salivation or dry mouth, blurred vision, flushing, hiccoughs, shivering, increased temperature, diaphoresis, hypertension, hypotension, dizziness, excitement, headache, anorexia, nausea, weakness, and tremors. An allergic response with urticaria and rash is a rare side effect.

Composition and Supply
Injection   50 mg ampuls

Legal Status
Nonprescription

Benzthiazide (Exna®)

See DIURETICS.

Benztropine mesylate (Cogentin®)

Action and Use
Anticholinergic skeletal muscle relaxant used in all forms of parkinsonism.

Dosage and Administration
1 to 2 mg (dosage ranges from 500 μg to 6 mg), orally or parenterally (IV or IM).

Cautions
Atropine-like side effects may occur. Glaucoma may be aggravated. Parenteral use should be reserved for patients who cannot take oral medications or for emergency situations.

Adverse Reactions
Long-term therapy may produce tardive dyskinesia. See **Atropine sulfate** for further adverse reactions.

Composition and Supply
Injection   1 mg/ml, in 2 ml ampuls
Tablets   500 μg, 1 mg, and 2 mg

Legal Status
Prescription

Benzyl alcohol/benzocaine (Foille®)

See ANTIPRURITICS, topical preparations.

Benzyl alcohol/menthol/camphor (Topic®)

See ANTIPRURITICS, topical preparations.

Benzyl benzoate compound

See ANTI-INFECTIVES, LOCAL, scabicide-pediculicides.

Benzyl benzoate lotion

Action and Use
Scabicide-pediculicide.

Dosage and Administration
Apply to entire body (except face) after thorough washing; wash off after 24 hours.

Cautions
Avoid contact with face and eyes.

Adverse Reactions
Transient, slight burning sensations sometimes occur after application. Skin irritation may also occur.

Composition and Supply
Lotion   26 to 30%

Legal Status
Prescription

Bephenium hydroxynaphthoate (Alcopara®)

Action and Use
Anthelmintic effective in the treatment of hookworm and in mixed infections of hookworm and roundworm.

Dosage and Administration
5 g twice a day, orally.

Cautions
Use with caution in patients with severe renal, hepatic, or cardiac disease.

Adverse Reactions
Side effects include mild and temporary looseness of stool, and possibly nausea, vomiting, and abdominal pain.

Composition and Supply
Granules   5 g per foil packet (equivalent to 2.5 g bephenium ion)

Legal Status
Prescription

Berocca® Tablets

See VITAMINS, MULTIPLE, oral.

Berocca®-C

See VITAMINS, MULTIPLE, parenteral.

Berocca®-C 500

See VITAMINS, MULTIPLE, parenteral.

Betadine®

See **Povidone-iodine.**

Betalin® Complex

See VITAMINS, MULTIPLE, parenteral.

Betalin® Complex F.C.

See VITAMINS, MULTIPLE, parenteral.

Betamethasone (Benisone®, Celestone®, Diprosone®, Flurobate®, Valisone®)

Action and Use
Corticosteroid, anti-inflammatory.

Dosage and Administration
Individualized according to condition being treated; used orally, parenterally (except IV), or topically.

Cautions
Essentially the same as for cortisone acetate (see). Contraindicated in systemic fungal infections.

Adverse Reactions
Essentially the same as for cortisone acetate (see), but with less potential for retention of sodium and water.

Composition and Supply
Tablets   600 µg (Celestone®)
Injection   3 mg/ml each of betamethasone sodium phosphate and
   betamethasone acetate (Celestone® Soluspan®)

Cream   0.05% betamethasone dipropionate (Diprosone®)
Cream and gel   0.025% betamethasone benzoate (Benisone®, Fluro-
   bate®)
Cream, lotion, and ointment   0.1% betamethasone valerate (Vali-
   sone®)
Syrup   600 μg/5 ml

Legal Status
Prescription

Betapar® (meprednisone)

See CORTICOSTEROIDS.

Betazole hydrochloride (Histalog®)

Action and Use
Stimulates production of gastric acid and thus is a diagnostic aid in
the clinical testing of gastric secretions.

Dosage and Administration
500 mg/kg SC.

Cautions
Use cautiously in patients with severe allergies or bronchial asthma.

Adverse Reactions
Lower incidence of toxicity than occurs with histamine phosphate.
The most common side effects are diaphoresis, flushed face, and a
feeling of warmth. Headache, urticaria, and bronchoconstriction
occur rarely.

Composition and Supply
Injection   50 mg/ml, in 1 ml ampuls

Legal Status
Prescription

Bethanechol chloride (Urecholine®)

Action and Use
Anticholinergic for abdominal stasis, intestinal distention, and urinary retention.

Dosage and Administration
5 to 30 mg 3 or 4 times a day, orally; or 2.5 mg every 15 to 30 minutes,
SC (continued until response or side effects occur).

Cautions
Side effects are frequent following SC injections; never administer IV or IM. A syringe with atropine sulfate should always be on hand when bethanechol chloride is given by injection.

Adverse Reactions
Increased salivation, nausea, vomiting, and diarrhea may occur. Other possible side effects include muscle twitching, flushing, dyspnea, diaphoresis, urinary urgency, tachycardia, hypotension, headache, and difficulty in visual accommodation.

Composition and Supply
Injection   5 mg/ml, in 1 ml ampuls
Tablets   5 mg, 10 mg, and 25 mg

Legal Status
Prescription

Biavax® (rubella and mumps virus vaccine)

See BIOLOGICALS, vaccines.

Bicillin®

See **Penicillin G benzathine.**

Bicillin® C-R

See **Penicillin G benzathine/penicillin G procaine.**

Bicillin® L-A

See **Penicillin G benzathine.**

Bilopaque® (tyropanoate sodium)

See DIAGNOSTICS, roentgenography.

Biotin

See VITAMINS, water-soluble, vitamin B complex.

Biozyme® (neomycin palmitate/trypsin/chymotrypsin)

See DEBRIDEMENT ENZYMES.

Biperiden hydrochloride (Akineton®)

Action and Use
Anticholinergic skeletal muscle relaxant used as an adjunct in parkinsonism and in the control of drug-induced extrapyramidal disorders.

Dosage and Administration
2 mg 3 or 4 times a day, orally; 5 to 10 mg IV slowly, daily.

Cautions
Drowsiness may occur. Use with caution in patients with glaucoma, prostatism, or cardiac arrhythmias.

Adverse Reactions
Possible side effects include gastric irritation, dry mouth, blurred vision, and decreased urinary output. Euphoria and disorientation are rare side effects.

Composition and Supply
Injection (as the lactate)   5 mg/ml, 1 ml ampuls
Tablets   2 mg

Legal Status
Prescription

Bisacodyl (Dulcolax®)

Action and Use
Laxative that reflexly stimulates peristaltic contractions via cholinergic nerve fibers. It is indicated in acute and chronic constipation, in postoperative and antepartum care, and in preparation for delivery, colostomies, radiography, sigmoidoscopy, and proctoscopy.

Dosage and Administration
Tablets: 2 or 3 to effect one or two soft, formed stools; up to 6 for special procedures.
Suppositories: 1 at time movement is required.

Cautions
Contraindicated in patients with pain, nausea, or vomiting. The tablets must be swallowed whole, not chewed or crushed (to avoid possible emesis) and should not be taken within 1 hour after administration of antacids or milk.

Adverse Reactions
Abdominal cramps have been noted occasionally.

Composition and Supply
Suppositories   10 mg
Tablets, enteric-coated   5 mg

Legal Status
Nonprescription

Bishydroxycoumarin

See **Dicumarol.**

Bivax® (rubella and mumps virus vaccine, live)

See under BIOLOGICALS, vaccines.

Blenoxane®

See **Bleomycin sulfate.**

Bleomycin sulfate (Blenoxane®)

Action and Use
Antibiotic antineoplastic useful in the treatment of squamous cell carcinoma, lymphomas, and testicular carcinoma.

Dosage and Administration
0.25 to 0.50 units per kg weekly or twice weekly SC, IM, IV, or intra-arterially.

Cautions
A highly toxic drug; pulmonary toxicities occur in 10% of treated patients. Idiosyncratic reactions similar to anaphylaxis are possible. Damage to the kidneys and liver may occur also.

Adverse Reactions
Frequent side effects are skin and nail changes, mouth ulcers, alopecia, nausea, vomiting, anorexia, and weight loss. Other possible adverse effects include fever, chills, pain at tumor site, and phlebitis.

Composition and Supply
Injection   15 unit ampuls

Legal Status
Prescription

Bluboro® Powder (aluminum acetate, modified)

See ASTRINGENTS.

Bonine®

See **Meclizine hydrochloride.**

Borate/phenol/phenolate (Chloraseptic®)

See MOUTHWASHES.

Boric acid

Action and Use
Mild antiseptic used in skin and ocular infections.

Dosage and Administration
Administered topically.

Cautions
Apply only to intact skin. Boric acid has caused poisoning and death when applied to large denuded areas. Serious poisonings and deaths have resulted from ingestion.

Adverse Reactions
None with proper use.

Composition and Supply
Ointment   5% and 10%
Solutions   2%, 4%, and 5%

Legal Status
Nonprescription

Botulism antitoxin

Action and Use
Provides antibodies (antitoxins) against the toxins of *Clostridium botulinum;* the bivalent antitoxin provides protection against types A and B, and the trivalent against types A, B, and E. The antitoxin is most useful to protect those exposed to contaminated food who are as yet asymptomatic. All exposed persons should be treated immediately.

Dosage and Administration
Bivalent antitoxin: Contents of 1 vial diluted (1 : 10), preferably with dextrose 10%, and given at 4-hour intervals until the toxic condition is alleviated. First 10 ml (1 ml antitoxin) is injected very slowly over a 5 minute period; then, after an interval of 15 minutes, the remainder may be given more rapidly.
Trivalent antitoxin: Usually given as 8 ml IV and 8 ml IM, repeated in 2 to 4 hours if symptoms persist.

Cautions
Test for sensitivity to horse serum; desensitization should be attempted only when antitoxin is considered necessary to save the patient's life. Epinephrine must be available in case untoward reactions occur.

Adverse Reactions
Serum sickness (with fever, urticaria, pruritus) may develop 5 to 13 days after administration of the antitoxin.

Composition and Supply
Bivalent antitoxin   1 vial containing 10,000 units each of types A
  and B

Note: available from Lederle Laboratories, Pearl River, NY; telephone (914) 735–5000. Monovalent (type E) and trivalent antitoxins are available at Communicable Disease Control Center, Atlanta, GA; telephone (day) (404) 633–3311, extension 3351 or 3684; telephone (night) (404) 633–2176 or (404) 633–8673.

Legal Status
Prescription

Brethine®

See **Terbutaline sulfate.**

Brevital®

See **Methohexital sodium.**

Bricanyl®

See **Terbutaline sulfate.**

Bristamycin®

See **Erythromycin stearate.**

Bromelains (Ananase®)

Action and Use
Proteolytic, anti-inflammatory enzyme.

Dosage and Administration
50,000 to 100,000 units 3 to 4 times a day, orally.

Cautions
Contraindicated in patients on anticoagulant therapy; in hemophiliacs; in patients with hepatic disease, renal disease, or systemic infections; and in those sensitive to pineapple or its products.

Adverse Reactions
Urticaria, skin rash, nausea, vomiting, or diarrhea may occur.

Composition and Supply
Tablets   50,000 units and 100,000 units.

Legal Status
Prescription

Bromodiphenhydramine (Ambodryl®)

See ANTIHISTAMINES.

Brompheniramine maleate (Dimetane®)

Action and Use
Antihistamine.

Dosage and Administration
4 to 8 mg 3 to 4 times a day, orally. 5 to 20 mg IM, SC, or IV.

Cautions
Should be discontinued prior to skin testing procedures since it may prevent otherwise positive reactions. Contraindicated in newborn and premature infants and nursing mothers; in patients with lower respiratory tract conditions (including asthma), narrow-angle glaucoma, stenosing peptic ulcer, and prostatic hypertrophy or other obstruction of the bladder neck; and in patients being treated with MAO inhibitors. Additive effects occur when taken with alcohol and other CNS depressants. Should be used with caution in patients with increased intraocular pressure, hyperthyroidism, cardiovascular disease, or hypertension.

Adverse Reactions
The main side effect is drowsiness. Dizziness, difficult concentration, and disturbed coordination may occur with the first few days of treatment. Other frequent side effects include dryness of mouth, nose, and throat; sedation and sleepiness; epigastric distress; and thickening of bronchial secretions (which may lead to dyspnea and wheezing in asthma). Other possible side effects include fatigue, confusion, restlessness, excitation, nervousness, insomnia, euphoria, anorexia, nausea, vomiting, diarrhea, constipation, urticaria, rash, anaphylactic shock, blurred vision, diplopia, vertigo, tinnitus, headache, hypotension, faintness, weakness, sweating, pallor, nasal stuffiness, urinary frequency, difficult urination or urinary retention, photosensitivity, hemolytic anemia, agranulocytosis, and leukopenia.

Composition and Supply
Elixir   2 mg/5 ml
Tablets   4 mg
Tablets, long-acting   8 mg and 12 mg
Expectorants
    Dimetane® Expectorant: each 5 ml contains brompheniramine maleate 2 mg, guaifenesin 100 mg, phenylephrine hydrochloride 5 mg, and phenylpropanolamine hydrochloride 5 mg

Dimetane® Expectorant-DC: same as Dimetane® Expectorant plus 10 mg codeine phosphate (*Note:* codeine may be habit-forming.)

Dimetapp® Elixir: each 5 ml contains brompheniramine maleate 4 mg, phenylephrine hydrochloride 5 mg, and phenylpropanolamine hydrochloride 5 mg

Dimetapp® Extentabs®: each tablet contains brompheniramine maleate 12 mg, phenylephrine hydrochloride 15 mg, and phenylpropanolamine hydrochloride 15 mg *(Note:* dosage is 1 Extentab® morning and evening.)

Injection   10 mg/ml, 1 ml ampuls; 100 mg/ml, 2 ml ampuls

Legal Status
Prescription

Bromsulphalein®

See **Sulfobromophthalein sodium.**

Brondecon® (oxtriphylline/guaifenesin)

See ANTIASTHMATICS.

Bronkephrine® (ethylnorepinephrine hydrochloride)

See ADRENERGICS; ANTIASTHMATICS, adrenergics.

Bronkometer® (phenylephrine hydrochloride/isoetharine mesylate)

See ADRENERGICS; ANTIASTHMATICS, adrenergics.

BSP®

See **Sulfobromophthalein sodium.**

Bucladin®-S (buclizine hydrochloride)

See ANTIEMETICS.

Buclizine hydrochloride (Bucladin®-S)

See ANTIEMETICS.

Bufferin®

See under **Aspirin.**

Bupivacaine hydrochloride (Marcaine®)

Action and Use
Local anesthetic.

Dosage and Administration
Infiltration and nerve, caudal, and epidural block.

Cautions
Should be used with caution in patients with liver disease and in those who are receiving MAO inhibitors. Partially used vials are to be discarded since the solution does not contain preservatives.

Adverse Reactions
Duration of anesthesia is longer than for most other local preparations. Resuscitative equipment and drugs should be available. Side effects are essentially those of mepivacaine hydrochloride (see).

Composition and Supply
Ampuls and vials   0.25%, 0.5%, and 0.75%
Ampuls and vials   0.25%, 0.5%, and 0.75% with epinephrine
  1 : 200,000

Legal Status
Prescription

Burow's solution

See **Aluminum acetate solution.**

Busulfan (Myleran®)

Action and Use
Antineoplastic agent used to treat myelocytic (granulocytic) leukemia.

Dosage and Administration
1 to 6 mg daily, orally; initially, up to 12 mg may be used.

Cautions
Busulfan depresses bone marrow and should be discontinued for 10 to 20 days if this occurs. A weekly blood count is recommended. Busulfan should not be given if similar drugs or radiation has been administered in the recent past, or if the neutrophil or platelet count is depressed.

Adverse Reactions
The chief side effect is myelosuppression, especially of megakaryocytes. Rapid destruction of granulocytes may be accompanied by hyperuricemia and uric acid nephropathy; this result may be avoided by the use of allopurinol. Occasional side effects include nausea, vomiting, diarrhea, cheilosis, glossitis, impotence, sterility, amenorrhea, gynecomastia, generalized skin pigmentation, anhidrosis, alopecia, and interstitial pulmonary fibrosis.

Composition and Supply
Tablets   2 mg

Legal Status
Prescription

Butabarbital sodium (Butisol®)

Action and Use
Intermediate-acting barbiturate.

Dosage and Administration
Sedative: 15 to 30 mg 3 or 4 times a day, orally.
Hypnotic: 50 to 100 mg at bedtime, orally.

Cautions
Same as for amobarbital (see), except that butabarbital sodium is not contraindicated in liver disease.

Adverse Reactions
Same as for amobarbital (see).

Composition and Supply
Capsules   15 mg, 30 mg, 50 mg, and 100 mg (Buticaps®)
Elixir   30 mg/5 ml
Tablets   15 mg, 30 mg, 50 mg, and 100 mg

Legal Status
Schedule III

Butaperazine (Repoise®)

See PSYCHOTROPICS, antipsychotics.

Butazolidin®

See **Phenylbutazone.**

Butazolidin® Alka

See under **Phenylbutazone.**

Butethamine hydrochloride (Monocaine®)

See ANESTHETICS, local.

Buticaps®

See under **Butabarbital sodium.**

Butisol®

See **Butabarbital sodium.**

Cafergot®

See under **Ergotamine tartrate.**

Cafergot® P-B

See under **Ergotamine tartrate.**

Caffeine/sodium benzoate

Action and Use
Respiratory and cerebral stimulant.

Dosage and Administration
500 mg to 1 g, IM.

Cautions
High dosage provokes tachycardia and possibly extrasystoles.

Adverse Reactions
Possible reactions include nausea, vomiting, tremors, diuresis, restlessness, excitement, and headache.

Composition and Supply
Injection 250 mg/ml, in 2 ml ampuls and 10 ml vials

Legal Status
Prescription

Calamine lotion

Action and Use
Protectant and antipruritic.

Dosage and Administration
Apply to affected areas as needed.

Cautions
Should not be used in infected areas.

Adverse Reactions
Accumulation of lotion in hairy areas may cause discomfort and irritation.

137

Composition and Supply
Lotion   8% zinc oxide
Lotion, phenolated   8% zinc oxide with 1% phenol

Legal Status
Nonprescription

Calciferol™

See **Ergocalciferol.**

Calcimar® (calcitonin)

See BLOOD CALCIUM REGULATORS.

Calcitonin (Calcimar®)

See BLOOD CALCIUM REGULATORS.

Calcium carbonate/glycine (Titralac®)

See ANTACIDS.

Calcium chloride injection

Action and Use
Calcium replacement and urinary acidifier.

Dosage and Administration
Administered IV in individualized dosage.

Cautions
Inject slowly. Calcium chloride increases toxicity of digitalis; it should be used with caution in digitalized patients and should not be used in patients with seriously injured kidneys.

Adverse Reactions
Irritating to tissues when given parenterally other than intravenously. Tingling sensations, a sense of oppression, or heat waves may occur.

Composition and Supply
Injection   10%, in 10 ml ampuls
Syringes (prefilled for emergency use)

Legal Status
Prescription

Calcium disodium edetate (Calcium Disodium Versenate™)

Action and Use
Chelating antidote used in acute lead poisoning and lead encephalopathy.

Dosage and Administration
Injection: total daily dosage for mild cases should not exceed 50 mg/kg in adults (IV infusion) or in children (IM).
Tablets: 8 tablets daily in divided doses for adults and 2 tablets daily per 35 pounds (in divided doses) for children.

Cautions
This drug is capable of potentially fatal effects and should not be given during periods of anuria. Dosage should not exceed 75 mg/kg per day. Procaine to produce a concentration of 0.5% should be added to minimize pain at IM injection site. IV solution should be given over a period of at least 1 hour.

Adverse Reactions
Oral administration may cause vomiting, diarrhea, and abdominal cramps, and also may increase absorption of lead from the gastrointestinal tract and thereby increase toxicity. Pain may occur at the site of intramuscular injection. Frequent urinalysis is recommended to detect renal damage (tubular necrosis).

Composition and Supply
Injection   200 mg/ml, in 5 ml ampuls (diluted with 250 to 500 ml of isotonic sodium chloride or sterile 5% glucose)
Tablets   500 mg

Legal Status
Prescription

Calcium Disodium Versenate™

See **Calcium disodium edetate.**

Calcium gluceptate injection

See BLOOD CALCIUM REGULATORS.

Calcium gluconate

Action and Use
Calcium replacement.

Dosage and Administration
Tablets: 5 g 3 times a day 1 hour after meals, orally.
Injection: 5 to 20 ml, as indicated, IV.

Cautions
See **Calcium chloride injection.**

Adverse Reactions
Intramuscular injection may cause abscess formation in young children. Rapid IV administration may cause a tingling sensation, a sense of oppression, or heat waves.

Composition and Supply
Injection   10%, in 10 ml ampuls
Tablets   500 mg and 1 g

Legal status
Prescription

Calcium undecylenate (Caldesene®)

See ANTI-INFECTIVES, LOCAL, fungicides.

Caldesene® (calcium undecylenate)

See ANTI-INFECTIVES, LOCAL, fungicides.

Camalox® (magnesium hydroxide and aluminum hydroxide/calcium carbonate)

See ANTACIDS.

Camoquin®

See **Amodiaquine hydrochloride.**

Camphorated tincture of opium

See **Paregoric.**

Candeptin®

See **Candicidin.**

Candicidin (Candeptin®, Vanobid®)

Action and Use
Antifungal antibiotic for vaginal candidiasis.

Dosage and Administration
3 mg in the morning and at bedtime, intravaginally.

Cautions
The patient should be advised either to abstain from sexual intercourse or to have her partner use a condom during treatment.

Adverse Reactions
Relatively nontoxic; occasionally temporary irritation may occur.

Composition and Supply
Ointment, vaginal   0.6 mg/g
Suppositories, vaginal   3 mg
Tablets, vaginal   3 mg

Legal Status
Prescription

Cantharidin (Cantharone®)

See KERATOLYTICS.

Cantharone® (cantharidin)

See KERATOLYTICS.

Cantil® (mepenzolate bromide)

See ANTICHOLINERGICS.

Cantil®-PHB (mepenzolate bromide/phenobarbital)

See ANTIDIARRHEALS.

Capastat® (capreomycin sulfate)

See ANTITUBERCULOTICS.

Capreomycin sulfate (Capastat®)

See ANTITUBERCULOTICS.

Carbachol (Isopto® Carbachol)

Action and Use
A long-acting miotic, carbachol must be combined with a wetting agent, such as benzalkonium chloride, for increased corneal penetration.

Dosage and Administration
1 or 2 drops of solution in the eye 2 or 3 times a day.

Cautions
Contraindicated in asthma, hyperthyroidism, coronary insufficiency, and peptic ulcer.

Adverse Reactions
May cause momentary stinging. Early in therapy, there may be spasm of the ciliary body and iris sphincter as evidenced by aching of eyes,

brow pain, headache, photophobia, and blurred vision. Rarely, hypotension may occur.

Composition and Supply
Solution, ophthalmic   0.75%, 1.5%, and 3%

Legal status
Prescription

Carbamazepine (Tegretol®)

Action and Use
Anticonvulsant and analgesic specific to trigeminal neuralgia.

Dosage and Administration
200 to 1,200 mg daily (depending on use), orally.

Cautions
Fatal blood dyscrasias have been reported, including aplastic anemia, agranulocytosis, and thrombocytopenia. Blood studies are essential. Carbamazepine is not recommended for use in patients receiving MAO inhibitors, and should be used with caution in patients with heart disease, hepatic failure, or increased intraocular pressure.

Adverse Reactions
The most frequent side effects include dizziness, drowsiness, unsteadiness, nausea, and vomiting.

Composition and Supply
Tablets   200 mg

Legal Status
Prescription

Carbamide peroxide 6.5% (Debrox®)

See CERUMINOLYTICS.

Carbamide peroxide 10% (Gly-Oxide®)

See MOUTHWASHES.

Carbarsone

See ANTIPROTOZOALS, antiamebials.

Carbenicillin disodium (Geopen®, Pyopen®)

Action and Use
Broad-spectrum semisynthetic penicillin with high activity against *Pseudomonas aeruginosa* and *Proteus* species.

Dosage and Administration
Daily dose should not exceed 40 g; administered IM or IV.

Cautions
Contraindicated in patients with penicillin allergies. Use with caution in patients with asthma. See **Penicillin G potassium** for further cautions.

Adverse Reactions
See **Penicillin G potassium.**

Composition and Supply
Piggyback units   2 g, 5 g, and 10 g
Vials   1 g, 2 g, and 5 g

Legal Status
Prescription

Carbenicillin indanyl sodium (Geocillin®)

See ANTIBIOTICS, penicillins.

Carbidopa/levodopa (Sinemet®)

See **Levodopa.**

Carbocaine®

See **Mepivacaine hydrochloride.**

Carbol-fuchsin solution (Castellani's paint)

Action and Use
Fungicide.

Dosage and Administration
Apply once or twice a day.

Cautions
Do not use on acute lesions.

Adverse Reactions
May cause excessive drying if applied too frequently and may prove irritating or sensitizing. Stains clothing.

Composition and Supply
Solution   1,000 ml contains basic fuchsin 3 g, phenol 45 g, resorcinol 100 g, acetone 50 mg, and purified water

Legal Status
Prescription

Carboxymethylcellulose sodium (Dialose®)

See CATHARTICS.

Cardilate® (erythrityl tetranitrate)

See CARDIACS, vasodilators.

Cardiografin®

See under **Diatrizoate meglumine.**

Cardio-Green® (indocyanine green)

See DIAGNOSTICS, cardiac output.

Cardioquin® (quinidine polygalacturonate)

See CARDIACS, antiarrhythmics.

Cardrase® (ethoxzolamide)

See CARBONIC ANHYDRASE INHIBITORS.

Carisoprodol (Rela®, Soma®)

Action and Use
Skeletal muscle relaxant.

Dosage and Administration
250 to 350 mg 4 times a day, orally.

Cautions
Contraindicated in patients with porphyria and in those sensitive to meprobamate. Carisoprodol may impair mental or physical abilities required for performance of hazardous tasks.

Adverse Reactions
Similar to adverse reactions to meprobamate (see).

Composition and Supply
Capsules   250 mg
Tablets   250 mg

Legal Status
Prescription

Carmol® (urea preparation)

See EMOLLIENT-PROTECTANTS; KERATOLYTICS.

Carmustine (BCNU)

See ANTINEOPLASTICS, miscellaneous.

Casanthranol (Peristim® Forte)

See CATHARTICS.

Cascara sagrada

Action and Use
Mild laxative.

Dosage and Administration
Fluidextract: 2 to 12 ml at bedtime.
Tablets: 300 mg at bedtime.

Cautions
Contraindicated in inflammatory disorders of the alimentary tract, undiagnosed abdominal pain, pregnancy, severe anemia, debilitation, chronic and spastic constipation, bowel obstruction, hemorrhage, and intussusception. Also contraindicated in patients recovering from perineal or rectal operations.

Adverse Reactions
May affect nursing infant if taken by mother during lactation.

Composition and Supply
Aromatic cascara fluidextract
Cascara tablets   300 mg

Legal Status
Nonprescription

Castellani's paint

See Carbol-fuchsin solution.

Castor oil

Action and Use
Prompt cathartic.

Dosage and Administration
15 to 60 ml, orally.

Cautions
Contraindicated in nursing mothers and when patient is experiencing abdominal pain.

Adverse Reactions
Unflavored oil is unpleasant (may be mixed with juice). Cramping and exhaustion may occur in some persons.

Composition and Supply
Oil, plain and flavored

Legal Status
Nonprescription

Catapres®

See **Clonidine hydrochloride.**

CCNU

See **Lomustine.**

Cebral® (ethaverine hydrochloride)

See ANTISPASMODICS; VASODILATORS, PERIPHERAL.

Cedilanid® (lanatoside C)

See CARDIACS, cardiac glycosides.

Cedilanid®-D

See **Deslanoside.**

CeeNu®

See **Lomustine.**

Cefadyl® (cephapirin sodium)

See ANTIBIOTICS, cephalosporins.

Cefazolin (Ancef®, Kefzol®)

See ANTIBIOTICS, cephalosporins.

Celbenin®

See **Methicillin sodium.**

Celestone®

See **Betamethasone.**

Celestone® Soluspan®

See under **Betamethasone.**

Cellulose, oxidized regenerated (Surgicel™ Absorbable Hemostat)

Action and Use
Hemostatic.

Dosage and Administration
Only the minimum amount needed to control bleeding should be used. It should be removed once hemostasis is achieved.

Cautions
Should not be used as packing or implantation in fractures or laminectomies (since it interferes with bone regeneration and may cause cyst formation), as wrap in vascular surgery or around the optic nerve and optic chiasm, in hemorrhage from large arteries, or on oozing surfaces (since it is not effective in such circumstances). Should not be autoclaved or impregnated or moistened with any substance.

Adverse Reactions
Allergic reactions may occur. There may be necrosis of nasal mucous membranes or perforation of nasal septum (due to tight packing). Complications are possible in contaminated wounds that are closed without drainage. Occasional adverse reactions include intestinal obstruction, ureteral obstruction, headache, and stinging.

Composition and Supply
Knitted fabric strips:
$2'' \times 14''$
$4'' \times 8''$
$2'' \times 3''$
$\frac{1}{2}'' \times 2''$

Legal Status
Prescription

Celontin®

See **Methsuximide.**

Cendevax®

See **Rubella virus vaccine, live.**

Cēpacol® (cetylpyridinium chloride)

See MOUTHWASHES.

pain injection site

Cephalexin (Keflex®)

Action and Use
Cephalosporin antibiotic.

Dosage and Administration
250 to 500 mg every 6 hours, orally, to a maximum dose of 4 g per day.

Cautions
See **Cephalothin sodium.**

Adverse Reactions
See **Cephalothin sodium.**

Composition and Supply
Capsules   250 mg and 500 mg
Suspension   125 mg/5 ml and 250 mg/5 ml

Legal Status
Prescription

Cephaloglycin (Kafocin®)

See ANTIBIOTICS, cephalosporins.

Cephaloridine (Loridine®)

Action and Use
Cephalosporin antibiotic.

Dosage and Administration
250 mg to 1 g 4 times a day, IM or IV.

Cautions
See **Cephalothin sodium.**

Adverse Reactions
See **Cephalothin sodium.**

Composition and Supply
Injection   500 mg and 1 g ampuls

Legal Status
Prescription

Cephalothin sodium (Keflin®, Neutral®)

Action and Use
Cephalosporin antibiotic.

Dosage and Administration
Up to 12 g per day, IM or IV (by injection or by continuous or intermittent infusion).

Cautions
Contraindicated in persons hypersensitive to cephalosporin antibiotics. Cross-sensitivity with penicillin may occur. Cephalothin sodium is nephrotoxic, and periodic kidney function tests are recommended. Thrombophlebitis may possibly occur with intravenous injection. Should be used with caution in patients with impaired renal function. May produce false-positive Coombs' test and false-positive glycosuria with tests not specific for glucose.

Adverse Reactions
Hypersensitivity may occur, especially in patients with a history of allergy (particularly in cases of allergy to penicillin). Other adverse reactions include occasional blood dyscrasias; pain, induration, tenderness, and fever following repeated IM injections; transient rise in SGOT, alkaline phosphatase, and BUN; and decreased creatinine clearance.

Composition and Supply
Injection   1 g, 2 g, 4 g, and 20 g ampuls (for reconstitution) (*Note:* concentrated solution darkens, but a slight discoloration is permissible)

Legal Status
Prescription

Cephapirin sodium (Cefadyl®)

See ANTIBIOTICS, cephalosporins.

Cephradine (Anspor®, Velosef®)

See ANTIBIOTICS, cephalosporins.

Cephulac™ (lactulose syrup)

See ELECTROLYTE SOLUTIONS AND WATER-BALANCE AGENTS, ammonia detoxicants.

Cerespan®

See **Papaverine hydrochloride.**

Cerose® Compound Capsules

See COUGH-COLD PREPARATIONS, common cold preparations.

Cerose®-DM

See COUGH-COLD PREPARATIONS, cough preparations.

Cerose® Sedative Expectorant

See COUGH-COLD PREPARATIONS, cough preparations.

Cerumenex® (triethanolamine polypeptide oleate condensate)

See CERUMINOLYTICS.

Cetaphil® (cetyl alcohol/sodium lauryl sulfate)

See DETERGENTS.

Cetyl alcohol/sodium lauryl sulfate (Cetaphil®)

See DETERGENTS.

Cetylpyridinium chloride (Cēpacol®)

See MOUTHWASHES.

CG® (indocyanine green)

See DIAGNOSTICS, cardiac output.

Charcoal, activated

Action and Use
Adsorbent and general purpose antidote.

Dosage and Administration
100 g suspended in 6 ounces of water (to form a slurry); orally, following gastric lavage.

Cautions
The effectiveness of charcoal as an antidote is limited and should not preclude other measures in the emergency treatment of poisoning.

Adverse Reactions
None, if used properly.

Composition and Supply
Powder

Legal Status
Nonprescription

Cheracol®

See COUGH-COLD PREPARATIONS, cough preparations.

Chloral hydrate (Aquachloral®, Felsules®, Noctec®, Somnos®)

Action and Use
Sedative and hypnotic for short-term use.

Dosage and Administration
Sedative: 250 mg 3 times a day; orally or rectally.
Hypnotic: 500 mg to 1 g; orally or rectally.

Cautions
Should be used with caution in cardiac patients, mentally depressed patients with suicidal tendencies, or patients with a history of drug abuse. Contraindicated in patients with impaired hepatic or renal function. Interacts with other CNS depressants, with furosemide, and with coumarin anticoagulants.

Adverse Reactions
Possible side effects include nausea, vomiting, gastric distress, and rash. There is a wide margin of safety, but acute poisoning can occur (with symptoms similar to poisoning with other CNS depressants).

Composition and Supply
Capsules   250 mg and 500 mg
Suppositories   300 mg, 600 mg, and 1 g
Syrup   500 mg/5 ml

Legal Status
Schedule IV

Chlorambucil (Leukeran®)

Action and Use
Nitrogen mustard antineoplastic.

Dosage and Administration
Initial dose: 4 to 10 mg daily, orally.
Maintenance doses: determined according to clinical and hematologic response.

Cautions

Irreversible bone marrow damage may occur. Chlorambucil should not be given sooner than 4 weeks after a full course of radiation therapy or other chemotherapy.

Adverse Reactions

Usually well tolerated without nausea. Bone marrow depression is usually moderate, gradual, and rapidly reversible. Weekly blood studies are recommended, and the patient should be observed for infection and bleeding. Gastric distress sometimes occurs. Large doses cause nausea, vomiting, dermatitis, and hepatoxicity.

Composition and Supply

Tablets   2 mg

Legal Status

Prescription

Chloramphenicol (Chloromycetin®)

Action and Use

Broad-spectrum antibiotic. Drug of choice in typhoid fever.

Dosage and Administration

50 mg/kg per day, orally or IM. Chloramphenicol may also be applied topically as an ointment or solution.

Cautions

Not to be used for treatment of trivial infections or when not specifically indicated; prophylactic use is not recommended. Chloramphenicol can cause bone marrow depression and blood dyscrasias (periodic blood tests are recommended); it can antagonize activity of penicillin. Should be used with caution in renal and hepatic diseases.

Adverse Reactions

Occasional adverse effects include gastrointestinal disturbances (nausea, vomiting, diarrhea) and superinfection. Other possible effects include hypersensitivity; hemorrhage of skin, mouth, intestine, and bladder; depression; confusion; headache; and blurred vision. Cardiovascular collapse has been reported in infants, as a result of gray syndrome. Skin preparations may cause burning, itching, or other signs of sensitization.

Composition and Supply

Capsules   250 mg
Injection (as sodium succinate)   vials containing 1 g base
Suspension (as palmitate)   156.25 mg base/5 ml

Cream   1%
Ointment, ophthalmic   1%
Solution, ophthalmic   0.5%

Legal Status
Prescription

Chloraseptic® (borate/phenol/phenolate)

See MOUTHWASHES.

Chlordantoin (Sporostacin®)

Action and Use
Antifungal agent for vaginal and vulvovaginal candidiasis.

Dosage and Administration
The contents of 1 applicator are applied intravaginally twice daily for 2 weeks. This course is repeated as necessary.

Cautions
No known contraindications.

Adverse Reactions
Sensitization may occur.

Composition and Supply
Cream   1%

Legal Status
Prescription

Chlordiazepoxide hydrochloride (Librium®)

Action and Use
Minor tranquilizer.

Dosage and Administration
Oral: 15 to 40 mg daily in divided doses.
IM or IV: 50 to 100 mg.

Cautions
Intramuscular absorption is poor and requires higher dosage. The daily dose should not exceed 300 mg. Combined effects will occur when taken with alcohol or other CNS depressants.

Adverse Reactions
Adverse reactions include drowsiness, ataxia, and confusion; pain at injection site; constipation; skin eruptions; edema; minor menstrual

irregularities; extrapyramidal symptoms; increased or decreased libido; and syncope, hypotension, and tachycardia.

Composition and Supply
Capsules and tablets   5 mg, 10 mg, and 25 mg
Injection   100 mg ampuls
Tablets   5 mg with amitriptylene hydrochloride 12.5 mg (Limbitrol® 5-12.5); 10 mg with amitriptylene hydrochloride 25 mg (Limbitrol® 10-25)

Legal Status
Schedule IV

Chloresium® (chlorophyll derivatives)

See DEODORANTS.

Chlorhexidine gluconate (Hibiclens®)

See ANTI-INFECTIVES, LOCAL, miscellaneous antiseptic-disinfectants.

Chloromycetin®

See **Chloramphenicol.**

Chloromycetin® Palmitate

See under **Chloramphenicol.**

Chloromycetin® Sodium Succinate

See under **Chloramphenicol.**

Chlorophyll derivatives, oral (Derifil®)

See DEODORANTS.

Chlorophyll derivatives, topical (Chloresium®)

See DEODORANTS.

Chloroprocaine hydrochloride (Nesacaine®)

See ANESTHETICS, local.

Chloroquine (Aralen®)

Action and Use
Antiprotozoal useful in extraintestinal amebiasis and in treatment and suppression of malaria.

Dosage and Administration
Amebiasis: 250 mg 4 times per day for 2 days, followed by 250 mg daily for 2 weeks, orally.
Malaria suppression: 500 mg (single dose) per week.
Malaria treatment: 1 g initially; then 500 mg after 6 to 8 hours; then 500 mg per day for 2 days.

Cautions
Contraindicated in psoriasis. Avoid concomitant use with phenylbutazone or gold. Blood dyscrasias and retinal damage may occur, especially with prolonged therapy; periodic blood studies and eye examinations are recommended.

Adverse Reactions
Intravenous administration may produce effects on the heart similar to those produced by quinidine. High dosage may cause bleaching of hair, weight loss, and nerve deafness. Lichenoid skin eruptions may occur, but they disappear when drug is discontinued. Overdose may produce cardiopulmonary collapse, convulsions, and death.

Composition and Supply
Injection (as hydrochloride)   50 mg/ml, in 5 ml ampuls
Tablets (as phosphate)   125 mg and 250 mg

Legal Status
Prescription

Chlorothiazide (Diuril®)

Action and Use
Diuretic and antihypertensive.

Dosage and Administration
Diuretic: 500 mg to 1 g once or twice a day, orally or IV.
Antihypertensive: 250 g twice a day to 500 mg 3 times a day, orally.

Cautions
Contraindicated in patients with anuria or hypersensitivity to sulfonamide-derived drugs. Chlorothiazide may cause hypokalemia and may potentiate the potassium-depleting effect of corticosteroids. It also potentiates the action of other antihypertensive drugs and digitalis. The use of chlorothiazide interferes with a number of laboratory tests.

Adverse Reactions
Possible adverse reactions include electrolyte imbalance (with muscle weakness or cramps), drowsiness, dizziness, thirst, dry mouth, fatigue, paresthesias, anorexia, nausea, vomiting, diarrhea or constipation, oliguria, hypotension, convulsions, and coma. Hypokalemia may precipitate digitalis toxicity (the patient may need potassium sup-

plementation). Hyperglycemia and glycosuria may occur in patients with latent diabetes. Occasional effects include skin eruptions, transient blurred vision, headache, tinnitus, and tremors. Rare effects include hyperuricemia, photosensitivity, fever, pancytopenia, crystalluria, renal calculi, vasculitis, dyspnea, and anaphylaxis.

Composition and Supply
Injection (as sodium salt)   500 mg vials
Suspension, oral   250 mg/5 ml
Syrup   250 mg/5 ml
Tablets   250 mg and 500 mg

Legal Status
Prescription

Chlorotrianisene (TACE®)

Action and Use
Long-acting synthetic estrogen.

Dosage and Administration
Dosage is individualized, in the range of 12 to 72 mg, orally.

Cautions
See **Estradiol.**

Adverse Reactions
See **Estradiol.**

Composition and Supply
Capsules   12 mg, 25 mg, and 72 mg

Legal Status
Prescription

Chlorphenesin carbamate (Maolate®)

See SKELETAL MUSCLE RELAXANTS.

Chlorpheniramine maleate (Chlor-Trimeton®, Teldrin®)

Action and Use
Antihistamine.

Dosage and Administration
12 to 24 mg daily, orally; or 5 to 20 mg doses may be administered SC, IM, or IV.

Cautions
The ampuls of the 100 mg/ml concentration are not to be used intravenously. For other cautions, see **Brompheniramine maleate.**

Adverse Reactions
Weak pulse and transitory hypotension may occur after parenteral injection. There may be transitory stinging or burning sensation at injection site. See **Brompheniramine maleate** for further adverse reactions.

Composition and Supply
Capsules, long-acting (Teldrin® Spansules®)   8 mg and 12 mg
Injection   10 mg/ml, in 1 ml ampuls; and 100 mg/ml, in 2 ml ampuls
Syrup   2.5 mg/5 ml
Tablets   4 mg
Tablets (Repetabs®)   8 mg and 12 mg

Legal Status
Prescription

Chlorphentermine hydrochloride (Pre-Sate®)

See CEREBRAL STIMULANTS, anorectics.

Chlorpromazine hydrochloride (Thorazine®)

Action and Use
Major tranquilizer. Also useful as an antiemetic and in the control of intractable hiccups and acute intermittent porphyria.

Dosage and Administration
25 to 200 mg daily (individualized), administered orally, rectally, or IM.

Cautions
The intense sedative action of chlorpromazine constitutes a major hazard. Action of other CNS depressants is potentiated. Jaundice is not uncommon, and continual use may cause bone marrow depression. Injection site should be massaged to avoid abscesses.

Adverse Reactions
Adverse reactions include postural hypotension (which is common initially, especially after parenteral administration), drowsiness, jaundice (which usually is promptly reversible), blood dyscrasias (including agranulocytosis, eosinophilia, leukopenia, hemolytic anemia, and thrombocytopenic purpura), extrapyramidal (neuromuscular) reactions resembling parkinsonism, tardive dyskinesia, convulsive seizures, abnormality of cerebrospinal proteins, allergic reactions of a mild urticarial type, photosensitivity, lactation and moderate breast

engorgement, amenorrhea and gynecomastia, ocular changes, and skin pigmentation. Autonomic reactions, which are fairly common, include dry mouth, nasal congestion, constipation, urinary retention, miosis, and mydriasis. *Note:* contact dermatitis has been reported in nursing personnel; consequently, rubber gloves are recommended in dealing with liquid and injectable forms.

Composition and Supply
Capsules, long-acting   30 mg, 75 mg, 150 mg, and 200 mg
Injection   25 mg/ml, in 1 ml and 2 ml ampuls and in 100 ml multiple-dose vials
Liquid (concentrated)   30 mg/ml and 100 mg/ml
Suppositories   25 mg and 100 mg
Syrup   10 mg/5 ml
Tablets   10 mg, 25 mg, 50 mg, 100 mg, and 200 mg

Legal Status
Prescription

Chlorpropamide (Diabinese®)

Action and Use
Oral hypoglycemic for selected cases of diabetes mellitus.

Dosage and Administration
100 to 500 mg daily, orally.

Cautions
Contraindicated in patients with diabetes mellitus that is adequately controlled by diet, in patients with juvenile diabetes, and in patients with diabetes complicated by acidosis, coma, severe infection, major surgical procedures, or severe trauma. Should be used with caution in patients with hepatic, renal, or thyroid dysfunction. Chlorpropamide may prolong the action of barbiturates and other hypnotics and sedatives. It depresses thyroid uptake of radioactive iodine. Potency may be increased by MAO inhibitors, coumarin type anticoagulants, and anti-inflammatory agents (e.g., phenylbutazone). Thiazide type diuretics detract from the effectiveness of chlorpropamide.

Adverse Reactions
Possible adverse reactions include hypersensitivity with skin eruptions (itching, erythema, urticaria), photosensitivity, fever, eosinophilia, and pancytopenia (patient should be observed for sore throat); biliary stasis and jaundice with increased levels of alkaline phosphatase, SGOT, and SGPT (liver tests are recommended). Other reported effects include weakness, paresthesias, headache, tinnitus, intolerance to alcohol, anorexia, nausea, vomiting, and diarrhea. Cardiac abnormalities such as tachycardia and myocardial infarction have occurred. Overdosage may result in hypoglycemic reactions (e.g., nervousness,

pallor, tremors, diaphoresis, coma), which should be treated with glucose (e.g., orange juice). Such hypoglycemic reactions are especially likely in patients with kidney or liver disorders, in elderly patients, and in those who do not adhere to their diets. Patients who experience hypoglycemic reactions should be closely observed for several days.

Composition and Supply
Tablets   100 mg and 250 mg

Legal Status
Prescription

Chlortetracycline hydrochloride (Aureomycin®)

See ANTIBIOTICS, tetracyclines.

Chlorthalidone (Hygroton®)

Action and Use
Diuretic, antihypertensive.

Dosage and Administration
50 to 200 mg daily, orally, in the morning with food.

Cautions
May cause electrolyte imbalance and decreased glucose tolerance. Crosses placenta to cause fetal or neonatal jaundice and thrombocytopenia. Contraindications include anuria and use during pregnancy except when treating edema due to a pathological condition.

Adverse Reactions
See **Chlorothiazide.**

Composition and Supply
Tablets   50 mg and 100 mg

Legal Status
Prescription

Chlor-Trimeton®

See **Chlorpheniramine maleate.**

Chlorzoxazone (Paraflex®)

See SKELETAL MUSCLE RELAXANTS.

Choledyl®

See **Oxtriphylline.**

Cholera vaccine

Action and Use
Used for the protective vaccination of individuals traveling or living in areas where cholera is prevalent.

Dosage and Administration
Given SC or IM at weekly intervals as follows:
Age 6 months to 4 years: 0.1 ml, 0.3 ml, 0.3 ml.
Age 5 years to 9 years: 0.3 ml, 0.5 ml, 0.5 ml.
Age 10 years to adult: 0.5 ml, 0.5 ml (third dose is unnecessary).

Cautions
Booster injection is needed every 6 months for as long as exposure exists. Contraindicated in persons with a history of hypersensitivity to eggs or chicken.

Adverse Reactions
Discomfort and inflammation at injection site may persist for 1 to 2 days, possibly accompanied by fever, malaise, and headache. Serious reactions are rare.

Composition and Supply
Injection   1.5 ml ampuls and 20 ml vials

Legal Status
Prescription

Cholestyramine (Questran®)

Action and Use
Anion exchange resin that absorbs and combines with bile acids in the intestines. Cholestyramine is indicated as adjunctive therapy in elevated serum cholesterol (primary type II hyperlipidemia) and for the relief of pruritus associated with partial biliary obstruction.

Dosage and Administration
4 g 3 or 4 times a day, orally.

Cautions
Cholestyramine should not be taken in its dry form, but should always be mixed with water or other fluids before ingestion. Prevents absorption of fat-soluble vitamins and a number of drugs (thyroid and digitalis preparations, warfarin, aspirin, and others).

Adverse Reactions
Cholestyramine has an unpleasant taste. Nausea, vomiting, diarrhea, and anorexia may occur. Prolonged use may promote bleeding tendencies, which can be prevented by the administration of vitamin K. Rare effects include cardiovascular disorders, allergic reactions, headache, nervousness, drowsiness, and dizziness. Changes in weight may occur.

Composition and Supply
Packets   4 g

Legal Status
Prescription

Choline salicylate (Arthropan®)

See ANALGESICS, nonnarcotic.

Cholografin®

See **Iodipamide meglumine.**

Choloxin®

See **Sodium dextrothyroxine.**

Chorionic gonadotropin

See **Gonadotropin, chorionic.**

Chymoral® (trypsin/chymotrypsin)

See ANTI-INFLAMMATORY ENZYMES.

Chymotrypsin, ophthalmic (Alpha Chymar®)

See ENZYMES.

Chymotrypsin/trypsin/ceomycin (Biozyme®)

See DEBRIDEMENT ENZYMES.

Cimetidine (Tagament®)

Action and Use
H₂ receptor antagonist indicated in the short-term (up to 8 weeks) treatment of duodenal ulcer and in the treatment of pathological hypersecretory disorders, including Zollinger-Ellison syndrome, systemic mastocytosis, and multiple endocrine adenomas.

Dosage and Administration
Duodenal ulcer: 300 mg 4 times a day, orally, with meals and at bedtime.

Hypersecretory disorders: 300 mg 4 times a day, orally, with meals and at bedtime. In some cases it may be necessary to administer cimetidine more frequently (but not to exceed 2.4 g per day); continue as long as needed. *Note:* Cimetidine may be given by IV injection or IV infusion at a dosage of 300 mg every 6 hours (not to exceed 2.4 g per day).

Cautions
Not recommended in pregnant women, women of child-bearing potential, nursing mothers, or children under 16 unless anticipated benefits outweigh potential risks.

Adverse Reactions
The usual dosage may cause dizziness, diarrhea, muscular pain, rash, and mild gynecomastia. Increases in plasma creatinine and serum transaminase have been reported.

Composition and Supply
Injection   150 mg/ml, in 2 ml ampuls
Tablets   300 mg

Legal Status
Prescription

Citanest® (prilocaine hydrochloride)

See ANESTHETICS, local.

Citrate of magnesia

See **Magnesium citrate solution.**

Citrogen®

See FOOD FORMULATIONS.

Citrovorum factor

See **Leucovorin calcium.**

Cleocin®

See **Clindamycin.**

Cleocin® Pediatric

See under **Clindamycin.**

Cleocin® Phosphate

See under **Clindamycin.**

Clindamycin (Cleocin®)

Action and Use
Lincomycin analogue effective against most gram-positive organisms.

Dosage and Administration
Oral: 150 to 450 mg every 6 hours.
IM and IV: 600 mg to 4.8 g daily; single dose not to exceed 600 mg.

Cautions
Contraindicated in individuals hypersensitive to clindamycin or lincomycin. Use of parenteral clindamycin should be confined to hospitalized patients with serious infections caused by susceptible pathogens. May cause severe colitis (which may end in death) and should be used with caution in patients with renal or hepatic disease.

Adverse Reactions
Adverse reactions include nausea, vomiting, diarrhea, and fever. Thrombophlebitis may result from intravenous administration. Uncommon effects include rash, increased SGOT and SGPT, granulocytopenia, thrombocytopenia (patient should be observed for sore throat and bleeding), and anaphylaxis.

Composition and Supply
Capsules (as hydrochloride)   75 mg and 150 mg
Injection (as phosphate)   150 mg/ml, in 2 ml and 4 ml ampuls (Cleocin® Phosphate)
Suspension (as palmitate)   75 mg/5 ml (Cleocin® Pediatric)

Legal Status
Prescription

Clindinium bromide/chlordiazepoxide hydrochloride
(Librax®)

See ANTICHOLINERGICS.

Clinitest® tablets

See DIAGNOSTICS, urine (glucose).

Clofibrate (Atromid-S®)

Action and Use
Antilipemic that lowers both serum cholesterol and triglycerides.

Dosage and Administration
500 mg 4 times a day, orally.

Cautions
May potentiate the action of tolbutamide and anticoagulants. Contraindicated in renal or hepatic dysfunction and in pregnant and nursing women.

Adverse Reactions
Most common effects include nausea, vomiting, and diarrhea. Occasional effects include headache, muscle cramps, weakness, pruritus, urticaria, alopecia, arrhythmias, decreased libido, renal dysfunction, blood dyscrasias, and abnormal results in liver function studies.

Composition and Supply
Capsules   500 mg

Legal Status
Prescription

Clomid®

See **Clomiphene citrate.**

Clomiphene citrate (Clomid®)

Action and Use
Gonadotropin stimulant indicated for treatment of secondary anovulatory infertility.

Dosage and Administration
50 to 100 mg daily for 5 to 7 days, orally.

Cautions
Contraindicated in patients with liver disease.

Adverse Reactions
Adverse reactions include gastrointestinal disturbances similar to that in pregnancy, breakthrough bleeding, abdominal pain, weight gain, rash and hot flashes, ovarian enlargement with or without cyst formation, and visual disturbances. Occasionally, multiple pregnancies may occur.

Composition and Supply
Tablets   50 mg

Legal Status
Prescription

Clonazepam (Clonopin®)

See ANTICONVULSANTS.

Clonidine hydrochloride (Catapres®)

Action and Use
Antihypertensive.

Dosage and Administration
Dosage is individualized, with a maintenance range of 200 µg to 1.2 mg per day, orally.

Cautions
Rebound hypertension may occur when the drug is abruptly discontinued. Clonidine has a sedative effect and may enhance the CNS depressant action of alcohol, barbiturates, sedatives, and tranquilizers. Bradycardia may occur, thus enhancing the effects of guanethidine, propranolol, and digitalis glycosides. Not recommended in women who are or may become pregnant.

Adverse Reactions
Most common effects include dry mouth, sedation, constipation, headache, dizziness, and fatigue. Less common effects include gynecomastia, impotence, urinary retention, anorexia, nausea, vomiting, rash, pruritus, angioneurotic edema, weight gain, postural hypotension (the patient should use caution on rising), congestive heart failure, arrhythmias, abnormal results on liver function tests, hyperglycemia, increased serum creatinine phosphokinase, nightmares, insomnia, restlessness, and depression. Intravenous administration may produce hypertension in patients with accelerated hypertension. Effects of overdosage include hypotension and coma.

Composition and Supply
Tablets   100 µg (0.1 mg) and 200 µg (0.2 mg)

Legal Status
Prescription

Clonidine hydrochloride/chlorthalidone (Combipres®)

See ANTIHYPERTENSIVES, combinations.

Clonopin® (clonazepam)

See ANTICONVULSANTS.

Clorazepate dipotassium (Tranxene®)

Action and Use
A benzodiazepine minor tranquilizer indicated for the symptomatic relief of anxiety associated with psychoneuroses and as an adjunct in disease states in which anxiety is manifested.

Dosage and Administration
Dosage is adjusted gradually within the range of 15 to 60 mg daily, orally. The usual daily dose is 30 mg.

Cautions
See **Diazepam.**

Adverse Reactions
See **Diazepam.**

Composition and Supply
Capsules   3.75 mg, 7.5 mg, and 15 mg
Tablets   22.5 mg (Tranxene®-SD)
Tablets   11.25 mg (Tranxene®-SD Half Strength)

Legal Status
Prescription

Clorazepate monopotassium (Azene™)

See PSYCHOTROPICS, tranquilizers, minor.

Clortermine hydrochloride (Voranil®)

See CEREBRAL STIMULANTS, anorectics.

Clotrimazole (Lotrimin®)

See ANTI-INFECTIVES, LOCAL, fungicides.

Cloxacillin sodium (Tegopen®)

Action and Use
Synthetic penicillin for use in infections caused by penicillinase-producing staphylococci.

Dosage and Administration
250 to 500 mg every 6 hours, orally.

Cautions
Use of cloxacillin sodium may result in penicillin allergy. Food interferes with absorption; medication should be given 1 hour before or 2 hours after meals. See **Penicillin G potassium** for further cautions.

Adverse Reactions
See **Penicillin G potassium.**

Composition and Supply
Capsules   250 mg
Solution, oral   125 mg/5 ml

Legal Status
Prescription

Coal tar

Action and Use
Keratoplastic used to treat eczema.

Dosage and Administration
Apply cream or ointment to affected areas 2 or 3 times a day, or add 60 ml of appropriate solution to a tub of water.

Cautions
Contraindicated on infected or impetiginized lesions. Coal tar should not be applied to more than one-fourth of the body surface to minimize danger of phenol absorption. The skin should not be exposed to direct rays of the sun immediately after application of coal tar.

Adverse Reactions
Odiferous and irritating. Continuous contact with skin for long periods may result in dermatitis and skin cancer.

Composition and Supply
Cream and ointment   1 to 5%
Gel   5% (Estar®)
Solution   10 to 20%
Solution for dilution (L.C.D.™)

Legal Status
Prescription

Cocaine hydrochloride

Action and Use
Potent local anesthetic for mucous membranes.

Dosage and Administration
Eye: 4% instillation.
Nose and throat: 5 to 10% instillation.

Cautions
Habit-forming and dangerous if absorbed into blood. Should not be applied to abraded mucous membranes. Damage to cornea may occur.

Adverse Reactions
The cornea may become dry and thus possibly be damaged.

Composition and Supply
Solution   2%, 4%, 5%, and 10% to 20%

Legal Status
Schedule II

Coccidioidin

Action and Use
Antigen used in the diagnosis of coccidioidomycosis.

Dosage and Administration
0.1 ml (100 μl) of 1 : 100 dilution, intradermally.

Cautions
Accurate dilution, dosage, and administration are essential.

Adverse Reactions
Exaggerated reaction may occur in allergic individuals.

Composition and Supply
Injection   1 : 100 and 1 : 10

Legal Status
Prescription

Codeine phosphate
Codeine sulfate

Action and Use
Narcotic analgesic, antitussive (the only important difference between the two forms is in their solubility; codeine phosphate is more soluble in water).

Dosage and Administration
Analgesic: 15 to 60 mg every 3 to 4 hours, orally or SC.
Antitussive: 5 to 10 mg every 3 hours as needed.

Cautions
Narcotic analgesics have a potential toxicity and an addicting tendency. Contraindicated in head injuries and bronchial asthma.

Adverse Reactions
Similar to morphine sulfate but much less severe.

Composition and Supply
Injection (phosphate)   15 mg/ml and 30 mg/ml
Tablets (phosphate or sulfate)   15 mg, 30 mg, and 60 mg

Legal Status
Schedule II

Cogentin®

See **Benztropine mesylate.**

Colace®

See **Dioctyl sodium sulfosuccinate.**

ColBENEMID®

See under **Probenecid.**

Colchicine

Action and Use
Analgesic for acute gout.

Dosage and Administration
Tablets: 1 or 2 tablets initially followed by 1 tablet every 1 or 2 hours until pain is relieved or nausea, diarrhea, or vomiting develops.
Injection: 2 mg initially followed by 500 μg every 6 hours until pain is relieved, IV.

Cautions
Bone marrow depression may occur with long-term use. Colchicine may interfere with 17-hydroxycorticosteroid determinations. Special caution should be used in elderly or debilitated patients and in patients with renal, gastrointestinal, or heart disease.

Adverse Reactions
Common adverse reactions include vomiting, abdominal pain, diarrhea, and a burning sensation in the throat or stomach. Possible side effects include shock, muscle weakness with ascending paralysis, delirium, and convulsions. Death may occur from respiratory depression.

Composition and Supply
Injection   500 μg/ml, in 2 ml ampuls
Tablets   600 μg

Legal Status
Prescription

Colestid® (colestipol)

See ANTILIPEMICS.

Colestipol (Colestid®)

See ANTILIPEMICS.

Colistimethate sodium (Coly-Mycin® M Parenteral)
Colistin sulfate (Coly-Mycin® S [Oral and Otic])

Action and Use
Polypeptide antibiotic for treatment of infections caused by susceptible strains of *Pseudomonas aeruginosa* and certain other gram-negative bacilli.

Dosage and Administration
100 mg 3 times a day, orally; 1.3 to 5 mg/kg per day in divided doses, IM (daily dose should never exceed 5 mg/kg).

Cautions
Should not be used for minor infections that can be treated with less toxic drugs. These drugs are neurotoxic and nephrotoxic; they should not be used concomitantly with kanamycin, streptomycin, neomycin, or polymyxin B.

Adverse Reactions
Common adverse reactions include gastrointestinal disturbances, dermatitis, and pruritus. Leukopenia, granulocytopenia, or respiratory arrest (especially after parenteral administration) may occur. Pain may occur at the injection site; rotate sites and inject deeply. There may be suprainfection during treatment. These drugs are nephrotoxic and neurotoxic in high dosage.

Composition and Supply
Injection   150 mg vials
Suspension, oral   25 mg/5 ml
Suspension, otic   3 mg/ml with neomycin 3.3 mg and hydrocortisone acetate 10 mg

Legal Status
Prescription

Collagenase (Santyl®)

Action and Use
Debridement enzyme.

Dosage and Administration
Applied topically, once daily, to cleansed area, with surrounding healthy skin protected by petrolatum or a similar preparation.

Cautions
Contraindicated in patients who have shown local or systemic sensitivity.

Adverse Reactions
None reported when used as directed. If desired, the action of the enzyme may be stopped by application of aluminum acetate (Burow's) solution.

Composition and Supply
Ointment   250 units/g

Legal Status
Prescription

Collodion

Action and Use
Protectant and vehicle for application of medicines requiring prolonged contact with skin.

Dosage and Administration
Apply as indicated, topically.

Cautions
Extremely flammable.

Adverse Reactions
Enhancement of an infection may occur.

Composition and Supply
4% pyroxylin in ether and alcohol (collodion)
Collodion with 2% camphor and 3% castor oil (flexible collodion)

Legal Status
Nonprescription

Collosul® (sulfur, colloidal, preparation)

See KERATOLYTICS.

Colonil™

See **Diphenoxylate hydrochloride/atropine sulfate.**

Coly-Mycin® M Parenteral

See **Colistimethate sodium.**

Coly-Mycin® S (Oral and Otic)

See **Colistin sulfate.**

Combid® (isopropamide iodide/prochlorperazine)

See ANTICHOLINERGICS.

Combipres® (clonidine hydrochloride/chlorthalidone)

See ANTIHYPERTENSIVES, combinations.

Comfolax®

See **Dioctyl sodium sulfosuccinate.**

Compazine®

See **Prochlorperazine.**

Compleat®-B

See FOOD PREPARATIONS.

Compocillin®-VK

See **Penicillin V potassium.**

Conceptrol® (nonoxynol 9)

See CONTRACEPTIVES, TOPICAL.

Conray®

See **Iothalamate meglumine.**

Coparaffinate (Iso-Par®)

See ANTI-INFECTIVES, LOCAL, fungicides.

Co-Pyronil™

See **Pyrrobutamine compound.**

Coramine® (nikethamide)

See RESPIRATORY STIMULANTS.

Cordran®

See **Flurandrenolide.**

Cordran®-N

See under **Flurandrenolide.**

Cordran® Tape

See under **Flurandrenolide.**

Coricidin® "D" Decongestant Tablets

See COUGH-COLD PREPARATIONS, common cold preparations.

Corlutin®

See **Progesterone.**

Corn starch

See **Starch.**

Cor-Tar-Quin®

See KERATOPLASTICS.

Cort-Dome®

See **Hydrocortisone.**

Cortef®

See **Hydrocortisone.**

Corticotropin (ACTH) (Acthar®, H.P. Acthar®-Gel)

Action and Use
Adrenocorticotropic hormone with basically the same indications as for corticosteroids.

Dosage and Administration
Individualized according to the patient and disease; administered IM or IV. Dosage ranges from 10 to 100 units.

Cautions
See **Cortisone acetate.**

Adverse Reactions
See **Cortisone acetate.** Observe the patient for a few minutes after the injection for possible allergic reactions.

Composition and Supply
Injection (powder)   10 unit, 25 unit, and 40 unit vials (Acthar®)
Injection, repository (gel)   40 units/ml and 80 units/ml, in 1 ml ampuls and 5 ml vials (H.P. Acthar®-Gel)

Legal Status
Prescription

Cortisone acetate (Cortone®)

Action and Use
Standard corticosteroid.

Dosage and Administration
Dosage varies with patient and with disease being treated: 2.5 to 75 mg orally; 5 to 300 mg IM; used topically as 0.25% to 2.5% creams and ointments.

Cautions
Cortisone acetate is a potent drug with a wide range of side effects; it is contraindicated in patients with peptic ulcer, psychosis, Cushing's disease, glomerulonephritis, herpes simplex of the eye, and infections not controlled by antibiotics. It interferes with control of diabetes mellitus, congestive heart failure, hypertension, osteoporosis, diverticulitis, convulsive disorders, and myasthenia gravis. Vaccination should be avoided. Abrupt withdrawal could cause adrenal insufficiency. A drug history on new patients should be taken. Patients undergoing long-term or lifetime therapy with cortisone should carry identification, such as Medic Alert tags. A patient who must undergo surgery and who has received therapy with cortisone or a similar preparation should be prepared preoperatively with the administration of cortisone; its administration should be continued postoperatively in decreasing doses for several days.

Adverse Reactions
Common adverse reactions include fluid and electrolyte imbalance (potassium loss and retention of sodium and fluid), hypertension and congestive heart failure in susceptible individuals, negative nitrogen balance, Cushing's syndrome, impaired wound healing and infections due to immunosuppression, facial erythema, increased perspiration, changes in skin pigmentation, purpura, subcutaneous and cutaneous atrophy, osteoporosis, and muscle weakness. Neurological symptoms include euphoria, psychosis, and increased intracranial pressure with papilledema, vertigo, headache, and convulsions. Gastrointestinal symptoms include increased appetite, gastric bleeding and ulcers, pancreatitis, and ulcerative esophagitis. Endocrine symptoms include menstrual irregularities, suppression of growth in children, diabetes, and secondary adrenocortical and pituitary unresponsiveness (particularly in times of stress, as in trauma, surgery, or illness). Ocular effects include cataract, glaucoma, and exophthalmos.

Composition and Supply
Creams and ointments   0.25% to 2.5%
Injection   25 mg/ml and 50 mg/ml
Ophthalmic preparations   0.5% to 2.5%
Tablets   5 mg, 10 mg, and 25 mg

Legal Status
Prescription

Cortisporin® Ointment

See under **Polymyxin B sulfate.**

Cortisporin® Ointment Ophthalmic

See under **Polymyxin B sulfate.**

Cortisporin® Otic Drops

See under **Polymyxin B sulfate.**

Cortisporin® Suspension Ophthalmic

See under **Polymyxin B sulfate.**

Cortone®

See **Cortisone acetate.**

Cortril®

See **Hydrocortisone.**

Cortrosyn®

See **Cosyntropin.**

Cosmegen®

See **Dactinomycin.**

Cosyntropin (Cortrosyn®)

Action and Use
Synthetic, fast-acting corticotropin for diagnosis of adrenocortical insufficiency.

Dosage and Administration
250 µg, IM. Blood should be collected before and 60 and 90 minutes after injection for coritisol levels.

Cautions
Hydrocortisone should not be given to patients on days of testing. Estrogens (including oral contraceptives) and spironolactone cause erroneously high plasma cortisol levels.

Adverse Reactions
The patient should be observed for possible allergic reactions.

Composition and Supply
Injection   250 µg (25 unit) ampuls

Legal Status
Prescription

Cotazym®

See **Pancrelipase.**

Coumadin®

See **Sodium warfarin.**

Creamalin®

See **Magnesium hydroxide/aluminum hydroxide.**

Cromolyn sodium (Aarane®, Intal®)

Action and Use
Adjunct in the management of severe bronchial asthma. Inhibits the release of histamine and the slow-reacting substance of anaphylaxis.

Dosage and Administration
20 mg 4 times a day, inhalation.

Cautions
Cromolyn sodium is for prophylactic use only; it is of no value in treating acute attacks. Proper administration is necessary to obtain optimal results, and the patient needs careful instruction in its use.

Adverse Reactions
Rash and urticaria may occur. Occasional adverse reactions include cough and bronchospasm. Eosinophilic pneumonia has been reported.

Composition and Supply
Capsule for inhalation   20 mg

Legal Status
Prescription

Crotamiton (Eurax®)

See ANTI-INFECTIVES, LOCAL, scabicide-pediculicides.

Cryptenamine tannate (Unitensin®)

See ANTIHYPERTENSIVES, nondiuretic.

Crysticillin®

See **Penicillin G procaine.**

Crystodigin®

See **Digitoxin.**

Cuprimine®

See **Penicillamine.**

Cyanocobalamin injection (vitamin B_{12}) (Redisol®, Rubramin PC®)

Action and Use
One of the B-complex vitamins; administered to patients with vitamin B_{12} deficiency resulting from malabsorption (including pernicious anemia) and with conditions marked by increased needs, including pregnancy, hyperthyroidism, hemolytic anemia, hemorrhage, malignancy, and hepatic and renal disease.

Dosage and Administration
Dosage is adjusted to the patient and condition being treated. In the treatment of vitamin B_{12} deficiency 1,000 μg is given 2 to 4 times per week until condition is corrected; maintenance ranges from 100 to 1,000 μg monthly; administered IM and deep SC. In the Schilling test the flushing dose is 1,000 μg (1 mg).

Cautions
Refrigerate this drug and protect it from light.

Adverse Reactions
Cyanocobalamin is nontoxic with few side effects. An allergic reaction to impurities in some preparations may rarely occur.

Composition and Supply
Vials, multiple-dose   100 μg/ml and 1,000 μg/ml

Legal Status
Prescription

177

Cyantin®

See **Nitrofurantoin.**

Cyclaine®

See **Hexylcaine hydrochloride.**

Cyclandelate (Cyclospasmol®)

Action and Use
Musculotropic vasodilator for adjunctive therapy in intermittent claudication, arteriosclerosis obliterans, thrombophlebitis, nocturnal leg cramps, and Raynaud's phenomenon, and for selected cases of ischemic cerebral vascular disease.

Dosage and Administration
100 to 200 mg 4 times a day, orally.

Cautions
Should be used with extreme caution in patients with glaucoma, obliterative coronary artery disease, or cerebral vascular disease.

Adverse Reactions
Occasional side effects include gastrointestinal distress, flushing, headache, weakness, and tachycardia.

Composition and Supply
Capsules   200 mg and 400 mg
Tablets   100 mg

Legal Status
Prescription

Cyclizine hydrochloride (Marezine®)

Action and Use
Antiemetic for prevention and treatment of motion sickness, and for treatment of postoperative nausea.

Dosage and Administration
50 mg every 4 to 6 hours, orally or IM; 100 mg every 4 to 6 hours, rectally. For motion sickness, 50 mg taken ½ hour before departure.

Cautions
Contraindicated in pregnancy.

Adverse Reactions
Possible adverse reactions include drowsiness, dry mouth, and blurred vision.

Composition and Supply
Injection (as lactate)   50 mg/ml ampuls
Suppositories   50 mg and 100 mg
Tablets   50 mg

Legal Status
Prescription

Cyclobenzaprine hydrochloride (Flexeril™)

See SKELETAL MUSCLE RELAXANTS.

Cyclogyl®

See **Cyclopentolate hydrochloride.**

Cyclomethycaine sulfate (Surfacaine®)

Action and Use
Local anesthetic.

Dosage and Administration
Apply 3 or 4 times a day, topically.

Cautions
Should not be used in the eye or in vesicular lesions. Use with caution when applied extensively or for prolonged periods, and in patients with allergies.

Adverse Reactions
Transitory stinging or burning may occur, and occasionally dermatitis develops.

Composition and Supply
Lotion   0.5%
Ointment   0.5% and 1%

Legal Status
Nonprescription

Cyclopar®

See **Tetracycline hydrochloride.**

Cyclopentolate hydrochloride (Cyclogyl®)

Action and Use
Mydriatic and cycloplegic.

Dosage and Administration

2 drops of 0.5% or 1 drop of 1% solution, repeated in 5 minutes. Blacks and people with darkly pigmented irises are particularly resistant to this drug and may require a stronger solution and/or repeated instillations.

Cautions

See **Atropine sulfate.**

Adverse Reactions

Use care to minimize systemic absorption, especially in young children. See **Atropine sulfate.**

Composition and Supply

Solution, ophthalmic   0.5% and 1%

Legal Status

Prescription

Cyclophosphamide (Cytoxan®)

Action and Use

Alkylating antineoplastic.

Dosage and Administration

Initial loading dose: 40 to 50 mg per kg IV.
Maintenance dosage: 1 to 5 mg per kg, daily, orally.

Cautions

Bone marrow depression may occur. Insure ample fluid intake (3 liters per day) and frequent voiding to prevent development of cystitis. Discontinue use if dysuria or hematuria occurs.

Adverse Reactions

Incidence and severity of side effects is less than with nitrogen mustard. Alopecia occurs in 50% of patients (scalp tourniquet is helpful; hair grows back, but may be of a different color or texture). Skin and fingernails may become darker during therapy, and transverse ridging of nails is possible. Bone marrow depression may occur, but with less depression of platelets than with other mustards (the patient should be observed for infection and bleeding). Delayed anorexia, nausea, and vomiting are common, and antiemetics are helpful. Occasionally hemorrhagic colitis, oral mucosal ulceration, or jaundice may develop. Other possible adverse reactions include gonadal suppression resulting in amenorrhea or azoospermia (which is probably reversible), interstitial pulmonary fibrosis (which may develop with prolonged therapy), and dizziness of short duration.

Composition and Supply
Injection 100 mg, 200 mg, and 500 mg vials
Tablets   50 mg

Legal Status
Prescription

Cyclopropane

See ANESTHETICS, general.

Cycloserine (Seromycin®)

See ANTIBIOTICS, miscellaneous; ANTITUBERCULOTICS.

Cyclospasmol®

See **Cyclandelate.**

Cycrimine hydrochloride (Pagitane®)

See ANTIPARKINSONICS.

Cylert® (pemoline)

See CEREBRAL STIMULANTS.

Cyproheptadine hydrochloride (Periactin®)

Action and Use
Antihistamine and antipruritic.

Dosage and Administration
4 to 32 mg in divided doses, daily, orally.

Cautions
Cyproheptadine hydrochloride causes drowsiness; it is contrain-dicated in glaucoma.

Adverse Reactions
See **Brompheniramine.**

Composition and Supply
Syrup   2 mg/5 ml
Tablets   4 mg

Legal Status
Prescription

Cystografin®

See under **Diatrizoate meglumine.**

Cytarabine (Cytosar®)

Action and Use
Antineoplastic for treatment of acute leukemia.

Dosage and Administration
500 μg to 4 mg per kg, daily; administered SC or IV.

Cautions
Highly toxic. Bone marrow depression (with leukopenia, thrombocytopenia, and anemia) or liver dysfunction may occur. Teratogenic in animals.

Adverse Reactions
The main toxic effect is bone marrow suppression 7 to 14 days after dose (the patient should be observed for infection and bleeding; daily blood studies are recommended). Less serious responses, especially at high dosage, include nausea and vomiting (antiemetics are helpful), diarrhea, abdominal pain, stomatitis and oral ulceration, esophagitis, and occasionally fever. Hepatic or renal dysfunction is possible (periodic liver and kidney function studies are recommended). Infrequent adverse effects include anorexia, gastrointestinal hemorrhage, sepsis, cellulitis at the injection site, pneumonia, neuritis or neurotoxicity, rash, freckling, skin and mucosal bleeding, chest pain, and joint pain.

Composition and Supply
Injection   100 mg and 500 mg vials

Legal Status
Prescription

Cytellin®

See **Sitosterols.**

Cytomel®

See **Liothyronine sodium.**

Cytosar®

See **Cytarabine.**

Cytoxan®

See **Cyclophosphamide.**

Dacarbazine (DTIC-Dome®)

See ANTINEOPLASTICS, antimetabolites.

Dactinomycin (actinomycin D) (Cosmegen®)

Action and Use
Antineoplastic antibiotic useful in testicular cancer and Wilms' tumor.

Dosage and Administration
Dosage is individualized; administered IV. Usual dosage 500 μg daily for a maximum of 5 days.

Cautions
Highly toxic with a low therapeutic index. Extravasation produces severe local reactions.

Adverse Reactions
Bone marrow depression with pancytopenia may occur 1 to 7 days after completion of treatment (the patient should be observed for infection and bleeding). Other adverse effects include nausea, vomiting, anorexia, stomatitis (progressing to ulcerations), diarrhea, alopecia (a scalp tourniquet is helpful), mental depression, acne, malaise, fever, and myalgia.

Composition and Supply
Injection   500 μg vials

Legal Status
Prescription

Dakin's solution

See **Sodium hypochlorite solution, diluted.**

Dalidyne® (methylbenzethonium chloride)

See MOUTHWASHES.

Dalmane®

See **Flurazepam hydrochloride.**

Danazol (Danocrine®)

Action and Use
Danazol is an antigonadotropin that suppresses the output of both follicle-stimulating hormone (FSH) and luteinizing hormone (LH). It is indicated for the treatment of endometriosis amenable to hormonal management.

Dosage and Administration
400 mg twice a day, orally.

Cautions
Contraindications include pregnancy, breast-feeding, undiagnosed genital bleeding, and marked impairment of hepatic, renal, or cardiac function. Patients should be watched closely for signs of androgenic effects, some of which may not be reversible.

Adverse Reactions
Possible adverse reactions include acne, hirsutism, decrease in breast size, edema, flushing, sweating, vaginitis, and nervousness.

Composition and Supply
Capsules   200 mg

Legal Status
Prescription

Danocrine®

See **Danazol.**

Danthron (Dorbane®, Modrane®)

See CATHARTICS.

Dantrium®

See **Dantrolene sodium.**

Dantrolene sodium (Dantrium®)

Action and Use
Skeletal muscle relaxant used in patients with chronic spastic disorders, including spinal injury, stroke, cerebral palsy, and multiple sclerosis.

Dosage and Administration
Initial dosage 25 mg daily, orally, gradually increased; some patients require up to 200 mg 4 times a day.

Cautions
Long-term safety and efficacy have not been established. There are many side effects. Laboratory SGOT, alkaline phosphatase, BUN, and total serum bilirubin test results are increased. Contraindicated in nursing mothers, in patients with impaired pulmonary or cardiac function, and in patients in whom spasticity is used to sustain the upright position or maintain balance in locomotion.

Adverse Reactions
The major side effect is weakness. Common side effects include transient early symptoms of euphoria, lightheadedness, dizziness, drowsiness, and fatigue. The patient should move cautiously. Occasional effects include diarrhea, leukocytosis, and alteration of liver function tests (liver function studies are recommended before and during therapy). Other effects that have been reported include gastrointestinal bleeding, anorexia, difficulty in swallowing, tearing, feeling of suffocation, backache, speech disturbance, visual disturbance, alteration of taste, depression, confusion, nervousness, abnormal hair growth, rash, pruritus, diaphoresis, and urinary frequency.

Composition and Supply
Capsules   25 mg and 100 mg

Legal Status
Prescription

Dapsone (DDS)(Avolsulfon®)

See ANTILEPROTICS.

Daranide® (dichlorphenamide)

See CARBONIC ANHYDRASE INHIBITORS.

Daraprim®

See **Pyrimethamine.**

Darbid® (isopropamide iodide)

See ANTICHOLINERGICS.

Daricon® (oxyphencyclimine hydrochloride)

See CHOLINERGICS.

Darrow's solution (potassic saline injection, lactated)

See ELECTROLYTE SOLUTIONS AND WATER-BALANCE AGENTS, replacement solutions.

Darvocet®-N

See under **Propoxyphene hydrochloride.**

Darvocet®-N 100

See under **Propoxyphene hydrochloride.**

Darvon®

See **Propoxyphene hydrochloride.**

Darvon® with A.S.A.

See **Propoxyphene hydrochloride.**

Darvon® Compound

See under **Propoxyphene hydrochloride.**

Darvon® Compound-65

See under **Propoxyphene hydrochloride.**

Darvon®-N

See under **Propoxyphene hydrochloride.**

Darvon®-N with A.S.A.

See **Propoxyphene hydrochloride.**

Datril®

See **Acetaminophen.**

Daunorubicin

See ANTINEOPLASTICS, antibiotics.

Daxolin® (loxapine succinate)

See PSYCHOTROPICS, antipsychotics.

Dayalets®

See VITAMINS, MULTIPLE, oral.

Dayalets® plus Iron

See VITAMINS, MULTIPLE, oral.

DDS (dapsone)

See ANTILEPROTICS.

Deaner®

See **Deanol acetamidobenzoate.**

Deanol acetamidobenzoate (Deaner®)

Action and Use
Mild cerebral stimulant and adjunct in treatment of children with learning problems and hyperkinetic behavior.

Dosage and Administration
25 to 300 mg daily, orally.

Cautions
Contraindicated in patients with grand mal epilepsy; should not be used to treat severe depression.

Adverse Reactions
Headache may occur during early therapy. Other adverse reactions include constipation, tense muscles, insomnia, pruritus, and rash. Hypotension is a rare side effect.

Composition and Supply
Tablets   25 mg and 100 mg

Legal Status
Prescription

Debrox® (carbamide peroxide 6.5%)

See CERUMINOLYTICS.

Decadron®

See **Dexamethasone.**

Decadron®-LA

See under **Dexamethasone.**

Deca-Durabolin® (nandrolone decanoate)

See ANDROGENS.

Decapryn® (doxylamine succinate)

See ANTIHISTAMINES.

Decavitamin capsules and tablets

See VITAMINS, MULTIPLE, oral.

Decholin®

See **Dehydrocholic acid.**

Decholin® Sodium

See under **Dehydrocholic acid.**

Declomycin®

See **Demeclocycline hydrochloride.**

Deferoxamine mesylate (Desferal®)

Action and Use
Chelating agent useful as an adjunctive measure in acute iron intoxication.

Dosage and Administration
1 g IM or slow IV infusion followed by 500 mg at 4-hour intervals for 2 doses.

Cautions
Total daily dose should not exceed 6 g. IV infusion should not exceed 15 mg/kg per hour and IM route should not be used in shock.

Adverse Reactions
Rapid infusion may produce urticaria and shock. Occasional side effects include cataract, leg cramps, exacerbation of iron poisoning symptoms in renal infection, pain, and swelling at injection site.

Composition and Supply
Injection   500 mg ampuls

Legal Status
Prescription

Dehydrocholic acid (Decholin®)

Action and Use
Hydrocholeretic and diagnostic aid in circulation time, cholecystography, and cholangiography.

Dosage and Administration
250 to 500 mg 2 or 3 times a day, orally; 3 to 10 ml, IV, depending on use.

Cautions
Injection should not be made until skin tests for allergies have been done. Severe reactions have occurred with IV administration. Contraindicated in patients with biliary tract obstruction and acute hepatitis.

Adverse Reactions

Diarrhea may occur. Parenteral administration may cause hypotension, bradycardia, and skeletal muscle hyperactivity.

Composition and Supply

Injection (sodium dehydrocholate)   200 mg/ml, in 3 ml, 5 ml and 10 ml ampuls (Decholin® Sodium)
Tablets   250 mg (Decholin®)
Tablets   250 mg with homatropine 10 mg (Hepahydrin®)

Legal Status

Prescription

Deladumone® (testosterone enanthate/estradiol valerate)

See ANDROGENS; ESTROGENS.

Delalutin®

See **Hydroxyprogesterone caproate.**

Delatestryl®

See **Testosterone enanthate.**

Delta-Cortef®

See **Prednisolone.**

Deltasone®

See **Prednisone.**

Demecarium bromide (Humorsol®)

Action and Use

Miotic used in treatment of open-angle glaucoma.

Dosage and Administration

1 to 2 drops in eye weekly to 1 to 2 drops twice a day.

Cautions

Demecarium bromide is a potent drug; all patients should be under continuous supervision. Contraindicated in narrow-angle glaucoma.

Adverse Reactions

See **Echothiophate iodide.**

Composition and Supply

Solution, ophthalmic   0.125% and 0.25%

Legal Status
Prescription

Demeclocycline hydrochloride (Declomycin®)

Action and Use
Broad-spectrum antibiotic (a tetracycline).

Dosage and Administration
600 mg daily, orally 1 hour before or 2 hours after meals.

Cautions
See **Tetracycline hydrochloride.**

Adverse Reactions
See **Tetracycline hydrochloride.**

Composition and Supply
Capsules   150 mg and 300 mg
Suspension   75 mg/5 ml

Legal Status
Prescription

Demerol®

See **Meperidine hydrochloride.**

Demulen® (ethynodiol diacetate ethinyl estradiol)

See CONTRACEPTIVES, ORAL.

Dendrid®

See **Idoxuridine.**

Depakene® (valproic acid)

See ANTICONVULSANTS.

Depo®-Estradiol Cypionate

See **Estradiol cypionate.**

Depo-Medrol®

See under **Methylprednisolone.**

Depo-Provera®

See **Medroxyprogesterone acetate.**

Depo®-Testosterone (testosterone cypionate)

See ANDROGENS.

Derifil® (chlorophyll derivatives)

See DEODORANTS.

Derma Medicone® (menthol preparation)

See ANTIPRURITICS, topical preparations.

Deronil®

See **Dexamethasone.**

DES

See **Diethylstilbestrol.**

Desenex®

See **Undecylenic acid/zinc undecylenate.**

Deserpidine (Harmonyl®)

See ANTIHYPERTENSIVES, nondiuretic.

Desferal®

See **Deferoxamine mesylate.**

Desipramine hydrochloride (Norpramin®, Pertofrane®)

Action and Use
Antidepressant.

Dosage and Administration
25 to 50 mg 3 or 4 times a day, orally; the maximum daily dose is 200 mg.

Cautions
May potentiate the action of thyroid and adrenergic drugs. Concurrent therapy with MAO inhibitors is contraindicated, and desipramine hydrochloride should not be given within 2 weeks after MAO inhibitor therapy. Contraindicated in children; use with caution in patients who are manic depressive or psychotic. See **Amitriptyline hydrochloride** for further cautions.

Adverse Reactions
See **Amitriptyline hydrochloride.**

Composition and Supply
Capsules   25 mg and 50 mg (Pertofrane®)
Tablets   25 mg, 50 mg, 75 mg, 100 mg, and 150 mg
(Norpramin®)

Legal Status
Prescription

Deslanoside (Cedilanid®-D)

Action and Use
Digitalis glycoside for rapid digitalization.

Dosage and Administration
Digitalization: 1.6 mg IM or IV (slowly).
Maintenance: institute therapy with oral preparation after 12 hours.

Cautions
Extremely poisonous. Effects may be additive with those of quinidine, procainamide, or propranolol. Caution should be used to avoid over-dosage.

Adverse Reactions
See **Digitalis.**

Composition and Supply
Injection   200 μg/ml, in 2 ml and 4 ml ampuls

Legal Status
Prescription

Desonide (Tridesilon®)

See CORTICOSTEROIDS.

Desoximetasone (Topicort®)

See CORTICOSTEROIDS.

Desoxycorticosterone acetate (Doca®, Percorten®)
Desoxycorticosterone pivalate (Percorten® Pivalate)

Action and Use
Mineralocorticoid for partial replacement in adrenocortical insuffi-ciency (Addison's disease).

Dosage and Administration
Acetate: 1 to 5 mg daily, IM.
Pivalate: 25 to 100 mg every 4 weeks, IM.
Buccally: 2 to 10 mg daily.

Cautions
Do not administer more than 10 mg at once. Contraindicated in patients with hypersensitivity to the drug and in those with hypertension or cardiac disease.

Adverse Reactions
Similar to the adverse reactions to cortisone acetate, but with greater potential for salt retention, increased blood volume, edema, elevation of blood pressure, and enlargement of heart shadow.

Composition and Supply
Injection (acetate)   5 mg/ml, in 10 ml vials
Injection (pivalate)   25 mg/ml, in 4 ml vials
Pellets (acetate)   125 mg (*Note:* 1 pellet is implanted for each 500 μg of daily injected maintenance dose of desoxycorticosterone acetate in oil)
Tablets, buccal   2 mg and 5 mg

Legal Status
Prescription

Desoxyribonuclease (Dornavac®)

See MUCOLYTICS.

Desquam-X® (benzoyl peroxide preparation)

See KERATOLYTICS.

Dexamethasone (Decadron®, Deronil®, Dexone™, Gammacorten®, Hexadrol®)

Action and Use
Synthetic glucocorticoid used primarily for anti-inflammatory and antiallergic action.

Dosage and Administration
Dosage is individualized to the patient and condition treated, and ranges from 500 μg to 6 mg daily, orally, IM, or IV (except that dexamethasone acetate should be used IM only). Also used topically.

Cautions
More potent than cortisone acetate (see).

Adverse Reactions
Essentially the same as adverse reactions to cortisone acetate and hydrocortisone, but dexamethasone almost completely lacks sodium-retaining property.

Composition and Supply

Aerosol (as sodium phosphate) 18 mg/cartridge (Respihaler®, Turbinaire®)

Injection (as acetate) 8 mg/ml, in 5 ml vials (Decadron®-LA)

Injection (as sodium phosphate salt) 4 mg/ml, in 1 ml, 5 ml, and 25 ml vials and 1 ml disposable syringes

Liquid, oral 500 g/5 ml

Ointment, ophthalmic (as sodium phosphate salt) 0.05%

Solution, ophthalmic 0.1%

Solution, ophthalmic 0.1% with methylcellulose (Maxidex®)

Tablets 250 μg, 500 μg, 750 μg, 1.5 mg, and 4 mg

Legal Status
Prescription

Dexamyl® (dextroamphetamine sulfate/amobarbital)

See CEREBRAL STIMULANTS.

Dexbrompheniramine maleate (Disomer®)

See ANTIHISTAMINES.

Dexbrompheniramine maleate/ d-isoephedrine sulfate (Drixoral®)

See ANTIHISTAMINES.

Dexchlorpheniramine maleate (Polaramine®)

See ANTIHISTAMINES.

Dexedrine®

See **Dextroamphetamine sulfate.**

Dexone™

See **Dexamethasone.**

Dexpanthenol (Ilopan®)

Action and Use
Coenzyme A precursor indicated in the treatment and prevention of postsurgical atony, distention, and flatulence.

Dosage and Administration
500 mg IM, repeated in 2 hours, and followed by comparable doses every 6 hours.

Cautions
Avoid concurrent use of cholinergic drugs. Bleeding times may be prolonged. Dexpanthenol should not be administered sooner than 12 hours after giving cholinergic drugs and 1 hour after giving succinyl-choline chloride.

Adverse Reactions
There have been rare instances of allergic reactions during concomitant use of antibiotics, narcotics, and barbiturates.

Composition and Supply
Injection   125 mg/ml, in ampuls, vials, and disposable syringes

Legal Status
Prescription

Dextran 40 (Rheomacrodex®)

See ELECTROLYTE SOLUTIONS AND WATER-BALANCE AGENTS, plasma extenders.

Dextran 70 (Macrodex®)

See ELECTROLYTE SOLUTIONS AND WATER-BALANCE AGENTS, plasma extenders.

Dextroamphetamine sulfate (Dexedrine®)

Action and Use
Cerebral stimulant for treatment of patients with narcolepsy and minimal brain dysfunction, and as an adjunctive treatment in exogenous obesity.

Dosage and Administration
2.5 to 5 mg 1 to 3 times a day ½ hour before meals, orally.

Cautions
Dextroamphetamine sulfate is habit-forming and has a high potential for abuse. Contraindicated in hyperexcitability, hyperthyroidism, nephritis, diabetes mellitus, and severe hypertension, angina pectoris, and other cardiovascular diseases.

Adverse Reactions
Relatively common adverse reactions include dry mouth, metallic taste, restlessness, insomnia, dizziness, talkativeness, irritability, bruxism, anxiety, a sense of intoxication, euphoria, nausea, vomiting, diarrhea, and anorexia. Bone marrow depression may occur. Abrupt withdrawal may cause depression, lethargy, hunger, and prolonged sleep. Overdosage may cause weakness, chest pain, hallucinations,

excoriation of skin, increased reflex activity, confusion, and panic states. Coma, convulsions, and cerebral hemorrhage are also possible results of overdosage.

Composition and Supply
Capsules, long-acting   10 mg and 15 mg
Elixir   5 mg/5 ml
Tablets   5 mg

Legal Status
Schedule II

Dextroamphetamine sulfate/amobarbital (Dexamyl®)

See CEREBRAL STIMULANTS.

Dextromethorphan hydrobromide

See ANTITUSSIVES AND EXPECTORANTS, antitussives.

Dextrose injections 2.5%, 5%, 10%, 20%, and 50%

See PARENTERAL ALIMENTATION.

Dextrose 5% in lactated Ringer's injection

See PARENTERAL ALIMENTATION.

Dextrose 5% in Ringer's injection

See PARENTERAL ALIMENTATION.

Dextrose 5%/alcohol 5%

See PARENTERAL ALIMENTATION.

Dextrose/sodium chloride injections

See PARENTERAL ALIMENTATION.

Diabinese®

See **Chlorpropamide.**

Di-Alminate® (aluminum glycinate/magnesium carbonate)

See ANTACIDS.

Dialog® (acetaminophen/allobarbital)

See ANALGESICS, nonnarcotic.

Dialose® (carboxymethylcellulose sodium)

See CATHARTICS.

Diamox®

See **Acetazolamide.**

Dianabol® (methandrostenolone)

See ANDROGENS.

Dianeal®/Dextrose (peritoneal dialysis solution)

See DIALYZING SOLUTIONS.

Diapid® (lypressin)

See PITUITARY HORMONES.

Diasone® (sulfoxone sodium)

See ANTILEPROTICS.

Diatrizoate meglumine

Action and Use
Radiopaque contrast agent formulated in various ways for particular
roentgenographic procedures:

Diatrizoate meglumine injection 85% (Cardiografin®): used in angiocardiography and thoracic aortography.

Diatrizoate meglumine injection 76%: used in excretory urography,
aortography, pediatric angiocardiography, and peripheral arteriography.

Diatrizoate meglumine injection 60% (Reno-M-60®): used in excretory urography, cerebral angiography, peripheral arteriography,
venography, transhepatic cholangiography, splenoportography, ar-
thrography, and discography.

Diatrizoate meglumine injection 30% (Cystografin®, Reno-M-30®):
used in retrograde cytourethrography (Cystografin®) and retrograde
pyelography (Ren-M-30®).

*Diatrizoate meglumine 66% with diatrizoate sodium 10% solution
(Gastrografin®):* used in radiography of gastrointestinal tract.

*Diatrizoate meglumine 66% with diatrizoate sodium 10% injection
(Renografin®-76):* used in selective renal arteriography, selective vis-

ceral arteriography, selective coronary arteriography, and left ventriculography.

Diatrizoate meglumine 52% with diatrizoate sodium injection 8% (Renografin®-60): same uses as for Reno-M-60®.

Dosage and Administration
Dosage is adjusted to the particular procedure.

Cautions
During first ½ hour after diatrizoate meglumine is administered, patient is observed for allergic response. Diatrizoate is contraindicated in patients with hypersensitivity to the drug, in advanced kidney disease and in iodine allergy. It should be administered with caution in patients with multiple myeloma, liver disease, or kidney disease. The potential for anaphylaxis exists with any intravascular radiopaque agent, and emergency facilities should be available for at least an hour. Use with extreme caution in patients with any kind of allergy or history of sensitivity.

Adverse Reactions
Allergic reactions include sneezing, wheezing, urticaria, and dyspnea. Hypotension or reflex tachycardia may occur.

Composition and Supply
Diatrizoate meglumine injection 85% (Cardiografin®): 50 ml vials
Diatrizoate meglumine injection 76%: 20 ml and 50 ml vials
Diatrizoate meglumine injection 60% (Reno-M-60®): 10 ml, 30 ml, 50 ml, and 100 ml bottles
Diatrizoate meglumine injection 30%: 200 ml and 500 ml bottles containing 100 ml and 300 ml of diatrizoate (Cystografin®); and 50 ml and 100 ml vials (Reno-M-30®)
Diatrizoate meglumine 66% with diatrizoate sodium 10%: flavored oral solution in bottles 120 ml (Gastrografin®), 20 ml and 50 ml vials, and 100 ml and 200 ml IV bottles (Renografin®-76)
Diatrizoate meglumine 52% with diatrizoate sodium 8% injection (Renografin®-60): 10 ml, 30 ml, and 50 ml vials and 100 ml bottles

Legal Status
Prescription

Diatrizoate sodium (Hypaque® Sodium)
See DIAGNOSTICS, roentgenography.

Diazepam (Valium®)

Action and Use
Tranquilizer and adjunct in treatment of alcohol withdrawal, skeletal muscle spasm, status epilepticus, and severe recurrent seizures.

Dosage and Administration
2 to 10 mg 3 or 4 times a day (depending on indications and severity of problem), orally; 2 to 20 mg doses, IM or IV.

Cautions
Do not mix parenteral preparation with other solutions or drugs. Care should be taken to avoid possible venous thrombosis, phlebitis, local irritation, vascular impairment, apnea, and cardiac arrest with intravenous injection. There is a possibility of dependence, and diazepam may potentiate CNS depressants. The dosage of narcotic analgesics should be reduced by at least one-third when used with diazepam. Contraindicated in patients with acute narrow-angle glaucoma and in infants; also contraindicated in shock, coma, and acute alcohol intoxication. Should be used with caution in patients who are depressed or suicidal, in pregnant women, and in nursing mothers.

Adverse Reactions
The most commonly reported side effects include drowsiness, fatigue, and ataxia. Reactions that are more infrequently encountered include hypotension, changes in libido, dysarthria, skin rash, constipation, incontinence, changes in salivation, slurred speech, tremor, vertigo, urinary retention, blurred vision, diplopia, syncope, bradycardia, cardiovascular collapse, and nystagmus.

Composition and Supply
Injection   5 mg/ml, in 2 ml ampuls and 10 ml vials
Tablets   2 mg, 5 mg, and 10 mg

Legal Status
Schedule IV

Diazoxide (Hyperstat®)

Action and Use
Antihypertensive for emergency lowering of blood pressure.

Dosage and Administration
300 mg IV in 30 seconds or less; give a second dose if an adequate response is not produced within 30 minutes.

Cautions
Diazoxide is a potent agent that requires close monitoring of the patient; it should not be given intramuscularly or subcutaneously

199

because it is extremely alkaline. Its safety for children is not yet established.

Adverse Reactions
Frequent side effects include edema, hyperuricemia, and hyperglycemia. Alteration of taste, nausea, vomiting, diarrhea, constipation, flushing, headache, diaphoresis, increased salivation, lacrimation, orthostatic hypotension (the patient should use caution on rising), tachycardia or bradycardia, and dyspnea are possible adverse reactions. Infrequent effects include arrhythmias, myocardial and/or cerebral ischemia, convulsions, paralysis, coma, rash, leukopenia, fever, and cellulitis and/or phlebitis if extravasation occurs. An overdose can cause marked hypotension and shock.

Composition and Supply
Injection   15 mg/ml, in 20 ml vials

Legal Status
Prescription

Dibenzyline®

See **Phenoxybenzamine hydrochloride.**

Dibucaine (Nupercainal®)

Dibucaine hydrochloride (Nupercaine®)

Action and Use
Local anesthetic.

Dosage and Administration
Applied topically or intrathecally.

Cautions
Much more potent than cocaine hydrochloride (see). The dose should never exceed 12 mg. Contraindicated in patients with diseases of the cerebrospinal system or with infection at or near the site of puncture. Tissue sloughs may occur with subcutaneous injection.

Adverse Reactions
Essentially the same as adverse reactions to tetracaine hydrochloride (see).

Composition and Supply
Areosol   0.25% (Nupercainal®)
Cream   0.5% (Nupercainal®)

200

Injection   1 : 1,500, in 20 ml ampuls; 1 : 200, in 2 ml ampuls; 1 : 400
   in 5% dextrose (Heavy Solution Nupercaine®)
Ointment   1% (Nupercainal®)
Suppositories   2.5 mg (Nupercainal®)

Legal Status
Prescription (Nupercaine®)
Nonprescription (Nupercainal®)

Dical-D® (ergocalciferol/dibasic calcium phosphate)

See BLOOD CALCIUM REGULATORS.

Dichlorphenamide (Daranide®)

See CARBONIC ANHYDRASE INHIBITORS.

Dicloxacillin sodium (Dynapen®, Pathocil®, Veracillin®)

Action and Use
Penicillin analogue for infections caused by penicillinase-producing
staphylococci.

Dosage and Administration
125 to 500 mg every 6 hours, orally.

Cautions
There may be cross-sensitivity with penicillin and cephalosporins.
Food interferes with absorption. See **Penicillin G potassium** for fur-
ther cautions.

Adverse Reactions
See **Penicillin G potassium.**

Composition and Supply
Capsules   125 mg and 250 mg
Suspension   62.5 mg/5 ml

Legal Status
Prescription

Dicumarol (bishydroxycoumarin)

Action and Use
Anticoagulant.

Dosage and Administration
Dosage is individualized and ranges from 25 to 200 mg daily, orally.
First day, 200 to 300 mg orally; maintenance, 25 to 200 mg.

Cautions
Should be used with caution in subacute bacterial endocarditis, liver disease, pregnancy, and congestive heart failure. Drugs diminishing the response of dicumarol include barbiturates, ethchlorvynol, glutethimide, and vitamin K; drugs enhancing the response include chloral hydrate, mefenamic acid, phenylbutazone, chloramphenicol, broadspectrum antibiotics, and salicylates. See **Sodium warfarin.**

Adverse Reactions
Occasional side effects include anorexia, nausea, vomiting, and diarrhea. See **Sodium warfarin.**

Composition and Supply
Capsules   25 mg, 50 mg, and 100 mg
Tablets   25 mg, 50 mg, and 100 mg

Legal Status
Prescription

Dicurin® (merethoxylline procaine)

See DIURETICS.

Dicyclomine hydrochloride (Bentyl®)

Action and Use
Antispasmodic.

Dosage and Administration
10 to 20 mg 3 or 4 times a day, orally; 20 mg every 4 to 6 hours, IM.

Cautions
Not for intravenous use. Contraindicated in patients with urinary retention, paralytic ileus, pyloric or duodenal obstruction, and myasthenia gravis. Should be used with caution in hepatic or renal disease, ulcerative colitis, hyperthyroidism, prostatic hypertrophy, and glaucoma.

Adverse Reactions
Occasional side effects include euphoria, dizziness, drowsiness, fatigue, and headache. Fever and heat stroke can occur due to decreased perspiration in the presence of a high environmental temperature. In high doses or in susceptible persons, dry mouth, blurred vision, and other visual disturbances may develop.

Composition and Supply
Capsules   10 mg
Capsules   10 mg with phenobarbital 15 mg
Injection   10 mg/ml, in 2 ml ampuls and 10 ml vials

Syrup   10 mg/5 ml
Syrup   10 mg/5 ml with phenobarbital 15 mg/5 ml
Tablets   20 mg
Tablets   20 mg with phenobarbital 15 mg

Legal Status
Prescription

Didrex™ (benzphetamine hydrochloride)

See CEREBRAL STIMULANTS, anorectics.

Diethylcarbamazine citrate (Hetrazan®)

Action and Use
Anthelmintic in treatment of filariasis, loiasis, and onchocerciasis.

Dosage and Administration
2 mg/kg 3 times a day for 7 to 21 days, orally.

Cautions
See **Piperazine citrate.**

Adverse Reactions
Common side effects include headache, general malaise, weakness, joint pains, anorexia, nausea, vomiting, leukocytosis, lymphadenopathy, and fever.

Composition and Supply
Tablets   50 mg

Legal Status
Prescription

Diethylpropion hydrochloride (Tenuate®, Tepanil®)

Action and Use
Anorectic used in treatment of obesity.

Dosage and Administration
25 mg 3 times a day before meals, orally.

Cautions
Contraindicated in patients with hyperthyroidism, hypertension, angina pectoris, and other serious cardiovascular diseases. Habituation may develop.

Adverse Reactions
Similar to but generally less pronounced than adverse reactions to dextroamphetamine sulfate (see).

Composition and Supply
Tablets   25 mg
Tablets, long-acting   75 mg

Legal Status
Schedule IV

Diethylstilbestrol (DES, stilbestrol)
Diethylstilbestrol diphosphate (Stilphostrol®)

Action and Use
Nonsteroidal estrogen.

Dosage and Administration
Dosage is individualized to the patient and condition being treated. For diethylstilbestrol, dosages range from 200 μg to 30 mg daily, orally or rectally. For diethylstilbestrol diphosphate, daily dosage ranges up to 600 mg or more (depending on tolerance) orally and up to 1 g by slow IV infusion.

Cautions
See **Estradiol.**

Adverse Reactions
See **Estradiol.**

Composition and Supply
Injection   250 μg in 5 ml ampuls (for dilution) (Stilphostrol®)
Suppositories   100 μg, 500 μg, and 1 mg (stilbestrol)
Tablets   100 μg, 250 μg, 500 μg, 1 mg, and 5 mg (stilbestrol)
Tablets   50 mg (Stilphostrol®)

Legal Status
Prescription

Diethylstilbestrol/methyltestosterone (Tylosterone®)

Action and Use
Tylosterone® is indicated for the management of the menopausal syndrome in those patients who do not respond to estrogen alone.

Dosage and Administration
Initial dosage: 1 tablet daily, orally.
Maintenance dosage: ½ tablet or less daily, orally.

Cautions
See **Estradiol.**

Adverse Reactions
See **Estradiol**.

Composition and Supply
Tablets   diethylstilbestrol 250 µg/methyltestosterone 5 mg

Legal Status
Prescription

Digitaline Nativelle®

See **Digitoxin**.

Digitalis

Action and Use
Cardiotonic.

Dosage and Administration
Digitalization: 1.5 g daily in divided doses, orally.
Maintenance: 100 mg daily, orally.

Cautions
Apical pulse (with notation of rate and rhythm) should be taken prior
to each dose. The drug should be withheld if the apical rate is below
60 in adults, or 90 to 110 in children. Digitalis is extremely poisonous,
with a narrow margin of safety, and may potentiate the action of
quinidine, procainamide, or propranolol. Record urinary output and
weight daily. Use cautiously in hypokalemic patients and in patients
concurrently receiving insulin, corticosteroids, or diuretics. Use caution in patients receiving thyroid drugs. Digitalis acts synergistically
with reserpine, ephedrine, epinephrine, and certain other adrenergic
agents.

Adverse Reactions
Early side effects include anorexia, nausea, vomiting, increased salivation, and gastric irritation; these effects could be a sign of digitalis
toxicity. Later effects include diarrhea, headache, visual disturbances,
drowsiness, fatigue, weakness, restlessness, and irritability. Pain simulating trigeminal neuralgia may occur, which could be the first sign
of digitalis toxicity. Elderly patients may evidence confusion, disorientation, and delirium. Toxic effects include bradycardia with an
apical rate below 60, which can lead to atrioventricular block, poor
cerebral or coronary circulation with dizziness, weakness, faintness,
and possibly congestive heart failure. Other possible toxic effects include tachycardia, ectopic beats or extrasystoles (especially in children), premature ventricular contraction (especially bigeminy in
adults), atrial fibrillation, trigeminy, and pulse deficit. Ventricular
tachycardia can result in ventricular fibrillation. Digitalis toxicity

may be precipitated by hypoxia, disturbance in acid-base balance, hypercalcemia, hypomagnesemia, hypokalemia, kidney disease, liver disease, or severe heart disease.

Composition and Supply
Tablets (dried leaf of *Digitalis purpurea*)   100 mg

Legal Status
Prescription

Digitoxin (Crystodigin®, Digitaline Nativelle®, Purodigin®)

Action and Use
Cardiotonic digitalis glycoside with a slow onset of action.

Dosage and Administration
Digitalization: 1.2 to 1.6 mg in divided doses, orally, IM, or IV.
Maintenance: 100 μg daily, orally.

Cautions
1,000 times more potent than digitalis (see).

Adverse Reactions
See **Digitalis.**

Composition and Supply
Injection   200 μg/ml, in 1 ml ampuls
Tablets   50 μg, 100 μg, and 200 μg

Legal Status
Prescription

Digoxin (Lanoxin®)

Action and Use
Cardiotonic digitalis glycoside with prompt action.

Dosage and Administration
Digitalization: 2 to 3 mg orally, 1 to 1.5 mg IV, or 1 to 2 mg IM, in divided doses.
Maintenance: 125 to 500 μg daily, orally.

Cautions
1,000 times more potent than digitalis (see).

Adverse Reactions
Digoxin is eliminated rapidly from the body. See **Digitalis** for further cautions.

Composition and Supply
Elixir   50 μg/ml
Injection   250 μg/ml, in 2 ampuls and 500 μg/ml, in 2 ml ampuls
Tablets   125 μg, 250 μg, and 500 μg

Legal Status
Prescription

Dihydroergotoxine mesylates (Hydergine®)*

Action and Use
Antiserotonin alkaloids (chemically related to ergot alkaloids, or *Claviceps purpurea*) indicated for the treatment of certain symptoms in elderly patients—namely confusion, unsociability, depression, dizziness, and failure to care for himself or herself. The mechanism by which the drug achieves its mental effects is unknown.

Dosage and Administration
1 mg sublingually tablets 3 times a day.

Cautions
Contraindicated in patients hypersensitive to any component of the drug. Careful diagnosis should be attempted, since the symptoms treated by this drug are of unknown etiology.

Adverse Reactions
Sublingual irritation, transient nausea, and gastric disturbances may occur.

Composition and Supply
Tablets, sublingual   500 μg and 1 mg

Legal Status
Prescription

Dihydrotachysterol (Hytakerol®)

Action and Use
Parathyroid-like sterol metabolized in the liver to 25-hydroxydihydrotachysterol, the active analogue of 1,25-dihydroxy vitamin D. Used in the treatment of postoperative tetany, idiopathic tetany, and hypoparathyroidism.

Dosage and Administration
750 μg to 2.5 mg daily initially, decreased as indicated by blood calcium determinations.

*Dihydroergotoxine designates the chemical class to which the three constituents of the drug belong. Hydergine® has no official generic designation as yet.

Cautions
The toxic and therapeutic doses are very close. Contraindicated in hypercalcemia, abnormal sensitivity to effects of vitamin D, and hypervitaminosis D. Adequate dietary calcium is necessary for clinical response. Treatment should always be controlled by regular determination of blood calcium level.

Adverse Reactions
Essentially those of ergocalciferol (see). The effects can persist for up to 1 month after cessation of treatment.

Composition and Supply
Capsules   125 μg
Solution (in oil)   250 μg/ml

Legal Status
Prescription

Dihydroxyaluminum aminoacetate (Alglyn®, Alzinox®, Robalate®)

See ANTACIDS.

Diiodohydroxyquin (Diodoquin®)

See ANTIPROTOZOALS, antiamebials.

Dilantin®

See **Phenytoin sodium.**

Dilaudid®

See **Hydromorphone hydrochloride.**

Dimenhydrinate (Dramamine®)

Action and Use
Antinauseant used in motion sickness.

Dosage and Administration
50 to 100 mg every 4 hours, orally or IM.

Cautions
Drowsiness often occurs. Dimenhydrinate is capable of masking drug-induced otoxicity.

Adverse Reactions
See **Cyclizine hydrochloride.**

Composition and Supply
Injection   50 mg/ml, in 1 ml ampuls and 5 ml vials
Liquid   12.5 mg/4 ml
Tablets   50 mg

Legal Status
Prescription (injection)
Nonprescription (tablets and elixir)

Dimercaprol (BAL)

Action and Use
Antidote for heavy metal poisoning (namely, arsenic, mercury, and gold).

Dosage and Administration
3 to 5 mg/kg, IM (deep).

Cautions
Dimercaprol is contraindicated in hepatic insufficiency and should be discontinued if renal insufficiency develops during therapy. Local pain and possibly sterile abscess may occur at the site of injection.

Adverse Reactions
Common side effects include hypertension, tachycardia, and hypersensitivity; nausea and vomiting; burning sensation in the mouth, throat, and eyes; headache; a constricting feeling in the chest; conjunctivitis, lacrimation, rhinorrhea, and salivation; and muscle aches.

Composition and Supply
Injection   100 mg/ml, in 3 ml ampuls and 50 ml bottles

Legal Status
Prescription

Dimetane®

See **Brompheniramine maleate.**

Dimetane® Expectorant

See under **Brompheniramine maleate.**

Dimetane® Expectorant-DC

See under **Brompheniramine maleate.**

Dimetapp® Elixir

See under **Brompheniramine maleate.**

Dimetapp® Extentabs®

See under **Brompheniramine maleate.**

Dimethicone (Silicote®)

See EMOLLIENT-PROTECTANTS.

Dimethindene maleate (Forhistal®, Triten®)

See ANTIHISTAMINES.

Dimethisoquin hydrochloride (Quotane®)

Action and Use
Local anesthetic.

Dosage and Administration
Apply 4 or 5 times a day.

Cautions
Contraindicated for use in the eye or in bleeding hemorrhoids.

Adverse Reactions
Overuse results in irritation and erythema.

Composition and Supply
Lotion
Ointment   0.5%

Legal Status
Nonprescription

Dioctyl calcium sulfosuccinate (Surfak®)
Dioctyl sodium sulfosuccinate (DSS) (Colace®, Comfolax®, Doxinate®)

Action and Use
Surface-active stool softener.

Dosage and Administration
50 to 250 mg daily, orally.

Cautions
None.

Adverse Reactions
None, except that mild, transitory cramping pain may rarely occur.

Composition and Supply
Capsules   50 mg (Colace®, Surfak®)
Capsules   100 mg (Colace®, Comfolax®)
Capsules   240 mg (Doxinate®, Surfak®)
Liquid   10 mg/ml (Colace® Liquid)
Syrup   20 mg/5 ml (Colace® Syrup)

Legal Status
Nonprescription

Dioctyl sodium sulfosuccinate/casanthranol (Peri-Colace®)

See CATHARTICS.

Diodoquin® (diiodohydroxyquin)

See ANTIPROTOZOALS, antiamebials.

Diothane® (diperodon)

See ANESTHETICS, local.

Dioxyline phosphate (Paveril®)

See ANTISPASMODICS.

Dipaxin® (diphenadione)

See ANTICOAGULANTS.

Diperodon (Diothane®)

See ANESTHETICS, local.

Diphenadione (Dipaxin®)

See ANTICOAGULANTS.

Diphenhydramine hydrochloride (Benadryl®)

Action and Use
Antihistamine.

Dosage and Administration
12.5 to 50 mg 3 or 4 times a day, orally; 25 to 50 mg doses, IM or IV.

Cautions
Causes drowsiness. Avoid single doses greater than 100 mg.

Adverse Reactions
See **Brompheniramine maleate.**

Composition and Supply
Capsules   25 mg and 50 mg
Elixir   12.5 mg/5 ml
Injection   10 mg/ml, in 10 ml and 30 ml vials; and 50 mg/ml, in 1
   ml ampuls and 1 ml disposable syringes

Legal Status
Prescription

Diphenidol (Vontrol®)

See ANTIEMETICS.

Diphenoxylate hydrochloride/atropine sulfate (Lomotil®)

Action and Use
Antidiarrheal.

Dosage and Administration
5 mg 3 or 4 times a day, orally.

Cautions
Contraindicated in children under 2 years of age. Jaundice and ulcerative colitis may occur. Overdosage produces atropinism. Not to be
used in patients with diarrhea caused by poisoning until toxic material
has been removed. Physical dependence may occur. CNS depressants
may be potentiated.

Adverse Reactions
Common side effects include dryness of the skin and mucous membranes, flushing, hyperthermia, tachycardia, and urine retention. Occasional adverse reactions include anorexia, abdominal discomfort,
nausea, vomiting, paralytic ileus, toxic megacolon, swelling of gums,
respiratory depression, numbness of extremities, drowsiness, malaise,
headache, dizziness, euphoria or restlessness, angioneurotic edema,
urticaria, and pruritus. Overdose may result in severe, possibly fatal,
respiratory depression.

Composition and Supply
Liquid   diphenoxylate 2.5 mg/5 ml with atropine sulfate 25 μg/5 ml
Tablets   diphenoxylate 2.5 mg with atropine sulfate 25 μg

Legal Status
Schedule V

Diphenylpyraline hydrochloride (Hispril®)

See ANTIHISTAMINES.

Diphtheria antitoxin

Action and Use
Used in the prevention and treatment of diphtheria.

Dosage and Administration
20,000 to 40,000 units, IM; in severe cases one-half of the dose may be given IV.

Cautions
Recipients must be tested for sensitivity to horse serum before therapy begins. In the event of sensitivity, the indications for antitoxin should be reevaluated; if used, the antitoxin should be given carefully at 20-minute intervals in gradually increasing doses as follows:

    0.1 ml (100 μl) of a 1 : 20 dilution, SC
    0.1 ml (100 μl) of a 1 : 10 dilution, SC
    0.1 ml (100 μl) undiluted, SC
    0.3 ml (300 μl) undiluted, IM
    0.5 ml (500 μl) undiluted, IM

If no reaction has occurred, the remaining dose is injected IM. In the event of a reaction, the subsequent dose is reduced. Signs of acute anaphylaxis call for immediate intravenous injection of 0.2 to 0.5 ml (200 to 500 μl) of 1 : 1,000 epinephrine solution.

Adverse Reactions
A febrile reaction may occur.

Composition and Supply
Injection   10,000 units in 5 ml vials; and 20,000 units in 10 ml vials

Legal Status
Prescription

Diphtheria toxin for Schick Test

Action and Use
Used to determine susceptibility to diphtheria. In susceptible persons, a small amount of redness and perhaps induration occurs at the injection site within 24 to 72 hours.

Dosage and Administration
0.1 ml (100 μl) intradermally (on the volar surface of the forearm).

Cautions
Inject intradermally only.

Adverse Reactions
Desquamation may occur, and brownish pigmentation may persist for a month or more.

Composition and Supply
1 ml, 5 ml, and 10 ml vials, 10 tests/ml

Legal Status
Prescription

Diphtheria toxoid

See BIOLOGICALS, toxoids.

Diphtheria toxoid/tetanus toxoid, adsorbed

Action and Use
Used to achieve active immunization against diphtheria and tetanus.

Dosage and Administration
2 doses (0.5 ml [500 μl] or 1 ml, as specified) 1 to 2 months apart, and a third dose 1 year later, IM.

Cautions
Use only adult preparation in persons 6 years or over.

Adverse Reactions
Mild pain and possibly induration may occur at the injection site.

Composition and Supply
Injection   2 dose and 5 dose vials

Legal Status
Prescription

Diphtheria toxoid

See BIOLOGICALS, toxoids.

Diphtheria toxoid/tetanus toxoid/pertussis vaccine, adsorbed
(DPT) (Tri-Immunol®, Triogen®, Tri-Solgen®)

Action and Use
Used to achieve active immunization against diphtheria, tetanus, and pertussis.

Dosage and Administration
Primary immunization: 0.5 ml (500 μl) or 1 ml IM 3 times at intervals of 4 to 6 weeks, with a fourth reinforcing dose 12 months later. *Booster:* 0.5 ml (500 μl) at the time of school entrance.

Cautions
Contraindicated in persons with cerebral damage or active infections, or in those over 6 years of age.

Adverse Reactions
Occasionally local pain, tenderness, and induration at the injection site may occur.

Composition and Supply
Injection   3 and 5 dose vials and disposable syringes (*Note:* should be stored between 2° and 8°C; avoid freezing)

Legal Status
Prescription

Diplovax®

See **Poliovirus vaccine, live oral.**

Diprosone®

See **Betamethasone.**

Dipyridamole (Persantine®)

Action and Use
Coronary vasodilator used in long-term therapy of patients with chronic angina pectoris.

Dosage and Administration
50 mg 3 times a day, orally before meals.

Cautions
Use cautiously in patients with hypotension.

Adverse Reactions
Some side effects include nausea, vomiting, and diarrhea, especially if not taken before meals. Other possible adverse reactions include headache, vertigo, flushing, syncope, and weakness.

Composition and Supply
Tablets   25 mg

Legal Status
Prescription

Disipal®

See **Orphenadrine hydrochloride.**

Disomer® (dexbrompheniramine maleate)

See ANTIHISTAMINES.

Disopyramide phosphate (Norpace®)

Action and Use
Disopyramide phosphate is a class I antiarrhythmic drug (similar in action to procainamide and quinidine) indicated for treatment and suppression of unifocal premature (ectopic) ventricular contractions, premature (ectopic) ventricular contractions of multifocal origin, paired premature ventricular contractions, and episodes of ventricular tachycardia.

Dosage and Administration
The usual dosage range is 400 to 800 mg orally in divided doses 4 times daily. The usual loading dosage is 300 mg followed by 150 mg every 6 hours.

Cautions
Disopyramide phosphate is contraindicated in the presence of cardiogenic shock, preexisting second- or third-degree atrioventricular block (if no pacemaker is present) or known hypersensitivity to the drug. It should not be used in the presence of poorly compensated or uncompensated congestive heart failure unless the failure is exacerbated by or caused by an arrhythmia and proper treatment is instituted. Because of its anticholinergic action, disopyramide phosphate should not be used in patients with glaucoma or in patients with urinary retention unless these conditions are adequately controlled by appropriate therapeutic measures. The safety of the drug in pregnancy, nursing mothers, and children has not been established.

Adverse Reactions
The most serious, although relatively uncommon, adverse reaction is urinary retention, which occurs as a result of the drug's anticholinergic action. More common anticholinergic effects are dry mouth, urinary hesitancy, constipation, and blurred vision.

Composition and Supply
Capsules 100 mg and 150 mg

Legal Status
Prescription

Disulfiram (Antabuse®)

Action and Use
Adjunct in treatment of chronic alcoholism; disulfiram interferes with metabolism of alcohol, resulting in accumulation of acetaldehyde and symptoms of toxicity.

Dosage and Administration
The maintenance dose is 250 to 500 mg once daily, orally.

Cautions
Disulfiram is a dangerous drug and should never be administered to a patient in a state of alcohol intoxication or without his full knowledge. The patient must be told not to ingest alcohol in any form, including alcohol-containing medications. This advice should also be explained to the patient's relatives. Disulfiram should not be given to patients who are receiving or who have recently received CNS depressants or metronidazole. The supervised alchol-drug reaction test is potentially dangerous and should never be carried out in patients over 50 years of age.

Adverse Reactions
Occasional and usually transient side effects include fatigue, tremors, restlessness, headache, urticaria, acne, gastrointestinal disturbances, and garlic-like or metallic aftertaste. Other possible adverse reactions include optic neuritis, peripheral neuritis, and polyneuritis.

Composition and Supply
Tablets   250 mg and 500 mg

Legal Status
Prescription

Ditropan® (oxybutynin chloride)

See ANTISPASMODICS.

Diucardin® (hydroflumethiazide)

See DIURETICS.

Diupres® (reserpine/chlorothiazide)

See ANTIHYPERTENSIVES, combinations.

Diuril®

See **Chlorothiazide.**

Doca®

See **Desoxycorticosterone acetate.**

Dodecaethyleneglycol monolaurate (Ramses® Vaginal Jelly)

See CONTRACEPTIVES, TOPICAL.

Dolene®

See **Propoxyphene hydrochloride.**

Dolene® AP-65

See under **Propoxyphene hydrochloride.**

Dolene® Compound-65

See under **Propoxyphene hydrochloride.**

Dolophine®

See **Methadone hydrochloride.**

Domeboro® Powder (aluminum acetate solution, modified)

See ASTRINGENTS.

Donnagel® (kaolin/pectin/belladonna alkaloids)

See ANTIDIARRHEALS.

Donnasep® (methenamine mandelate/phenazopyridine hydrochloride/belladonna alkaloids/phenobarbital)

See URINARY ANTISEPTICS.

Donnatal® (belladonna alkaloids/phenobarbital)

See under **Atropine sulfate.**

Donnazyme® (pepsin/pancreatin/bile salts/belladonna alkaloids/phenobarbital)

See DIGESTANTS.

Dopamine hydrochloride (Intropin®)

Action and Use
Adrenergic agent (beta stimulator) useful in the treatment of shock caused by myocardial infarction, trauma, septicemia, open heart surgery, renal failure, or congestive heart failure.

Dosage and Administration
Dosage is individualized and ranges from 2 to 50 μg/kg per minute, IV infusion.

Cautions
Contraindicated in patients with pheochromocytoma, uncorrected tachyarrhythmias, or ventricular fibrillation. MAO inhibitors prolong the effects of the drug. Effects are antagonized by beta-adrenergic blocking agents. Solution must be diluted before use and should not be mixed with alkaline solutions. Infusion rate must be monitored. Local extravasation may cause ischemia and necrosis of tissues in elderly patients with preexisting vascular damage (for example, from arteriosclerosis or diabetes). Use cautiously with halogenated anesthetics.

Adverse Reactions
The most frequent responses include ectopic beats, nausea, vomiting, tachycardia, anginal pain, palpitations, dyspnea, headache, hypotension, and vasoconstriction. Occasionally bradycardia, piloerection, widened QRS complex, azotemia, or elevated blood pressure may occur. Overdose may produce hypertension.

Composition and Supply
Injection   40 mg/ml, in 5 ml ampuls

Legal Status
Prescription

Dopar®

See **Levodopa.**

Dopram®

See **Doxapram hydrochloride.**

Dorbane® (danthron)

See CATHARTICS.

Doriden®

See **Glutethimide.**

Dornavac® (desoxyribonuclease)

See MUCOLYTICS.

Doxapram hydrochloride (Dopram®)

Action and Use
Respiratory stimulant and general CNS stimulant used in anesthesiology and in the management of drug-induced CNS depression.

Dosage and Administration
When used to treat respiratory depression: 5 mg/min initially until satisfactory response, then 1 to 3 mg per minute by IV infusion; recommended maximum dose is 2 mg/kg.
When used to hasten arousal: 1 to 1.5 mg/kg in one dose or divided doses, IV.
When used in management of CNS depression: follow manufacturer's specific instructions.

Cautions
Contraindicated in patients with hypertension, seizure disorders, and incompetence of the ventilatory mechanism. Not recommended in patients 12 years of age or under. Incompatible with alkaline solutions (such as thiopental sodium). Monitor vital signs to prevent overdose.

Adverse Reactions
The most common effects are burning or itching. Other possible effects include hypertension, tachycardia, arrhythmias, tachypnea, sneezing, coughing, nausea, vomiting, restlessness, tremors, muscle rigidity, convulsions, perspiration, flushing, and hyperpyrexia.

Composition and Supply
Injection   20 mg/ml, in 20 ml vials

Legal Status
Prescription

Doxepin hydrochloride (Adapin®, Sinequan®)

Action and Use
Tricyclic antidepressant used to treat patients with anxious, agitated depression.

Dosage and Administration
25 to 300 mg daily, orally, carefully individualized.

Cautions
MAO inhibitors may potentiate the toxic effects of the drug; a 2 week medication-free period is required before transferring patients from MAO inhibitors to doxepin. Contraindicated in patients with glaucoma or urinary retention, and in children under 12 years of age.

Adverse Reactions
See **Amitriptyline hydrochloride.**

Composition and Supply
Capsules   10 mg, 25 mg, 50 mg, and 100 mg
Solution, oral   10 mg/ml

Legal Status
Prescription

Doxinate®

See **Dioctyl sodium sulfosuccinate.**

Doxorubicin hydrochloride (Adriamycin®)

See ANTINEOPLASTICS, antibiotics.

Doxycycline (Vibramycin®)

Action and Use
Broad-spectrum antibiotic. Doxycycline is the drug of choice when a tetracycline is indicated for treatment of extrarenal infections in patients with renal failure.

Dosage and Administration
200 mg on the first day and 100 to 200 mg per day thereafter, orally or IV infusion.

Cautions
See **Tetracycline hydrochloride.**

Adverse Reactions
See **Tetracycline hydrochloride.**

Composition and Supply
Capsules (as hyclate)   50 mg and 100 mg
Injection (as hyclate)   100 mg and 200 mg vials
Suspension (as monohydrate)   25 mg/5 ml
Syrup (as calcium salt)   50 mg/5 ml

Legal Status
Prescription

Doxylamine succinate (Decapryn®)

See ANTIHISTAMINES.

Doxylamine succinate/pyridoxine hydrochloride (Bendectin®)

See ANTIEMETICS.

DPT

See **Diphtheria toxoid/tetanus toxoid/pertussis vaccine, adsorbed.**

Dralzine™

See **Hydralazine hydrochloride.**

Dramamine®

See **Dimenhydrinate.**

Drisdol®

See **Ergocalciferol.**

Drixoral® (dexbrompheniramine maleate/*d*-isoephedrine)

See ANTIHISTAMINES.

Drolban® (dromostanolone propionate)

See ANTINEOPLASTICS, steroids, androgens.

Dromostanolone propionate (Drolban®)

See ANTINEOPLASTICS, steroids, androgens.

Droperidol (Inapsine®)

Action and Use
Tranquilizer and antiemetic used as an adjunct in surgical and diagnostic procedures and in the maintenance of general and regional anesthesia. Combined with a narcotic, such as fentanyl citrate (see), it induces neuroleptanalgesia.

Dosage and Administration
2.5 to 10 mg (depending on use), IM or IV.

Cautions
Droperidol is a potent depressant and may potentiate the action of other CNS depressants.

Adverse Reactions

The most common adverse reactions include hypotension, tachycardia, and postoperative drowsiness. Less common reactions include dizziness, chills and shivering, restlessness, hallucinations, depression, and extrapyramidal symptoms (namely, dystonia, akathisia, and oculogyric crisis).

Composition and Supply

Injection   2.5 mg/ml, in 2 ml and 5 ml ampuls and 10 ml vials

Legal Status

Prescription

Drysol™ (aluminum chloride)

See ASTRINGENTS.

DSS

See **Dioctyl sodium sulfosuccinate.**

DTIC-Dome® (dacarbazine)

See ANTINEOPLASTICS, antimetabolites.

DTO

See **Opium, deodorized tincture of.**

Dulcolax®

See **Bisacodyl.**

Duphaston® (dydrogesterone)

See PROGESTOGENS.

Durabolin® (nandrolone phenpropionate)

See ANDROGENS.

Duracillin® A.S.

See **Penicillin G procaine.**

Dyazide®

See under **Triamterene/hydrochlorothiazide.**

Dyclone®

See **Dyclonine hydrochloride.**

Dyclonine hydrochloride (Dyclone®)

Action and Use
Local anesthetic.

Dosage and Administration
Applied topically.

Cautions
May cause irritation at site of application.

Adverse Reactions
Sensitivity reaction may occur.

Composition and Supply
Cream 1%
Solution 0.5%

Legal Status
Prescription

Dydrogesterone (Duphaston®, Gynorest®)

See PROGESTOGENS.

Dymelor®

See **Acetohexamide.**

Dynapen®

See **Dicloxacillin sodium.**

Dyrenium®

See **Triamterene.**

Echothiophate iodide (Phospholine Iodide®)

Action and Use
Miotic (long-acting cholinesterase inhibitor) for use in glaucoma.

Dosage and Administration
Dosage is individualized to patient and severity of condition, instilled in the eye.

Cautions
Contraindicated in patients with narrow-angle glaucoma and uveal inflammation. Echothiophate iodide is absorbed through the conjunctival sac. It potentiates other cholinesterase inhibitors and succinylcholine and may potentiate the effects of CNS depressants. Should be

used with caution in pregnant women, in patients under general anesthesia, and in those with history of retinal detachment. Keep refrigerated.

Adverse Reactions
Momentary stinging ceases in a few seconds. Local effects, such as browache, headache, pain and redness of eyes, lacrimation and blurring or dimming of vision, disappear within 7 to 10 days. Application of the drops at bedtime may minimize photophobia and blurring of vision. Systemic side effects include nausea, diarrhea, bronchospasm, respiratory difficulty, salivation, diaphoresis, hypotension, urinary incontinence, muscle weakness, cardiac irregularities, lid muscle twitching, and increased intraocular pressure. Occasionally, cysts develop at pupillary margin of the iris.

Composition and Supply
Solution, ophthalmic   0.06%, 0.125%, and 0.25%

Legal Status
Prescription

Edecrin®

See **Ethacrynic acid.**

Edrophonium chloride (Tensilon®)

Action and Use
Cholinergic useful in the diagnosis of myasthenia gravis and as an antidote for curariform drugs.

Dosage and Administration
10 mg, IV (as antidote or for diagnosis).

Cautions
Not more than 30 mg is to be given. Not to be used as an antidote for succinylcholine. The patient should report any muscle weakness promptly if encountered 30 to 60 minutes after administration. It is important to differentiate between cholinergic crisis, which calls for drug withdrawal, and myasthenic crisis, which requires more medication. The patient may need respiratory assistance, and the physician should be notified immediately. The patient's airway must be kept clear of secretions, and cardiovascular functions should be monitored.

Adverse Reactions
The most important side effects include nausea, vomiting, diarrhea, bronchial constriction, increased bronchial secretions, increased salivation, lacrimation, diaphoresis, bradycardia, and hypotension. Other

effects include pupillary constriction, increased urinary frequency, dysarthria, dysphonia, dysphagia, laryngospasm, and convulsions. Respiratory failure may result from skeletal muscle paralysis and respiratory center depression.

Composition and Supply
Injection   10 mg/ml, in 10 ml vials

Legal Status
Prescription

E.E.S.™

See **Erythromycin ethylsuccinate.**

Effersyllium®

See **Psyllium hydrophilic mucilloid.**

Efudex®

See **Fluorouracil.**

Elase®

See **Fibrinolysin/desoxyribonuclease.**

Elase-Chloromycetin® Ointment

See under **Fibrinolysin/desoxyribonuclease.**

Elavil®

See **Amitriptyline hydrochloride.**

Electrolyte solution, oral (Pedialyte®)

See ELECTROLYTE SOLUTIONS AND WATER-BALANCE AGENTS, replacement solutions.

Elixophyllin® (theophylline)

See ANTIASTHMATICS, xanthine preparations.

Elspar® (asparaginase)

See ANTINEOPLASTICS, miscellaneous.

Emete-con®

See **Benzquinamide hydrochloride.**

Emetine hydrochloride

See ANTIPROTOZOALS, antiamebials.

Empirin® Compound

See **Aspirin/phenacetin/caffeine.**

Empirin® Compound with Codeine

See under **Aspirin/phenacetin/caffeine.**

Empracet® with Codeine No. 3

See under **Acetaminophen.**

Emprazil® Tablets

See COUGH-COLD PREPARATIONS, common cold preparations.

E-Mycin®

See **Erythromycin.**

Endep®

See **Amitriptyline hydrochloride.**

Enduron® (methyclothiazide)

See ANTIHYPERTENSIVES, diuretics.

Enfamil®

See INFANT FORMULAS.

Enovid®-E (norethynodrel/mestranol)

See CONTRACEPTIVES, ORAL.

Ensure®

See FOOD PREPARATIONS.

Entozyme® (pepsin/pancreatin/bile salts)

See DIGESTANTS.

Entsulfon sodium (pHisoDerm®)

See DETERGENTS.

Ephedrine sulfate (I-sedrin®)

Action and Use
Adrenergic and nasal decongestant.

Dosage and Administration
Capsules: 12.5 to 50 mg every 2 to 4 hours, orally.
Injection: 10 to 50 mg, SC or IM, not to exceed 150 mg in 24 hours.
Solution (nose drops): 2 or 3 of solution 2 or 3 times a day.

Cautions
Use cautiously in patients with organic heart disease, hypertension, hyperthyroidism, prostatic hypertrophy, and diabetes. May cause depression of cardiac muscle and arrhythmias in the digitalized patient and may set off a sharp rise in blood pressure in patients taking tricyclic and MAO inhibitor antidepressants. Ephedrine sulfate interferes with the action of guanethidine and is incompatible with pentobarbital, thiopental, phenobarbital, hydrocortisone, and secobarbital. Should not be mixed with fluids for infusions but may be injected through the Y-tube of the administration set.

Adverse Reactions
Hypertension, dysuria, nervousness, insomnia, headache, and palpitations may occur. A large dose or an overdose may produce diaphoresis, nausea, vomiting, precordial pain, vertigo, glycosuria, tremors, and fainting. Contact dermatitis may occur with topical application.

Composition and Supply
Capsules   25 mg and 50 mg
Injection   25 mg/ml
Solution   1% and 3% (I-sedrin®)
Syrup   10 mg/5 ml and 20 mg/5 ml

Legal Status
Prescription

Epinephrine (Adrenalin®)
Epinephrine Bitartrate (Epitrate®)

Action and Use
Epinephrine is an adrenergic, antiallergic, and hemostatic agent; epinephrine bitartrate is used for the control of open-angle glaucoma.

Dosage and Administration
1 : 100 solution: inhalation.
1 : 500 injection: 0.2 to 0.5 ml (200 to 500 μl) IM.
1 : 1,000 injection: 0.1 ml (100 μl) to 1 ml, SC or IM; 0.05 to 0.1 ml (50 to 100 μl), diluted, injected IV cautiously; or 1 ml intracardially.

1 : 1,000 topical solution: a pledget of gauze or cotton is soaked and applied with pressure.

Ophthalmic solution: 1 drop doses; the frequency is individualized from once every 2 or 3 days to twice daily.

Cautions

Contraindicated in cerebral arteriosclerosis, hypertension, shock, pulmonary edema, and narrow-angle glaucoma. May cause cardiac arrhythmias when used concurrently with halogenated anesthetics and when given to patients with cardiac disease. Use with caution in patients with angina pectoris or diabetes. Epinephrine may cause a hypertensive crisis in patients receiving MAO inhibitors, and should not be used in patients being treated with digitalis. Incompatible with hyaluronidase, sodium warfarin, and protein hydrolysates. Should not be mixed with fluids for infusion, but may be injected through the Y-tube of the administration set.

Adverse Reactions

The usual dosage may produce restlessness, anxiety, headache, tremors, dizziness, weakness, palpitations, and insomnia. A moderate overdose is marked by pallor, heart palpitations, and feelings of anxiety, nervousness, and fear. Severe toxicity may involve mydriasis, acute cardiac dilatation and irregularities, pulmonary edema, and respiratory difficulty.

Composition and Supply

Inhalation   1 : 100 solution
Injection   1 : 1,000, in 1 ml ampuls
Solution, ophthalmic   2% (Epitrate®)
Suspension, sterile (in oil)   1 : 500 (2 mg/ml), in 1 ml ampuls
Solution, topical   1 : 1,000, in 30 ml vials

Legal Status

Prescription

Epitrate®

See **Epinephrine bitartrate.**

Epsom salt

See **Magnesium sulfate.**

Equagesic® (ethoheptazine/aspirin/meprobamate)

See ANALGESICS, nonnarcotic.

Equanil®

See **Meprobamate.**

Ergocalciferol (vitamin D₂) (Calciferol™, Drisdol®)

Action and Use
Vitamin D supplement and therapeutic agent used to treat refractory rickets and hypoparathyroidism.

Dosage and Administration
Daily requirement: See Appendix 9.
Refractory rickets: 200,000 to 400,000 units per day, orally or IM.
Uncomplicated rickets: 160 units per day, orally.
Hypoparathyroidism: 50,000 to 200,000 units per day, orally or IM.

Cautions
Should not be administered concomitantly with mineral oil. Use cautiously in coronary disease, decreased renal function, and arteriosclerosis. Large doses are potentially dangerous, and frequent determinations of blood calcium are mandatory.

Adverse Reactions
Dosage of more than 100,000 units may produce hypercalcemia along with such early symptoms as weakness, anorexia, nausea, vomiting, diarrhea, drowsiness, fatigue, hypertension, and headache. A later effect is the loss of calcium from bones and calcium deposits in soft tissues.

Composition and Supply
Capsules   50,000 units (Drisdol®)
Injection   500,000 units/ml, in 10 ml vials (Calciferol™)
Tablets   50,000 units (Calciferol™)

Legal Status
Prescription

Ergocalciferol/dibasic calcium phosphate (Dical-D®)

See BLOOD CALCIUM REGULATORS.

Ergonovine maleate (Ergotrate®)

Action and Use
Oxytocic used to prevent postpartum bleeding.

Dosage and Administration
200 to 400 μg orally, IM or IV.

Cautions
Administer only after infant and placenta have been delivered. Subcutaneous injection irritates tissue and should be avoided. Prolonged use, especially in hypertensive patients, may lead to gangrene and other symptoms of ergotism.

Adverse Reactions
Early effects include nausea, vomiting, cramps, headache, confusion, flushing, faintness, urinary urgency, and uterine bleeding. The effects of prolonged use include edema, pallor, decreased temperature, rapid and weak pulse, diarrhea, thirst, tingling, itching, coldness of skin, anginal pain, muscle pain, convulsions, and blindness.

Composition and Supply
Injection   200 μg/ml and 500 μg/ml
Tablets   200 μg

Legal Status
Prescription

Ergostat™

See **Ergotamine tartrate.**

Ergotamine tartrate (Ergostat™, Gynergen®)

Action and Use
Analgesic used to treat migraine headache.

Dosage and Administration
Orally: 2 or 3 mg at once followed by 1 or 2 mg hourly, up to a total of 9 mg
Intramuscularly: 250 μg, followed by 500 μg after 2 to 3 hours, to a maximum of 1 mg
Sublingually: 1 tablet initially, repeated at ½ hour intervals, if needed, for a total of 3 tablets

Cautions
Total weekly dosage should not exceed 10 mg. Prolonged use and excessive dosage can lead to ergotism. Should be used cautiously in patients with arterial disease.

Adverse Reactions
Adverse reactions include nausea, vomiting, diarrhea, localized edema and itching, diuresis, insomnia, and anxiety. More severe effects include numbness and tingling of fingers and toes, muscle pain in extremities, weakness in legs, anginal pains, transient tachycardia or bradycardia, palpitations, and gangrene.

Composition and Supply
Injection   500 μg/ml
Suppositories   2 mg with caffeine 200 mg (Cafergot®)
Tablets   1 mg
Tablets   1 mg with caffeine 100 mg (Cafergot®)
Tablets   1 mg with caffeine 100 mg, Bellafoline® 125 μg, and pentobarbital 30 mg (Cafergot® P-B)
Tablets   1 mg with caffeine 50 mg and cyclizine 25 mg (Migral®)
Tablets, sublingual   2 mg (Ergostat™)

Legal Status
Prescription

Ergotrate®

See **Ergonovine maleate.**

Erythrityl tetranitrate (Cardilate®)

See CARDIACS, vasodilators.

Erythrocin®

See **Erythromycin.**

Erythrocin® Ethyl Succinate-I.M.

See **Erythromycin ethylsuccinate.**

Erythrocin® Lactobionate-I.V.

See **Erythromycin lactobionate.**

Erythrocin® Stearate

See **Erythromycin stearate.**

Erythromycin (Erythrocin®, E-Mycin®, Ilotycin®)

Action and Use
Antibiotic similar in spectrum to penicillin. Also used in treatment of intestinal amebiasis and infections due to *Listeria monocytogenes.*

Dosage and Administration
250 mg to 1 g every 6 hours, orally.

Cautions
Gastrointestinal disturbances are the chief side effects. Overgrowth of fungi and yeast may be promoted. Use cautiously in patients with hepatic impairment.

Adverse Reactions
Occasional side effects include abdominal cramps, nausea, vomiting, diarrhea, urticaria, and fever. Anaphylaxis is possible.

Composition and Supply
Drops   100 mg/dropperful (2.5 ml)
Liquid   200 mg/5 ml and 400 mg/5 ml
Ointment   10 mg/g
Ointment, ophthalmic   5 mg/g
Suppositories   125 mg (Erythrocin®)
Tablets   125 mg, 250 mg, and 500 mg
Tablets, enteric-coated   250 mg

Legal Status
Prescription

Erythromycin estolate (Ilosone®)

See ANTIBIOTICS, erythromycins.

Erythromycin ethylsuccinate (E.E.S.™, Erythrocin® Ethyl Succinate-I.M., Pediamycin®)

Action and Use
Same as erythromycin.

Dosage and Administration
400 mg every 6 hours, orally; 100 mg every 4 to 6 hours, deep IM.

Cautions
Should not be administered intravenously or subcutaneously. Must not be mixed with other medications in the same syringe. Give deep IM injection and rotate injection site. Intramuscular administration is not recommended in small children because they do not have the large muscle mass required for deep placement of injection.

Adverse Reactions
Same as adverse reactions to erythromycin.

Composition and Supply
Drops   100 mg/dropperful (2.5 ml)
Injection   2 ml ampuls, 50 mg/ml (Erythrocin® Ethyl Succinate-I.M.)
Suspension, oral   200 mg/5 ml and 400 mg/5 ml
Tablets   400 mg (E.E.S. 400™)
Tablets, chewable   200 mg

Legal Status
Prescription

Erythromycin gluceptate (Ilotycin® Gluceptate)

See ANTIBIOTICS, erythromycins.

Erythromycin lactobionate (Erythrocin® Lactobionate-I.V.)

Action and Use
Same as erythromycin.

Dosage and Administration
15 to 20 mg/kg per day, IV infusion.

Cautions
IV injection may be followed by thrombophlebitis. See **Erythromycin** for further cautions.

Adverse Reactions
See **Erythromycin.**

Composition and Supply
Injection   500 mg and 1 g vials

Note: supplied in the form of lyophilized powder that should be dissolved in plain sterile water only. Solution should be used within 8 hours.

Legal Status
Prescription

Erythromycin stearate (Bristamycin®, Erythrocin® Stearate, Ethril®, Pfizer-E®)

Action and Use
Same as erythromycin.

Dosage and Administration
250 to 500 mg every 6 hours, orally.

Cautions
See **Erythromycin.**

Adverse Reactions
See **Erythromycin.**

Composition and Supply
Tablets   125 mg, 250 mg, and 500 mg

Legal Status
Prescription

Eserine

See **Physostigmine salicylate.**

Esidrix®

See **Hydrochlorothiazide.**

Esimil®

See under **Guanethidine sulfate.**

Eskalith®

See **Lithium carbonate.**

Estar®

See under **Coal tar.**

Estinyl®

See **Ethinyl estradiol.**

Estradiol (Progynon®)

Action and Use
Estrogen.

Dosage and Administration
25 mg pellet implanted subcutaneously and repeated when necessary.

Cautions
Contraindicated in pregnancy and in patients with familial or personal history of carcinoma and precancerous lesions (unless specifically indicated as treatment for carcinoma). Usually contraindicated in patients with known or suspected cancer of the breast, endometrium, or cervix; chronic cystic mastitis; thromboembolic disorders; liver impairment; undiagnosed abnormal vaginal bleeding; epilepsy; migraine; asthma; cardiac or renal disease (because of salt and water retention); psychic depression; diabetes; metabolic bone diseases associated with hypercalcemia; or renal insufficiency (because estrogen influences the metabolism of calcium and phosphorus). Antagonizes the cholesterol-lowering effect of clofibrate and diminishes the response to oral anticoagulants. Estradiol (and all other estrogens) may increase the risk of endometrial carcinoma, and one study raises the possibility that during the menopause estrogen may increase the risk of developing cancer of the breast many years later. The use of estrogens also increases the risk of gallbladder disease.

Adverse Reactions
The most frequent side effects include nausea and vomiting, diarrhea, skin rash, edema, and hypercalcemia. Other possible side effects include vaginal bleeding, breast tenderness, and gynecomastia and loss of libido in men.

Composition and Supply
Pellets   25 mg

Legal Status
Prescription

Estradiol benzoate

Action and Use
Estrogen.

Dosage and Administration
Dosage individualized to patient and conditions; given IM.

Cautions
See **Estradiol.**

Adverse Reactions
See **Estradiol.**

Composition and Supply
Injection   3.3 mg/ml

Legal Status
Prescription

Estradiol cypionate (Depo®-Estradiol Cypionate)

Action and Use
Estrogen.

Dosage and Administration
Dosage is individualized, IM.

Cautions
See **Estradiol.**

Adverse Reactions
See **Estradiol.**

Composition and Supply
Injection (in oil)   1 mg/ml and 5 mg/ml

Legal Status
Prescription

Estradurin® (polyestradiol phosphate)

See ANTINEOPLASTICS, steroids, estrogens.

Estrogens, conjugated (Femest®, Premarin®)

Estrogens, esterified (Amnestrogen®, Evex®, Femogen®, Menest™)

Action and Use
Estrogen.

Dosage and Administration
Dosage is individualized to patient and condition being treated, administered orally, intravenously, or topically.

Cautions
See **Estradiol.**

Adverse Reactions
See **Estradiol.**

Composition and Supply
Injection package   25 mg ampuls with 5 ml diluent (Premarin®)
Tablets   300 μg, 625 μg, 1.25 mg, and 2.5 mg
Vaginal cream   625 μg/g

Legal Status
Prescription

Estrone/estradiol/estriol (Hormonin®)

See ESTROGENS.

Eta-Lent® (ethaverine hydrochloride)

See ANTISPASMODICS; VASODILATORS, PERIPHERAL.

Ethacrynic acid (Edecrin®)

Action and Use
Potent diuretic.

Dosage and Administration
Oral:
Day One—50 mg after a meal.
Day Two—50 mg twice daily after meals.

Day Three—100 mg in the morning and 50 to 100 mg following the afternoon or evening meal, depending upon response to morning dose.

For maintenance—reduce dosage and frequency of administration until dry weight is achieved.

Injection: usual dose, 50 mg.

Cautions

Contraindicated in patients with anuria or cirrhosis, in pregnant women, and in nursing mothers. Concomitant use with kanamycin and other aminoglycoside antibiotics should be avoided. Ethacrynic acid may cause electrolyte depletion and thereby potentiate the action of digitalis; it potentiates coumarin anticoagulants, antihypertensives, and oral hypoglycemics. The addition of 5% dextrose solution with a pH below 5 to the injectable form of the drug may result in a hazy solution that should not be used. Do not give subcutaneously or intramuscularly, since that causes local pain and irritation in some patients. Should be used cautiously in patients with liver disease and in those receiving high doses of salicylates.

Adverse Reactions

May cause weakness, muscle cramps, paresthesias, thirst, anorexia, nausea, malaise, abdominal discomfort or pain, dysphagia, vertigo, deafness, tinnitus, and skin rash. In some patients, a severe, watery diarrhea may result.

Composition and Supply

Injection (ethacrynate sodium)   50 mg vials

Tablets   25 mg and 50 mg

Legal Status

Prescription

Ethambutol hydrochloride (Myambutol®)

Action and Use

Antituberculotic.

Dosage and Administration

Initial treatment: 15 mg/kg per day as a single dose, orally.

Retreatment: 25 mg/kg per day as a single dose, orally.

Cautions

Contraindicated in patients with optic neuritis. Should always be used with other antituberculotics. Use with caution in patients with renal damage.

Adverse Reactions
Reported side effects include gastrointestinal upset (with abdominal pain, nausea, vomiting, and anorexia), fever, malaise, headache, dizziness, mental confusion, disorientation, hallucinations, peripheral neuropathy (with numbness and tingling), hypersensitivity (with pruritic dermatitis), joint pain, and anaphylaxis. Optic neuritis and impaired liver function may occur in patients taking high doses.

Composition and Supply
Tablets   100 mg and 400 mg

Legal Status
Prescription

Ethanol (alcohol)

See ANTI-INFECTIVES, LOCAL, miscellaneous antiseptic-disinfectants.

Ethaquin® (ethaverine hydrochloride)

See ANTISPASMODICS; VASODILATORS, PERIPHERAL.

Ethaverine hydrochloride (Cebral®, Eta-Lent®, Ethaquin®, Isovex-100®)

See ANTISPASMODICS; VASODILATORS, PERIPHERAL.

Ethchlorvynol (Placidyl®)

Action and Use
Hypnotic.

Dosage and Administration
100 mg to 1 g at bedtime, orally.

Cautions
Ethchlorvynol may be habit-forming. Use with caution in patients with depression or suicidal tendencies and in those with impaired hepatic function. Enhances effect of CNS depressants and MAO inhibitors. Decreases the anticoagulation response of oral anticoagulants. Contraindicated in patients with porphyria and in pregnant women.

Adverse Reactions
The more common adverse effects include hypotension, nausea, vomiting, aftertaste, facial numbness, urticaria, and headache. Unusual side effects include fatigue, prolonged hypnosis, muscle weakness, excitement, hysteria, confusion, nightmares, and syncope.

Composition and Supply
Capsules   100 mg, 250 mg, 500 mg, and 750 mg

Legal Status
Schedule IV

Ether (ethyl ether)

See ANESTHETICS, general.

Ethinamate (Valmid®)

See SEDATIVE-HYPNOTICS, nonbarbiturates.

Ethinyl estradiol (Estinyl®, Feminone®)

Action and Use
Estrogen.

Dosage and Administration
Dosage is individualized to the patient's needs and the condition being treated, administered orally. Range: 10 μg to 1 mg daily.

Cautions
See **Estradiol.**

Adverse Reactions
See **Estradiol.**

Composition and Supply
Tablets   20 μg, 50 μg, and 500 μg

Legal Status
Prescription

Ethionamide (Trecator®-SC)

See ANTITUBERCULOTICS.

Ethoheptazine (Zactane®)

Action and Use
Analgesic for mild to moderate pain.

Dosage and Administration
75 to 150 mg 3 or 4 times a day, orally.

Cautions
Contraindicated in patients with peptic ulcer.

Adverse Reactions
Occasionally epigastric distress, dizziness, or pruritus may occur.

Composition and Supply
Tablets   75 mg

Legal Status
Prescription

Ethoheptazine/aspirin/meprobamate (Equagesic®)

See ANALGESICS, nonnarcotic.

Ethopropazine hydrochloride (Parsidol®)

Action and Use
Antiparkinsonian and parasympatholytic agent.

Dosage and Administration
10 mg 4 times a day initially, orally, gradually increased (up to 600 mg) until optimal effect.

Cautions
There is a high incidence of side effects, and many patients will not tolerate therapeutic doses. Agranulocytosis may occur.

Adverse Reactions
Common side effects include dizziness and drowsiness. Less common effects include lassitude, blurred vision, dry mouth, epigastric distress, ataxia, paresthesias, hypotension, headache, and confusion. Administration with food or fluids may decrease epigastric distress.

Composition and Supply
Tablets   10 mg, 50 mg, and 100 mg

Legal Status
Prescription

Ethosuximide (Zarontin®)

Action and Use
Anticonvulsant used in petit mal epilepsy.

Dosage and Administration
250 mg to 1.5 g daily, orally.

Cautions
Use with caution in patients with liver or kidney disease, psychological abnormalities, or mixed types of epilepsy. Blood dyscrasias are possible.

Adverse Reactions
Relatively common side effects include anorexia, nausea, vomiting, cramps, abdominal pain, weight loss, diarrhea, CNS depression (with drowsiness, headache, dizziness, euphoria, lethargy, fatigue, and ataxia), urticaria, and pruritic erythematous rash. Occasional side effects include myopia, vaginal bleeding, swelling of the tongue, gum hypertrophy, and hirsutism.

Composition and Supply
Capsules   250 mg

Legal Status
Prescription

Ethotoin (Peganone®)

See ANTICONVULSANTS.

Ethoxzolamide (Cardrase®)

See CARBONIC ANHYDRASE INHIBITORS.

Ethril®

See **Erythromycin stearate.**

Ethyl alcohol (alcohol)

See ANTI-INFECTIVES, LOCAL, miscellaneous antiseptic-disinfectants.

Ethyl biscoumacetate (Tromexan®)

See ANTICOAGULANTS.

Ethyl chloride

Action and Use
Local anesthetic.

Dosage and Administration
Applied topically.

Cautions
Highly flammable. Excessive cooling may produce necrosis.

Adverse Reactions
Adverse reactions include edema, erythema, and painful thawing.

Composition and Supply
Spray bottles   120 ml

Legal Status
Prescription

Ethyl ether (ether)

See ANESTHETICS, general.

Ethylnorepinephrine hydrochloride (Bronkephrine®)

See ADRENERGICS; ANTIASTHMATICS, adrenergics.

Ethynodiol diacetate/ethinyl estradiol (Demulen®)

See CONTRACEPTIVES, ORAL.

Ethynodiol diacetate/mestranol (Ovulen®)

See CONTRACEPTIVES, ORAL.

Etrafon®

See **Perphenazine/amitriptyline hydrochloride.**

Eugenol

See ANESTHETICS, local.

Eurax® (crotamiton)

See ANTI-INFECTIVES, LOCAL, scabicide-pediculicides.

Euthroid® (liotrix)

See THYROID PREPARATIONS.

Eutonyl®

See **Pargyline hydrochloride.**

Eutron®

See under **Pargyline hydrochloride.**

Evex®

See **Estrogens, esterified.**

Excedrin® (aspirin/salicylamide/acetaminophen/caffeine)

See ANALGESICS, nonnarcotic.

Exna® (benzthiazide)

See DIURETICS.

Exsel®

See **Selenium sulfide.**

Falvin® (intrinsic factor/cyanocobalamin/ferrous fumarate/ascorbic acid)

See HEMATINICS.

Felsules®

See **Chloral hydrate.**

Femest®

See **Estrogens, conjugated.**

Feminone®

See **Ethinyl estradiol.**

Femogen®

See **Estrogens, esterified.**

Fenfluramine hydrochloride (Pondimin®)

See CEREBRAL STIMULANTS, anorectics.

Fenoprofen calcium (Nalfon®)

Action and Use
Nonsteroidal anti-inflammatory agent used to relieve rheumatoid arthritis.

Dosage and Administration
600 mg 4 times a day, initially, then adjusted in accordance with patient's needs (daily dosage over 3.2 g not recommended), orally, 30 minutes before or 2 hours after meals.

Cautions
Contraindicated in patients who have shown hypersensitivity to fenoprofen and in patients in whom aspirin and other nonsteroidal, anti-inflammatory drugs induce asthma, rhinitis, or urticaria. Should be used with caution in patients with a history of disease of the upper gastrointestinal tract (because severe bleeding may occur) and in patients with impaired renal function. May possibly enhance the action and toxicity of hydantoins, sulfonamides, sulfonureas, and coumarin-type anticoagulants. In the event that steroid dosage is reduced or eliminated, the change should be made slowly to avoid complications. Periodic liver function tests and ophthalmologic studies are recommended.

Adverse Reactions

The most common adverse reactions are gastrointestinal, namely, heartburn, dyspepsia, constipation, nausea, vomiting, abdominal pain, diarrhea, flatulence, dry mouth, melena, and gastrointestinal bleeding. Other reactions include pruritus, skin eruptions, drowsiness, dizziness, tinnitus, palpitations, edema, headache, fatigue, malaise, and dysuria.

Composition and Supply

Tablets (Pulvules®)   300 mg

Legal Status

Prescription

Fentanyl citrate (Sublimaze®)

Action and Use

Strong preoperative narcotic analgesic with quick onset and short duration. Also used as an adjunct to general and regular anesthesia and in the recovery room.

Dosage and Administration

25 to 100 μg, IM or IV, individualized.

Cautions

Strong respiratory depressant. Contraindicated in patients with head injuries, increased intracranial pressure, and respiratory problems. Has the same potential for toxicity as other narcotic analgesics. Fentanyl citrate is potentiated by other CNS depressants and by MAO inhibitors. Following administration of fentanyl citrate, the dosage of other CNS depressants (if being used) should be reduced.

Adverse Reactions

Common side effects include bradycardia, respiratory depression, apnea, and muscle rigidity, especially involving breathing muscles; without treatment, respiratory arrest, circulatory depression, or cardiac arrest can occur. Less common effects include hypotension, dizziness, miosis, nausea, vomiting, laryngospasm, diaphoresis, euphoria, and bronchoconstriction. Hypotension is common when fentanyl citrate is combined with droperidol (in the preparation Innovar®).

Composition and Supply

Injection   50 μg/ml, in 2 ml and 5 ml ampuls
Injection   50 μg/ml with 2.5 mg/ml droperidol, in 2 ml and 5 ml ampuls (Innovar®)

Legal Status

Schedule II

Fentanyl citrate/droperidol (Innovar®)

See under **Fentanyl citrate.**

Feosol®

See **Ferrous sulfate.**

Feosol® Spansules®

See under **Ferrous sulfate.**

Feostat® (ferrous fumarate)

See HEMATINICS.

Fergon®

See **Ferrous gluconate.**

Fergon®c̄ C

See under **Ferrous gluconate.**

Fergon® Plus

See under **Ferrous gluconate.**

Fer-In-Sol®

See **Ferrous sulfate.**

Fermalox®

See under **Ferrous sulfate.**

Fero-Folic-500® (folic acid/ferrous sulfate/ascorbic acid)

See HEMATINICS.

Fero-Grad-500® (ferrous sulfate/ascorbic acid)

See HEMATINICS.

Fero-Gradumet® (ferrous sulfate)

See HEMATINICS.

Ferro-Sequels® (ferrous fumarate/dioctyl sodium sulfosuccinate)

See HEMATINICS.

Ferrous fumarate (Feostat®)

See HEMATINICS.

Ferrous fumarate/dioctyl sodium sulfosuccinate
(Ferro-Sequels®)

See HEMATINICS.

Ferrous gluconate (Fergon®)

Action and Use
Hematinic used for the prevention and treatment of microcytic, hypochromic anemias resulting from iron deficiency.

Dosage and Administration
1 to 2 g daily, orally.

Cautions
Iron interacts with and inactivates tetracycline, and the two drugs should not be taken within 2 hours of each other. Food and antacids reduce the absorption of iron. Liquid preparations may stain teeth and should be diluted with water and preferably taken through a glass straw. All iron preparations produce black stools.

Adverse Reactions
Ferrous gluconate has a lower incidence of side effects than ferrous sulfate (see), but it contains less iron.

Composition and Supply
Caplets   500 mg plus ascorbic acid and vitamin B_{12} (Fergon® Plus)
Capsules   435 mg
Elixir   300 mg/5 ml
Tablets   325 mg
Tablets   450 mg with ascorbic acid 200 mg (Fergon® c̄ C)

Legal Status
Nonprescription

Ferrous sulfate (Feosol®, Fer-In-Sol®)

Action and Use
Hematinic used for the prevention and treatment of microcytic, hypochromic anemias resulting from iron deficiency.

Dosage and Administration
750 mg to 1.5 g daily, orally.

Cautions
See **Ferrous gluconate.**

Adverse Reactions
Possible adverse reactions include anorexia, gastric pain, nausea, vomiting, diarrhea, and constipation.

Composition and Supply
Capsules, prolonged release   250 mg (Feosol® Spansules®)
Capsules, sustained release   390 mg with vitamin C and vitamin B complex (Mol-Iron® Panhemic™ Chronosule®)
Drops   125 mg/ml (Fer-In-Sol®)
Elixir   220 mg/5 ml (Feosol®)
Tablets   325 mg (Feosol®)
Tablets   200 mg with magnesium hydroxide/aluminum hydroxide (Fermalox®)
Tablets, controlled release   525 mg with vitamin C and vitamin B complex (Iberet®, Iberet®-500)
Tablets, controlled release   525 mg with vitamin C and vitamin B complex including folic acid

Legal Status
Nonprescription

Ferrous sulfate/ascorbic acid (Fero-Grad-500®)

See HEMATINICS.

Festal® (lipase/amylase/protease/hemicellulase/bile constituents)

See ANTIFLATULENTS.

Fetamin® (methamphetamine hydrochloride)

See CEREBRAL STIMULANTS, anorectic.

Fibrinogen, human (Parenogen®)

See HEMOSTATICS.

Fibrinolysin/desoxyribonuclease (Elase®)

Action and Use
Enzyme debridement agent for necrotic tissue.

Dosage and Administration
Applied topically as an ointment or solution.

Cautions
Should be used cautiously in patients who are sensitive to materials of bovine origin. Solutions should be refrigerated and should not be used after 24 hours.

Adverse Reactions
High concentrations may cause hyperemia.

Composition and Supply
Ointment (10 g)   fibrinolysin 10 units, desoxyribonuclease 6,666 units (with chloromycetin, Elase-Chloromycetin®)

Ointment (30 g)   fibrinolysin 30 units, desoxyribonuclease 20,000 units (with chloromycetin, Elase-Chloromycetin®)

Dried form for solution (30 ml vials)   fibrinolysin 25 units, desoxyribonuclease 15,000 units

Legal Status
Prescription

Fiorinal®

See under **Aspirin/phenacetin/caffeine.**

Fiorinal® with Codeine

See under **Aspirin/phenacetin/caffeine.**

Flagyl®

See **Metronidazole.**

Flavoxate hydrochloride (Urispas®)

Action and Use
Antispasmodic used in the treatment of such symptoms as dysuria, urgency, nocturia, and suprapubic pain.

Dosage and Administration
100 to 200 mg 3 or 4 times a day, orally.

Cautions
Use cautiously in patients with glaucoma. Contraindicated in patients with obstructive gastrointestinal lesions, hemorrhage, or obstructive uropathies.

Adverse Reactions
Occasional side effects include nausea and vomiting, dry mouth, nervousness, vertigo, headache, drowsiness, blurred vision, tachycardia, and palpitations.

Composition and Supply
Tablets   100 mg

Legal Status
Prescription

Fleet® Brand Enema (sodium phosphate and biphosphate enema)

See CATHARTICS.

Fleet® Brand Phospho®-Soda (sodium phosphate and biphosphate oral solution)

See CATHARTICS.

Flexeril™ (cyclobenzaprine hydrochloride)

See SKELETAL MUSCLE RELAXANTS.

Florantyrone (Zanchol®)

Action and Use
Hydrocholeretic.

Dosage and Administration
250 mg 3 or 4 times a day, orally.

Cautions
Contraindicated in the presence of complete mechanical biliary obstruction, acute cholecystitis, or severe hepatitis.

Adverse Reactions
Diarrhea may occur.

Composition and Supply
Tablets   250 mg

Legal Status
Prescription

Florinef®

See **Fludrocortisone acetate.**

Floropryl® (isoflurophate)

See MIOTICS.

Florotic®

See under **Fludrocortisone acetate.**

Floxuridine (FUDR)

See ANTINEOPLASTICS, antimetabolites.

Flucytosine (Ancobon®)

Action and Use
Antifungal used for the treatment of serious infections involving *Candida albicans* and/or *Cryptococcus neoformans.*

Dosage and Administration
50 to 150 mg/kg per day every 6 hours, orally.

Cautions
Close medical supervision is required. May cause bone marrow depression. Should be used with caution in patients with kidney or renal disease. Before therapy is instituted, the patient's hematologic and renal status should be determined.

Adverse Reactions
Common side effects include nausea, vomiting, diarrhea, and rash. Less frequent reactions include confusion, hallucinations, headache, sedation, and vertigo.

Composition and Supply
Capsules   250 mg and 500 mg

Legal Status
Prescription

Fludrocortisone acetate (Florinef®)

Action and Use
Anti-inflammatory corticosteroid (with both glucocorticoid and mineralocorticoid action) useful in treatment of Addison's disease and salt-losing adrenogenital syndrome.

Dosage and Administration
100 μg to 2 mg daily, orally.

Cautions
Causes greatly increased sodium retention. Dietary salt restriction and potassium supplementation may be necessary. See **Cortisone acetate.**

Adverse Reactions
Essentially the same as adverse reactions to cortisone acetate (see).

251

Composition and Supply

Suspension, otic 0.1% with neomycin and polymyxin B
(Florotic®)
Tablets 100 µg

Legal Status

Prescription

Flumethasone pivalate (Locorten®)

See CORTICOSTEROIDS.

Fluocinolone acetonide (Fluonid®, Synalar®, Synemol®)

Fluocinonide (Lidex®)

Action and Use

Anti-inflammatory corticosteroid used for treatment of various dermatoses.

Dosage and Administration

Applied topically.

Cautions

Systemic absorption can occur if used over large areas for prolonged periods. Use with caution on lesions that are infected. Occlusive dressings should not be used when infection is present. Contraindicated in patients with vaccinia, varicella, and hypersensitivity to this agent.

Adverse Reactions

Possible effects include burning, itching, irritation, dryness, folliculitis, hypertrichosis, acne, and hypopigmentation. Occlusive dressings may result in maceration, infection, skin atrophy, striae, and miliaria.

Composition and Supply

Cream 0.025% (Synemol®)
Cream 0.025% with neomycin 0.5%, 5 g and 15 g
(Neo-Synalar®)
Cream and ointment 0.01% and 0.025% (Fluonid®, Synalar®)
Solution 0.01% (Synalar®)

Legal Status

Prescription

Fluonid®

See **Fluocinolone acetonide.**

Fluorescein sodium

Action and Use
Used in the diagnosis of corneal lesions and the detection of minute foreign bodies embedded in the cornea. Denuded areas of the epithelium are stained a bright green color when fluorescein sodium is applied to the cornea. Foreign bodies arc surrounded by a green ring. Loss of substance in the conjunctiva is indicated by a yellow stain.

Dosage and Administration
Paper strip: applicator is moistened with sterile water and placed in lower cul-de-sac close to the punctum.
Solution: 2 or 3 drops are instilled into conjunctival sac and washed out before observation.

Cautions
Solutions are easily contaminated by *Pseudomonas aeruginosa.*

Adverse Reactions
Fluorescein sodium has no adverse reactions with proper use.

Composition and Supply
Ophthalmic solution   2%
Paper strips, impregnated (Fluor-I-Strip® Applicators)

Legal Status
Prescription

Fluor-I-Strip® Applicators

See under **Fluorescein sodium.**

Fluoritab®

See **Sodium fluoride.**

Fluoromar® (fluroxene)

See ANESTHETICS, general.

Fluoroplex®

See **Fluorouracil.**

Fluorouracil (5-FU)(Efudex®, Fluoroplex®, Fluorouracil Roche®)

Action and Use
Antineoplastic used to treat certain solid tumors not amenable to surgery or radiation. It is used topically to treat multiple actinic (solar) keratoses.

Dosage and Administration
Injection: dosage is individualized, based on the patient's weight and response; daily dose should not exceed 800 mg. Should be given IV only.
Cream and solution: applied with gloved finger or nonmetal applicator.

Cautions
Fluorouracil is highly toxic, particularly to bone marrow and the gastrointestinal tract. Contraindicated for patients in poor nutritional state, with depressed bone marrow function, or those with serious infections.

Adverse Reactions
Early symptoms of developing toxicity include redness and dryness of the lips and soreness of mouth and stomatitis, followed by ulceration of the lips and buccal mucosa. More serious signs and symptoms include severe diarrhea, extensive ulceration of the mouth, alopecia (reported to be reversible), anorexia, nausea, and vomiting. Other possible reactions include a pruritic maculopapular rash, photosensitivity (as manifested by erythema or increased pigmentation), photophobia, epistaxis, and acute cerebellar syndrome. During first 2 to 4 weeks of treatment, the skin may develop redness, blistering, ulcer formation, and necrosis; these topical effects are necessary preliminaries to healing. Occlusive dressing should be avoided. The patient should avoid exposure to sunlight during treatment. Wash hands immediately after applying cream or ointment.

Composition and Supply
Cream   2% and 5%
Ointment   5%
Injection   50 mg/ml, in 10 ml ampuls (Fluorouracil Roche®)

Legal Status
Prescription

Fluorouracil Roche®
See **Fluorouracil.**

Fluothane® (halothane)
See ANESTHETICS, general.

Fluoxymesterone (Halotestin®)

Action and Use
Androgen used for replacement therapy in testicular hormone deficiencies and for the treatment of various conditions in females, including inoperable breast cancer.

Dosage and Administration
Dosage is individualized to the patient's needs, and ranges from 2 to 30 mg daily, orally.

Cautions
Fluoxymesterone is more potent than testosterone. Contraindicated in prostatic or breast cancer and in benign hypertrophy with obstructive symptoms. Edema may develop. Use with caution in patients with renal or cardiac disease.

Adverse Reactions
Masculinization in women may occur, with symptoms such as hirsutism and hoarsening or deepening of voice. With prolonged therapy, the patient may develop excessive body hair (which may be irreversible), male pattern of baldness, prominent musculature and veins, and hypertrophy of the clitoris. Priapism with initial therapy and azoospermia with prolonged use may occur. Other possible effects include impotence, gynecomastia, hypercalcemia in immobilized patients and in patients with breast cancer (which may indicate progression of bony metastases), hypersensitivity, precocious puberty in young boys, cessation of growth resulting from early closure of the epiphyses, and occasionally nausea and vomiting. Rarely, hepatic carcinoma may occur. PBI levels may be decreased without significance and the results of glucose tolerance tests may be altered. Serum cholesterol values may rise.

Composition and Supply
Tablets   2 mg, 5 mg, and 10 mg

Legal Status
Prescription

Fluphenazine (Permitil®, Prolixin®)

Action and Use
A major tranquilizer, fluphenazine is especially useful in treatment of patients with psychomotor agitation associated with schizophrenia.

Dosage and Administration
As hydrochloride: 500 μg to 10 mg daily, orally or IM.
As decanoate: 12.5 to 25 mg SC or IM initially; maintenance dose is given at 4 week intervals.
As enanthate: 25 mg SC or IM every 2 weeks.

Cautions
Contraindicated in patients with renal insufficiency. Use cautiously in patients with peptic ulcer. The maximum oral daily dose should not exceed 20 mg, and the weekly dose should not exceed 100 mg. Intramuscular doses greater than 10 mg daily should be used cautiously.

Adverse Reactions

Hypotension, sedation, ataxia, and extrapyramidal symptoms are the most common side effects. Other adverse reactions include dry mouth, constipation, dermatitis, blood dyscrasias, jaundice, antiemesis, nasal congestion, and edema.

Composition and Supply

Elixir (as hydrochloride)   500 μg/ml and 2.5 mg/ml
Injection (as hydrochloride)   2.5 mg/ml
Injection (as decanoate)   25 mg/ml, in 1 ml cartridge-needle units and 5 ml vials
Injection (as enanthate)   25 mg/ml, in 1 ml cartridge-needle units and 5 ml vials
Oral concentrate (as hydrochloride)   5 mg/ml
Tablets (as hydrochloride)   250 μg, 1 mg, 2.5 mg, 5 mg, and 10 mg

Legal Status
Prescription

Flurandrenolide (Cordran®)

Action and Use
Topical corticosteroid.

Dosage and Administration
Applied topically as cream, ointment, lotion, or dressing. (*Note:* Cordran® Tape must be replaced after 12 hours)

Cautions
Prolonged administration over large areas, especially when used occlusively or when the skin is broken, can lead to absorption. Can mask infection.

Adverse Reactions
Essentially the same as adverse reactions to fluocinolone acetonide (see). Cordran® Tape may cause purpura and stripping of the epidermis.

Composition and Supply
Cream and ointment   0.025% and 0.05%
Dressing   4 μg/cm^2 plastic tape (Cordran® Tape)
Lotion   0.05%
Ointment   0.05% with neomycin sulfate (Cordran®-N)

Legal Status
Prescription

Flurazepam hydrochloride (Dalmane®)

Action and Use
Hypnotic used for simple insomnia.

Dosage and Administration
15 to 30 mg at bedtime, orally.

Cautions
Interacts with other CNS depressants. There is a possibility of physical dependence with long-term use. Should be used cautiously in elderly or debilitated persons, in those with severe depression, and in patients with impaired renal or hepatic function.

Adverse Reactions
Dizziness, drowsiness, lightheadedness, staggering, and ataxia may occur. More pronounced reactions include sedation, lethargy, disorientation, and coma. Rare reactions include headache, gastrointestinal disturbances, excitement, irritability, chest pains, body and joint pains, urinary complaints, leukopenia, and agranulocytopenia.

Composition and Supply
Capsules   15 mg and 30 mg

Legal Status
Schedule IV

Flurobate®

See **Betamethasone.**

Fluroxene (Fluoromar®)

See ANESTHETICS, general.

Foille® (benzyl alcohol/benzocaine)

See ANTIPRURITICS, topical preparations.

Folbesyn®

See VITAMINS, MULTIPLE, parenteral.

Folic acid (Folvite®)

Action and Use
Hematinic used to treat folic acid deficiencies.

Dosage and Administration
250 μg to 1 mg daily; orally or IM.

Cautions
Pernicious anemia may be masked. Increases the metabolism of phenytoin sodium, phenobarbital, and primidone and thereby decreases their effectiveness.

Adverse Reactions
Rare.

Composition and Supply
Injection (as sodium folate)   5 mg/ml, in 10 ml vials
Tablets   250 μg and 1 mg

Legal Status
Prescription

Folic acid/ferrous sulfate (Folvron®)
See HEMATINICS.

Folic acid/ferrous sulfate/ascorbic acid (Fero-Folic-500®)
See HEMATINICS.

Follutein®
See **Gonadotropin, chorionic.**

Folvite®
See **Folic acid.**

Folvron® (folic acid/ferrous sulfate)
See HEMATINICS.

Forhistal® (dimethindene maleate)
See ANTIHISTAMINES.

Fostex®
See KERATOLYTICS.

FreAmine® II (amino acid injection)
See PARENTERAL ALIMENTATION.

FreAmine® Kit (parenteral hyperalimentation kit [amino acids-dextrose])
See PARENTERAL ALIMENTATION.

Fructose 5% and 10% (Levugen®, Travert®)

See PARENTERAL ALIMENTATION.

5-FU

See **Fluorouracil.**

Fuadin® (stibophen)

See ANTHELMINTICS, schistosomiasis.

FUDR (floxuridine)

See ANTINEOPLASTICS, antimetabolites.

Fulvicin-U/V®

See **Griseofulvin.**

Fungizone®

See **Amphotericin B.**

Furacin®

See **Nitrofurazone.**

Furadantin®

See **Nitrofurantoin.**

Furazolidone (Furoxone®)

See ANTIDIARRHEALS.

Furazolidone/nifuroxime (Tricofuron®)

See ANTIPROTOZOALS.

Furosemide (Lasix®)

Action and Use
Potent diuretic.

Dosage and Administration
Diuresis: Usual oral dose 20 to 80 mg as a single dose in the morning; usual parenteral dose 20 to 40 mg as a single dose IM or IV.
Hypertension: 40 mg twice daily for both initiation of therapy and maintenance.

Cautions
May cause electrolyte and fluid imbalance. Ototoxicity has been reported; concomitant use with other ototoxic drugs should be avoided.

Interferes with the hypoglycemic effect of insulin and oral hypo-glycemic agents. Contraindicated in women of child-bearing potential and in patients with anuria. The effects of other diuretics are increased when used together. Caution should be used in patients with liver disease and in those treated with high dosages of salicylates.

Adverse Reactions
Rapid diuresis with dehydration may produce excessive loss of sodium, chloride, and potassium (with muscle cramps, weakness, thirst, and paresthesias) and reduction of blood volume (with resulting vascular collapse, thrombosis, and embolism). Hypokalemia may precipitate digitalis toxicity. Furosemide may lead to hepatic coma in patients with cirrhosis. Other possible effects include skin rash, urticaria, nausea, vomiting, diarrhea, anorexia, hyperglycemia, transient deafness, tinnitus, blurred vision, postural hypotension, bone marrow depression, and hyperuricemia.

Composition and Supply
Injection   10 mg/ml, in 2 ml ampuls and 10 ml vials
Liquid   10 mg/ml
Tablets   20 mg and 40 mg

Legal Status
Prescription

Furoxone® (furazolidone)

See ANTIDIARRHEALS.

Gamastan®

See **Globulin, immune human serum.**

Gamene®

See **Gamma benzene hexachloride.**

Gamma benzene hexachloride (Gamene®, Kwell®)

Action and Use
Scabicide and pediculicide.

Dosage and Administration
Applied topically as directed by the manufacturer.

Cautions
This agent is highly toxic and should be used with care. Avoid contact with the eyes. Lipoid solvents enhance the percutaneous absorption of gamma benzene hexachloride.

Adverse Reactions
Sensitization has been reported, with resulting eczematous eruptions.

Composition and Supply
Lotion, shampoo, and cream   1%

Legal Status
Prescription

Gammacorten®

See **Dexamethasone.**

Gammagee®

See **Globulin, immune human serum.**

Gamulin® Rh

See **Globulin, Rh$_0$(D) immune human.**

Gantanol®

See **Sulfamethoxazole.**

Gantrisin®

See **Sulfisoxazole.**

Garamycin®

See **Gentamicin sulfate.**

Gas gangrene antitoxin polyvalent

Action and Use
Used in the prevention and treatment of gas gangrene.

Dosage and Administration
1 to 4 vials initially, IV, followed by 1 vial every 4 hours IM, for several days if needed.

Cautions
Test for sensitivity prior to injection. Highly sensitized persons may react even to a skin-test dose.

Adverse Reactions
Neurologic reactions may occur.

Composition and Supply
Injection   vial with 1 therapeutic dose

Legal Status
Prescription

Gastrografin®

See under **Diatrizoate meglumine.**

Gelatin film, absorbable (Gelfilm®)

See HEMOSTATICS.

Gelatin sponge, absorbable (Gelfoam®)

Action and Use
Hemostatic used to control capillary bleeding.

Dosage and Administration
Apply sponge to bleeding area moistened with 1,000 to 2,000 units of thrombin or sterile saline.

Cautions
None.

Adverse Reactions
None.

Composition and Supply
Packs, cones, and sponges, in various sizes

Legal Status
Prescription

Gelfilm® (gelatin film, absorbable)

See HEMOSTATICS.

Gelfoam®

See **Gelatin sponge, absorbable.**

Gelusil®

See **Aluminum hydroxide/magnesium trisilicate.**

Gemonil® (metharbital)

See ANTICONVULSANTS.

Gentamicin sulfate (Garamycin®)

Action and Use
Aminoglycoside antibiotic.

Dosage and Administration
3 to 5 mg/kg in divided doses daily, IM or IV. Also applied topically as cream, ointment, or solution.

Cautions
Parenteral gentamicin sulfate should be reserved for serious infections caused by organisms resistant to other antibiotics, namely, *Pseudomonas aeruginosa, Escherichia coli,* and *Klebsiella, Enterobacter,* and *Serratia* species. It is ototoxic (and should not be used with other ototoxic drugs), nephrotoxic, and neurotoxic. Contraindicated in pregnant women. Patients should be well hydrated while on the drug. Avoid using this agent in patients who are being treated with ethacrynic acid or furosemide.

Adverse Reactions
Possible side effects include nausea, vomiting, and candidiasis. Skin applications may produce allergic skin reactions and photosensitivity. Ophthalmic preparations may produce transient burning or stinging. May increase alkaline phosphatase and serum transaminases.

Composition and Supply
Cream and ointment   0.1%
Injection, pediatric   10 mg/ml, in 2 ml vials, and 20 mg/ml, in 2 ml vials
Injection   40 mg/ml, in 2 ml vials
Ointment and solution, ophthalmic   0.3%
Syringes, disposable   60 mg and 80 mg

Legal Status
Prescription

Gentian violet (crystal violet)

Action and Use
Antifungal agent and anthelmintic used in pinworm infestation.

Dosage and Administration
Antifungal: topical preparations.
Anthelmintic: 60 mg 3 times a day, orally.

Cautions
Use carefully in patients with cardiac, hepatic, renal, or gastrointestinal disease.

Adverse Reactions
Stains clothing and skin.

Composition and Supply
Cream, vaginal   1.35%
Solution   1% and 2%
Suppositories, vaginal   2 mg
Tablets   10 mg and 25 mg
Tampons, vaginal   5 mg

Legal Status
Prescription

Geocillin® (carbenicillin indanyl sodium)

See ANTIBIOTICS, penicillins.

Geopen®

See **Carbenicillin disodium.**

Germanin® (suramin)

See ANTIPROTOZOALS, antitrypanosomals.

Gitaligin® (gitalin)

See CARDIACS, cardiac glycosides.

Gitalin (Gitaligin®)

See CARDIACS, cardiac glycosides.

Globulin, immune human serum (Gamastan®, Gammagee®, Immu-G®)

Action and Use
Used to effect passive immunization against measles, rubella, infectious hepatitis, agammaglobulinemia, hypogammaglobulinemia, and dysgammaglobulinemia.

Dosage and Administration
Individualized according to the patient's weight and the condition being treated.

Cautions
Anaphylaxis is possible. Inject only intramuscularly or subcutaneously.

Adverse Reactions

May infrequently cause pain and tenderness. Rarely, a local necrosis occurs, and it can develop into sterile abscesses and fibrosis. Nerve injury may result if the injection site' is near peripheral nerves.

Composition and Supply

Injection   2 ml and 10 ml vials

Legal Status

Prescription

Globulin, Rh$_o$(D) immune human (Gamulin® Rh, RhoGAM®)

Action and Use

Specific anti-Rh$_o$ gamma globulin, which prevents formation of destructive antibodies in Rh$_o$D^u negative, D^u negative individuals who have received Rh positive blood as a result of delivering an Rh$_o$(D) positive or D^u positive infant, or from a transfusion.

Dosage and Administration

Dosage depends on the volume of Rh positive blood that entered the patient's circulation. 1 vial completely suppresses the antigenic action of 15 ml of Rh positive packed cells. In the usual full term delivery 1 vial is adequate; it is given within 72 hours of delivery, IM. (*Note:* the mother's consent should be obtained.)

Cautions

Contraindicated in infants, in Rh$_o$(D) positive or D^u positive individuals, and in Rh$_o$(D) or D^u negative mothers previously sensitized to the Rh$_o$(D) or D^u blood factor. The precautions are the same as those that are followed when administering whole blood; two nurses should double-check the identifying numbers on the medication vial and the patient's name against laboratory slips.

Adverse Reactions

Reactions are rare. Local inflammation is possible at the injection site, and slight temperature elevation may occur. It may be helpful to check vital signs twice within the first 4 hours after administration of the medication.

Composition and Supply

Injection   single dose vials (*Note:* should be stored at 2° to 8°C—*do not freeze*)

Legal Status

Prescription

Glucagon for injection

Action and Use
An antihypoglycemic agent that acts by stimulating glycogenolysis; used in the treatment of insulin shock or coma.

Dosage and Administration
500 µg to 1 mg, SC, IM, or IV.

Cautions
Observe patient closely during and after administration. Glucagon is useful only if liver glycogen is available. Hypoglycemic patients with juvenile or unstable diabetes do not respond satisfactorily to treatment with glucagon.

Adverse Reactions
Occasionally nausea and vomiting may occur, and hypotension is possible.

Composition and Supply
Injection 1 mg glucagon in ampuls of dry powder with diluting solution

Legal Status
Prescription

Glucola®

See DIAGNOSTICS, glucose tolerance.

Glucosulfone sodium (Promin®)

See ANTILEPROTICS.

Glutamic acid hydrochloride (Acidulin®)

Action and Use
Releases hydrochloric acid on contact with water. Useful in the treatment of hypochlorhydria and a chlorhydria.

Dosage and Administration
1 to 3 capsules three times daily before meals.

Cautions
Contraindicated in patients with gastric hyperacidity or peptic ulcer.

Adverse Reactions
Overdosage may produce systemic acidosis.

Composition and Supply
Capsules   300 mg and 340 mg (Pulvules®)

Legal Status
Prescription

Glutethimide (Doriden®)

Action and Use
Hypnotic.

Dosage and Administration
250 mg to 1 g, orally.

Cautions
Glutethimide possesses anticholinergic activity and should be used cautiously in patients with problems that may be aggravated by such action. It also should be used cautiously with other CNS depressants, and it may enhance the anticholinergic effects of tricyclic antidepressants. The metabolism of coumarin anticoagulants is increased, and adjustments in anticoagulant dosage must be kept in mind. Dependence may occur with prolonged use; prolonged use also diminishes effectiveness.

Adverse Reactions
The most common side effects include nausea, anorexia, vomiting, and rash. Occasional side effects include confusion, headache, and drowsiness. Blood dyscrasias and porphyria are rare side effects.

Composition and Supply
Tablets   250 mg and 500 mg

Legal Status
Schedule III

Glycerin (glycerol)

Action and Use
Used orally, glycerin decreases intraocular pressure in glaucoma; it is also used rectally as a cathartic and topically as a lubricant and emollient.

Dosage and Administration
0.8 to 1.2 ml/kg, orally; 1 suppository as needed, rectally.

Cautions
See **Cascara sagrada** for cautions about use of cathartics.

Adverse Reactions
Can have drying and irritating effect when used in pure form (as a skin emollient and protectant).

Composition and Supply
Lotions, varying percents
Solution   50% (Osmoglyn®)
Suppositories

Legal Status
Nonprescription except oral forms

Glycerol

See **Glycerin.**

Glyceryl trinitrate

See **Nitroglycerin.**

Glycopyrrolate (Robinul®)

Action and Use
Anticholinergic used in the management of peptic ulcer and other gastrointestinal disorders amenable to cholinergic inhibition.

Dosage and Administration
1 mg 2 or 3 times a day, orally; 100 to 200 μg every 4 hours, IM.

Cautions
Use cautiously in patients with cardiac disease or glaucoma.

Adverse Reactions
Dry mouth, and occasionally other atropine-like effects, may occur.

Composition and Supply
Injection   200 μg/ml, in 1 ml ampuls and 5 ml vials
Tablets   1 mg and 2 mg (Robinul®, Robinul® Forte)
Tablets   1 mg with 16 mg phenobarbital (Robinul®-PH)
Tablets   2 mg with 16 mg phenobarbital (Robinul®-PH Forte)

Legal Status
Prescription

Gly-Oxide® (carbamide peroxide 10%)

See MOUTHWASHES.

Gold Au 198 (Aureotope®)

See ANTINEOPLASTICS, radioisotopes.

Gold sodium thiomalate (Myochrysine®)

Action and Use
Gold treatment of rheumatoid arthritis.

Dosage and Administration
10 mg IM per week for 2 weeks, then 25 mg per week for 2 weeks, then 50 mg per week for 10 weeks, then 25 mg per week for 10 weeks, to a total of 820 mg. Maintenance dosage is 30 to 50 mg every 2 to 3 weeks.

Cautions
Potentially toxic. See **Aurothioglucose.**

Adverse Reactions
See **Aurothioglucose.**

Composition and Supply
Injection 10 mg/ml, 25 mg/ml, and 100 mg/ml in 1 ml ampuls; 50 mg/ml in 1 ml ampuls and 10 ml vials

Legal Status
Prescription

Gonadotropin, chorionic (A.P.L.®, Follutein®)

Action and Use
Gonadotropic hormone indicated for use in prepubertal cryptorchidism, hypogonadotropic hypogonadism, and secondary anovulatory infertility.

Dosage and Administration
Dosage is individualized according to use. In cryptorchidism, the dosage is 1,000 to 2,000 units 2 to 3 times a week, IM.

Cautions
Contraindicated in patients with sensitivity to the drug, hypertrophy or tumor of the pituitary, or prostatic carcinoma, and in individuals experiencing precocious puberty. Excessive dosage may induce pseudopuberty.

Adverse Reactions
Adverse effects include headache, instability, restlessness, depression, fatigue, pain at injection site, edema, and gynecomastia. Drug should be discontinued if signs of precocious maturity appear.

Composition and Supply
Vials 5,000 units, 10,000 units, and 20,000 units

Legal Status
Prescription

Gravindex™ Slide Test

See DIAGNOSTICS, pregnancy.

Green soap tincture (medicinal soft soap liniment)

Action and Use
Detergent.

Dosage and Administration
Use as soap.

Cautions
Not for use on the face.

Adverse Reactions
Irritating to abraded or sensitive areas.

Composition and Supply
Tincture (containing green soap, lavender oil, and alcohol)

Legal Status
Nonprescription

Grifulvin V®

See **Griseofulvin.**

Grisactin®

See **Griseofulvin.**

Griseofulvin (Fulvicin-U/V®, Grifulvin V®, Grisactin®, Gris-PEG®)

Action and Use
Fungistatic antibiotic indicated for the treatment of ringworm of the skin, hair, and nails.

Dosage and Administration
Microsize crystals: 500 mg to 1 g daily, orally.
Ultramicrosize crystals: 250 to 500 mg daily, orally.

Cautions
Ineffective in candidiasis and systemic mycoses. Griseofulvin potentiates the effect of alcohol, reduces the absorption of phenobarbital, and decreases the effectiveness of sodium warfarin. It is contraindicated in porphyria and hepatic failure.

Adverse Reactions
Photosensitivity may occur in some patients. Some common effects include nausea, vomiting, diarrhea, flatulence, dry mouth, thirst, black furry tongue, stomatitis, and thrush. Other possible effects include dizziness, confusion, peripheral neuritis, lethargy, fatigue, syncope, blurred vision, and paresthesias. Hepatotoxicity and nephrotoxicity have been reported. Exfoliation and loosening of infected hair are therapeutic effects.

Composition and Supply
Capsules   125 mg, 250 mg, and 500 mg (microsize crystals)
Suspension   125 mg/5 ml (microsize crystals)
Tablets   125 mg, 250 mg, and 500 mg (microsize crystals)
Tablets 125 mg (ultramicrosize crystals—Gris-PEG®)
Note: an oral dose of Gris-PEG® (griseofulvin ultramicrosize) is biologically equivalent to 500 mg of griseofulvin microsize.

Legal Status
Prescription

Gris-PEG®

See **Griseofulvin.**

G-strophanthin

See **Ouabain.**

Guaifenesin (Robitussin®)

Action and Use
Expectorant.

Dosage and Administration
100 to 200 mg every 2 to 4 hours, orally.

Cautions
Doses above required expectorant levels may cause emesis. Guaifenesin may produce colorimetric aberrations with laboratory tests, for example in tests for levels of VMA and 5-HIAA.

Adverse Reactions
Rare.

Composition and Supply
Syrup   100 mg/5 ml
Combinations (*Note:* see COUGH-COLD PREPARATIONS for composition):
  Robitussin A-C®
  Robitussin-CF®
  Robitussin-DM®
  Robitussin-DM Cough Calmers®
  Robitussin-PE®

Legal Status
Schedule V (Robitussin A-C®)
Nonprescription (all other forms)

Guanethidine sulfate (Ismelin®)

Action and Use
Potent antihypertensive.

Dosage and Administration
Initial: 10 mg per day; increase dose every 5 to 7 days for the first 3 weeks.
Maintenance: 25 to 50 mg per day.

Cautions
The patient should be warned of the common occurrence of pronounced orthostatic hypotension. Should be used cautiously in patients with impaired renal function, coronary disease, or cerebral vascular disease. Amphetamines, mild stimulants, and tricyclic antidepressants may antagonize the drug's hypotensive effect. Should not be given to patients who are receiving MAO inhibitors.

Adverse Reactions
Orthostatic hypotension is accentuated by hot weather, alcohol ingestion, or exercise. Standing perfectly still for any length of time pools blood in extremities and may result in syncope. Hypotension could lead to kidney failure, coronary insufficiency, and cerebral insufficiency, and might precipitate congestive heart failure. Other side effects include abdominal distress, weight gain and edema, fatigue, and nasal stuffiness. Less common effects include dyspnea, nausea, vomiting, alopecia, blurred vision, depression, angina-like pain, and pancytopenia.

Composition and Supply
Tablets   10 mg and 25 mg
Tablets   10 mg with hydrochlorothiazide 25 mg (Esimil®)

Legal Status
Prescription

Gynergen®

See **Ergotamine tartrate.**

Gynorest® (dydrogesterone)

See PROGESTOGENS.

Halcinonide (Halog®)

See CORTICOSTEROIDS.

Haldol®

See **Haloperidol.**

Haldrone® (paramethasone acetate)

See CORTICOSTEROIDS.

Halog® (halcinonide)

See CORTICOSTEROIDS.

Haloperidol (Haldol®)

Action and Use
Major tranquilizer used for the management of manifestations of psychotic disorders and for the control of the tics and vocal utterances of Gilles de la Tourette's syndrome.

Dosage and Administration
Dosage is individualized to the patient and ranges from 500 μg to 100 mg daily, orally or IM.

Cautions
Contraindicated in patients who are severely depressed or comatose and in those who have Parkinson's disease. May potentiate other CNS depressants. Administer cautiously in patients receiving anticonvulsants and anticoagulants.

Adverse Reactions
Hypotension, which is aggravated by epinephrine, or tachycardia may occur. Other effects include extrapyramidal reactions, mild blood alterations, liver dysfunction (occasionally), skin reactions, lactation, mastalgia, breast engorgement, menstrual irregularities, gynecomastia, increased libido, impotence, hyperglycemia or hypoglycemia, anorexia, nausea, vomiting, constipation, diarrhea, hypersalivation, dyspepsia, blurred vision, dry mouth, urinary retention, diaphoresis,

laryngospasm, and bronchospasm. Effects of an overdose include severe extrapyramidal reactions, sedation, and hypotension.

Composition and Supply
Injection   5 mg/ml, in 1 ml ampuls and 10 ml vials
Solution   2 mg/ml
Tablets   500 μg, 1 mg, 2 mg, 5 mg, and 10 mg

Legal Status
Prescription

Haloprogin (Halotex®)

Action and Use
Topical fungistatic agent.

Dosage and Administration
1% cream or solution, applied topically.

Cautions
Keep out of the eyes.

Adverse Reactions
Occasional side effects include irritation, pruritus, burning, vesiculation, increased maceration, and sensitization (or exacerbation of lesion), especially if treated area is heavily covered.

Composition and Supply
Cream   1%
Solution, topical   1%

Legal Status
Prescription

Halotestin®

See **Fluoxymesterone.**

Halotex®

See **Haloprogin.**

Halothane (Fluothane®)

See ANESTHETICS, general.

Harmonyl® (deserpidine)

See ANTIHYPERTENSIVES, nondiuretic.

Hepahydrin®

See under **Dehydrocholic acid.**

Heparin sodium injection (Lipo-Hepin®, Liquaemin®, Panheprin®)

Action and Use
Anticoagulant.

Dosage and Administration
Deep subcutaneous: initially, 10,000 to 20,000 units; then 8,000 to 10,000 units every 8 hours or 15,000 to 20,000 units every 12 hours; given undiluted.

Intermittent intravenous: initially, 10,000 units; then 5,000 to 10,000 units every 4 to 6 hours, depending on coagulation time; given undiluted or diluted with 50 to 100 ml of isotonic sodium chloride injection.

Continuous intravenous: loading dose of 5,000 units should be used; for most patients, rate of flow is adjusted to 20,000 to 40,000 units in 24 hours; given at a dilution of 20,000 to 40,000 units per 1,000 ml of infusion.

Cautions
A trial dose is recommended to check for possible allergy. Clotting time and/or activated partial thromboplastin time must be carefully followed. Use with extreme caution in patients with disorders that involve an increased danger of hemorrhage. Use cautiously in pregnant women and in patients receiving salicylates. Digitalis, tetracyclines, nicotine, antihistamines, and penicillins may partially counteract the anticoagulant effect. Heparin is contraindicated in patients with blood dyscrasias, liver or kidney disease, peptic ulcer, chronic ulcerative colitis, active bleeding, threatened abortion, subacute bacterial endocarditis, suspected intracranial hemorrhage, visceral carcinoma, regional or lumbar block anesthesia, severe hypertension, tube drainage of stomach and small intestine, and shock. Heparin should be withheld during and after operations involving the eye, spinal cord, or brain. The patient should carry an identification card that lists the patient's and physician's names and phone numbers, and the name and dosage of the drug; the patient may also use a Medic Alert bracelet and wallet card. Treatment with heparin is incompatible with concurrent use of ascorbic acid, cephaloridine, chlordiazepoxide hydrochloride, dimenhydrinate, ergonovine maleate, erythromycin gluceptate, erythromycin lactobionate, gentamicin sulfate, human serum albumin, hyaluronidase, hydroxyzine hydrochloride, kanamycin sulfate, levarterenol bitartrate, meperidine hydrochloride, metaraminol bitartrate, methicillin sodium, narcotic salts, neomycin, penicillin G potassium, polymyxin B sulfate, prochlorperazine, promazine hydrochloride, promethazine hydrochloride, streptomycin sulfate, succinyl-

choline chloride, sulfisoxazole, tetracycline hydrochloride, thiopental sodium, vancomycin, and vitamin B complex.

Adverse Reactions
The most important adverse effects are related to bleeding tendencies, including gastrointestinal bleeding, epistaxis, ecchymosis, bleeding gums, and possibly hemarthrosis (urine and stools should be observed for bleeding). Rare responses include alopecia and osteoporosis. Intramuscular injection is usually avoided because bleeding and painful hematoma formation frequently occur at the injection site; also absorption may not be even, and tissue slough may rarely occur as a result of hematoma formation. Avoid rubbing the skin before and after when giving a subcutaneous injection in the abdomen. To prevent ecchymosis, do not pinch the skin and do not withdraw the plunger before administration.

Composition and Supply
Injection, USP   1,000 units/ml, in 1 ml ampuls and 10 ml vials; 10,000 units/ml, in 1 ml and 4 ml ampuls; 20,000 units/ml, in 2 ml, 5 ml, and 10 ml vials

Injection   5,000 units/ml, 10,000 units/ml, 20,000 units/ml, 40,000 units/ml, in 1 ml ampuls

Syringes, prefilled   units/0.5 ml: 1,000, 5,000, 7,500, 10,000, 15,000, and 20,000

Legal Status
Prescription

Herplex®

See **Idoxuridine.**

Hetrazan®

See **Diethylcarbamazine citrate.**

Hexa-Betalin®

See **Pyridoxine hydrochloride.**

Hexachlorophene detergent (pHisoHex®)

Action and Use
Topical germicidal cleansing agent.

Dosage and Administration
Applied topically.

Cautions
Rinse thoroughly after use, especially in sensitive areas. Caution should be used in infants; contraindicated in premature infants. Hexachlorophene is also contraindicated on burned or denuded skin and mucous membranes, on occlusive dressings, and for routine total body bathing. Systemic absorption from burn surfaces and the vaginal mucosa may result in CNS toxicity and death.

Adverse Reactions
Skin reactions and photosensitivity may occur.

Composition and Supply
Emulsion   3%

Legal Status
Prescription

Hexadrol®

See **Dexamethasone.**

Hexocyclium methylsulfate (Tral®)

See ANTICHOLINERGICS.

Hexylcaine hydrochloride (Cyclaine®)

See ANESTHETICS, local.

Hexylresorcinol

Action and Use
Anthelmintic effective against roundworm, hookworm, whipworm, and dwarf tapeworm.

Dosage and Administration
1 g swallowed whole with a glass of water.

Cautions
Pills should be swallowed whole to avoid irritating the mouth.

Adverse Reactions
Local irritation may occur.

Composition and Supply
Tablets   100 mg and 200 mg

Legal Status
Prescription

Hibiclens® (chlorhexidene gluconate)

See ANTI-INFECTIVES, LOCAL, miscellaneous antiseptic-disinfectants.

Hiprex®

See **Methenamine hippurate.**

Hispril® (diphenylpyraline hydrochloride)

See ANTIHISTAMINES.

Histadyl® (methapyrilene hydrochloride)

See ANTIHISTAMINES.

Histadyl® Fumarate (methapyrilene fumarate)

See ANTIHISTAMINES.

Histalog®

See **Betazole hydrochloride.**

Histamine phosphate injection

Action and Use
Used in the diagnosis of achlorhydria and pheochromocytoma.

Dosage and Administration
Achlorhydria: 10 µg/kg SC of histamine base.
Pheochromocytoma: 25 to 50 µg SC of histamine base.

Cautions
There are potentially dangerous side effects, including a severe drop in blood pressure. Frequent determinations of pulse rate and pressure must be made during and immediately following administration. Should be used cautiously in patients with bronchial disease or asthma.

Adverse Reactions
Simultaneous administration of epinephrine or other antagonist will provide an antidote for major reactions, such as headache, dizziness, asthmatic attack, hypotension, and shock.

Composition and Supply
Injection   275 µg/ml (equivalent to 100 µg of histamine base), in 1 ml and 5 ml ampuls

Legal Status
Prescription

Histoplasmin

Action and Use
Antigen used in the diagnosis of histoplasmosis. A positive reaction is demonstrated by an area of induration 5×5 mm or more at the injection site.

Dosage and Administration
0.1 ml (100 μl) of 1 : 100 dilution, injected intradermally on the flexor surface of the forearm. Reaction is read after 24 to 48 hours.

Cautions
Do not inject other than intradermally. Doses greater than those recommended may result in severe reactions. Reactivity to the test may be suppressed in patients recently immunized with live virus vaccines and in those receiving corticosteroids or immunosuppressive agents.

Adverse Reactions
Hypersensitivity may occur, with urticaria, shortness of breath, and perspiration.

Composition and Supply
Injection   0.01 ml (10 μl) in vials (to be mixed with 1 ml diluent)

Legal Status
Prescription

Homapin® (homatropine methylbromide)

See ANTICHOLINERGICS.

Homatropine hydrobromide

See MYDRIATICS.

Homatropine methylbromide (Homapin®)

See ANTICHOLINERGICS.

Homo-Tet®

See **Tetanus immune human globulin.**

Hormonin® (estrone/estradiol/estriol)

See ESTROGENS.

H.P. Acthar® Gel

See **Corticotropin.**

Humafac® (antihemophilic factor [human] VIII)

See HEMOSTATICS.

Humatin®

See **Paromomycin sulfate.**

Humorsol®

See **Demecarium bromide.**

Hyaluronidase (Alidase®, Hyazyme®, Wydase®)

Action and Use
Enzyme that hydrolyzes intercellular cement and facilitates tissue absorption of injected drugs and fluids.

Dosage and Administration
150 units added to drug solution or fluid to be administered.

Cautions
Should not be injected into or around areas of infection or carcinoma.

Adverse Reactions
Low level of toxicity. Hypersensitivity occasionally develops. Concomitant use with an anesthetic potentiates reactions to the anesthetic.

Composition and Supply
Injection   150 unit and 1,500 unit vials

Legal Status
Prescription

Hyazyme®

See **Hyaluronidase.**

Hycodan®

See **Hydrocodone bitartrate/homatropine methylbromide.**

Hycomine® Syrup

See COUGH-COLD PREPARATIONS, cough preparations.

Hycotuss® Expectorant

See COUGH-COLD PREPARATIONS, cough preparations.

Hydeltra®

See **Prednisolone.**

Hydergine®

See **Dihydroergotoxine mesylates.**

Hydralazine hydrochloride (Apresoline®, Dralzine™)

Action and Use
Antihypertensive.

Dosage and Administration
10 mg 4 times a day, orally, gradually increased to 50 mg 4 times a day; 20 to 40 mg, IM or IV every 4 to 6 hours as needed.

Cautions
Contraindicated in coronary heart disease and mitral valve rheumatic heart disease. Use with extreme caution in patients with advanced renal damage and in those with existing or incipient cerebral accidents. In a few patients hydralazine may produce a clinical picture simulating systemic lupus erythematosus.

Adverse Reactions
Common effects include headache, anxiety, mild depression, dizziness, tachycardia, angina pectoris, diarrhea, anorexia, nausea, and vomiting. Less frequent side effects include orthostatic hypotension, nasal congestion, flushing, lacrimation, paresthesias, tremors, and muscle cramps. Rare side effects include urticaria, pruritus, rash, gastrointestinal hemorrhage, pancytopenia, hepatitis, dysuria, dyspnea, polyneuritis, and paradoxical hypertension.

Composition and Supply
Capsules   25 mg with hydrochlorothiazide 25 mg (Apresazide™ 25/25)
Capsules   50 mg with hydrochlorothiazide 50 mg (Apresazide™ 50/50)
Capsules   100 mg with hydrochlorothiazide 50 mg (Apresazide™ 100/50)
Injection   20 mg/ml, in 1 ml ampuls
Tablets   10 mg, 25 mg, 50 mg, and 100 mg
Tablets   25 mg with hydrochlorothiazide 15 mg and reserpine 100 μg (Ser-Ap-Es®)

Note: for cautions and adverse reactions about hydrochlorothiazide and reserpine, see **Chlorothiazide** and **Rauwolfia serpentina,** respectively.

Legal Status
Prescription

Hydrea®

See **Hydroxyurea.**

Hydrochloric acid 10%

See DIGESTANTS; HEMATINICS.

Hydrochlorothiazide (Esidrix®, HydroDIURIL®, Oretic®)

Action and Use
Diuretic and antihypertensive.

Dosage and Administration
25 to 200 mg daily, orally.

Cautions
Contraindicated in renal decompensation and in pregnant women. See **Chlorothiazide** for further cautions.

Adverse Reactions
See **Chlorothiazide.**

Composition and Supply
Tablets   25 mg and 50 mg

Legal Status
Prescription

Hydrocodone bitartrate/homatropine methylbromide (Hycodan®)

Action and Use
Narcotic antitussive.

Dosage and Administration
5 to 10 mg 3 to 4 times a day, orally; a single dose should not exceed 15 mg.

Cautions
May be habit-forming. Contraindicated in patients with glaucoma. Potentiates the effect of tricyclic antidepressants and alcohol and other CNS depressants.

Adverse Reactions
Sedation, nausea, vomiting, and constipation are possible effects. Effects of an overdose include coma, shock, and respiratory depression.

Composition and Supply
Syrup   hydrocodone 5 mg/ml with homatropine 1.5 mg/ml
Tablets   hydrocodone 5 mg with homatropine 1.5 mg

Legal Status
Schedule III

Hydrocortisone (Cort-Dome®, Cortef®, Cortril®, Hydrocortone®, Solu-Cortef®)

Action and Use
Standard glucocorticoid.

Dosage and Administration
Dosage varies with patient and condition; hydrocortisone is administered topically, orally, intra-articularly, IM, or IV.

Cautions
See **Cortisone acetate.**

Adverse Reactions
See **Cortisone acetate.**

Composition and Supply
Injection (as sodium succinate)   100 mg, 500 mg, and 1 g vials
   (Solu-Cortef®)
Lotion and cream   0.125%, 0.25%, 0.5%, and 1% (Cort-Dome®)
Ointment   1% (Cortril®)
Tablets   5 mg, 10 mg, and 20 mg (Cortef®)

Legal Status
Prescription

Hydrocortone®

See **Hydrocortisone.**

HydroDIURIL®

See **Hydrochlorothiazide.**

Hydroflumethiazide (Diucardin®)

See **DIURETICS.**

Hydrogen peroxide

Action and Use
Anti-infective used as a gargle and as a cleanser for wounds.

Dosage and Administration
Gargle: dilute with equal volume of water.
Wounds: use undiluted.

Cautions
Effective only while actively releasing oxygen. The presence of pus and blood reduces the efficiency of hydrogen peroxide. Keep well stoppered and in cool, dark place.

Adverse Reactions
Prolonged use as a mouthwash may produce hypertrophied filiform papillae of the tongue ("hairy tongue"), which resolves when the drug is discontinued.

Composition and Supply
Solution 3%

Legal Status
Nonprescription

Hydromorphone hydrochloride (Dilaudid®)

Action and Use
Narcotic analgesic used in moderate to severe pain; also used as a cough suppressant.

Dosage and Administration
Pain: 2 to 4 mg every 4 to 6 hours, orally; 2 to 3 mg every 4 to 6 hours, SC; or 3 mg, rectally.
Cough: 1 mg every 3 to 4 hours.

Cautions
Tolerance and addiction are potential hazards. Respiratory depression may occur. Other CNS depressants are potentiated. Contraindicated in patients with increased intracranial pressure or status asthmaticus.

Adverse Reactions
The side effects are similar to those of morphine sulfate (see), but not as severe. Pain at the injection site and local tissue irritation may occur; the injection site should be rotated.

Composition and Supply
Injection   2 mg/ml and 4 mg/ml
Suppositories   3 mg
Syrup   1 mg/5 ml with guaifenesin 100 mg/5 ml
Tablets   1 mg, 2 mg, 3 mg, and 4 mg

Legal Status
Schedule II

Hydromox® (quinethazone)

See DIURETICS.

Hydrophilic ointment

See EMOLLIENT-PROTECTANTS.

Hydropres® (reserpine/hydrochlorothiazide)

See ANTIHYPERTENSIVES, combinations.

Hydroxocobalamin (alphaREDISOL®, Neo-Betalin® 12)

See HEMATINICS; VITAMINS, water-soluble.

Hydroxyamphetamine hydrobromide (Paredrine®)

See MYDRIATICS.

Hydroxychloroquine sulfate (Plaquenil®)

Action and Use
Antimalarial; also used in lupus erythematosus and rheumatoid arthritis.

Dosage and Administration
For malarial suppression: 500 mg per week, orally.
For malarial treatment: 1 g initially, orally, followed by 500 mg a day for 2 days.
For lupus erythematosus: 400 mg for several weeks or months, orally, followed by 200 to 400 mg daily for maintenance.
For rheumatoid arthritis: 400 to 600 mg daily initially, orally, followed by 200 to 400 mg daily, when a good response is obtained.

Cautions
See **Chloroquine.**

Adverse Reactions
The more common side effects are mild and transient headache, dizziness, anorexia, nausea, vomiting, and diarrhea. Occasional side effects include irritability, psychosis, tinnitus, nerve deafness, muscle weak-

ness, bleaching of hair, alopecia, pruritus, skin eruptions, and ocular reactions. Bone marrow depression with hemolysis may occur in individuals with glucose-6-phosphate dehydrogenase deficiency. Toxicity may involve headache, visual disturbances, drowsiness, cardiovascular collapse, convulsions, and sudden cardiopulmonary arrest.

Composition and Supply
Tablets   200 mg

Legal Status
Prescription

Hydroxyprogesterone caproate (Delalutin®)

Action and Use
Progestogen.

Dosage and Administration
125 to 250 mg, IM, according to indications.

Cautions
Contraindicated for use in patients with genital malignancies, carcinoma of the breasts, thrombophlebitis, thromboembolic disorders, cerebral apoplexy, and markedly impaired liver function.

Adverse Reactions
Essentially the same as adverse reactions to progesterone (see). Pain may occur at the injection site.

Composition and Supply
Injection   125 mg/ml, in 2 ml and 10 ml vials
Injection   250 mg/ml, in 5 ml vials

Legal Status
Prescription

Hydroxypropyl methylcellulose (Isopto® Tears, Ultra Tears®)

Action and Use
Ophthalmic lubricant and protectant.

Dosage and Administration
Applied topically.

Cautions
Consult physician in case of severe or persistent eye irritation.

Adverse Reactions
None when the medication is used as directed.

Composition and Supply
Solution   0.5% (Isopto® Tears)
Solution   1% (Ultra Tears®)

Legal Status
Nonprescription

Hydroxyurea (Hydrea®)

Action and Use
Antineoplastic.

Dosage and Administration
20 to 30 mg per kg daily, as a single dose, orally.

Cautions
Hydroxyurea is a potent drug and must be used under close medical supervision. It depresses bone marrow. Use cautiously in patients with impaired renal function.

Adverse Reactions
Leukopenia is generally the first and most common toxic manifestation, especially in patients who have previously been treated with radiotherapy or cytotoxic cancer drugs. Less frequent side effects include nausea, vomiting, gastrointestinal symptoms (such as stomatitis, anorexia, and diarrhea), maculopapular rash, pruritus, facial erythema, and possibly kidney impairment. Rare responses include dysuria, alopecia, dizziness, headache, disorientation, hallucinations, and convulsions.

Composition and Supply
Capsules   500 mg

Legal Status
Prescription

Hydroxyzine (Atarax®, Vistaril®)

Action and Use
Tranquilizer, sedative, and antiemetic.

Dosage and Administration
25 to 100 mg 3 to 4 times a day, orally or IM.

Cautions
May potentiate other CNS depressants. The action of anticoagulant drugs may be enhanced. False evaluations of urinary 17-hydroxycorticosteroids may occur.

Adverse Reactions
Occasionally impairment of mental alertness and dryness of mouth may occur. There have been rare instances of tremors and convulsions at higher doses.

Composition and Supply
Capsules (as pamoate)   25 mg, 50 mg, and 100 mg
Injection (as hydrochloride)   50 mg/ml, in 2 ml vials
Suspension (as pamoate)   25 mg/5 ml
Syrup   10 mg/5 ml
Tablets and capsules (as hydrochloride)   10 mg, 25 mg, 50 mg, and 100 mg

Legal Status
Prescription

Hygroton®

See **Chlorthalidone.**

Hyoscine

See **Scopolamine hydrobromide.**

Hyoscyamine sulfate (Levsin®)

See ANTICHOLINERGICS.

Hypaque® Sodium (diatrizoate sodium)

See DIAGNOSTICS, roentgenography.

Hyparotin® (mumps immune globulin)

See BIOLOGICALS, immune serums.

Hyperstat®

See **Diazoxide.**

Hyper-Tet®

See **Tetanus immune human globulin.**

Hypertussis® (pertussis immune human globulin)

See BIOLOGICALS, immune serums–antitoxins.

Hytakerol®

See **Dihydrotachysterol.**

Iberet®

See under **Ferrous sulfate.**

Ibuprofen (Motrin®)

Action and Use
Nonsteroidal anti-inflammatory agent indicated in the symptomatic treatment of osteoarthritis and rheumatoid arthritis.

Dosage and Administration
300 or 400 mg 3 or 4 times a day, orally, with a maximum dose of 2.4 g daily.

Cautions
Contraindicated in patients with hypersensitivity to the drug and in patients with nasal polyps, angioderma, and bronchospastic reaction to aspirin. Caution should be used in patients with cardiac decompensation or coagulation disorders, and in persons receiving anticoagulants.

Adverse Reactions
The most frequent side effects include gastrointestinal complaints such as cramps, pain, indigestion, heartburn, bloating, flatulence, nausea, vomiting, constipation, diarrhea, and occasionally bleeding. Occasional side effects include skin rash, pruritus, dizziness, and blurred vision. Periodic ophthalmologic examination is recommended.

Composition and Supply
Tablets   300 mg and 400 mg

Legal Status
Prescription

Ichthammol (Ichthyol®)

See **KERATOPLASTICS.**

Ichthyol® (ichthammol)

See **KERATOPLASTICS.**

Idoxuridine (Dendrid®, Herplex®, Stoxil®)

Action and Use
Topical antiviral agent effective in dendritic keratitis.

Dosage and Administration
Ointment: apply 5 times a day inside the conjunctival sac of the infected eye.
Solution: initially 1 drop in the infected eye hourly during the day and every 2 hours at night; followed by 1 drop every 2 hours during the day and every 4 hours at night after improvement has occurred.

Cautions
Should be used only under the close supervision of an ophthalmologist.

Adverse Reactions
Irritation, inflammation, pain, and pruritis may occur. Visual changes are possible.

Composition and Supply
Ointment, ophthalmic,   0.5%
Solution, ophthalmic   0.1%

Legal Status
Prescription

Iletin®, Lente®

See under **Insulin.**

Iletin®, NPH

See under **Insulin.**

Iletin®, Regular

See under **Insulin.**

Iletin®, Semilente®

See under **Insulin.**

Iletin®, Ultralente®

See under **Insulin.**

Ilopan®

See **Dexpanthenol.**

Ilosone® (erythromycin estolate)

See ANTIBIOTICS, erythromycins.

Ilotycin®

See **Erythromycin.**

Ilotycin® Gluceptate (erythromycin gluceptate)

See ANTIBIOTICS, erythromycins.

Ilozyme®

See **Pancrelipase.**

Imavate®

See **Imipramine hydrochloride.**

Imferon®

See **Iron dextran injection.**

Imipramine hydrochloride (Imavate®, Janimine®, Presamine®, Tofranil®)
Imipramine pamoate (Tofranil-PM®)

Action and Use
Tricyclic antidepressant; also useful in childhood enuresis.

Dosage and Administration
Dosage, which is individualized, ranges from 30 to 300 mg per day, orally or IM.

Cautions
Should be used cautiously in patients with glaucoma, heart disease, hyperthyroidism, or a history of seizures, and in those using alcoholic beverages or receiving electroshock therapy. Combined therapy with MAO inhibitors is not recommended. Imipramine may potentiate barbiturates and is contraindicated during the acute recovery period after a myocardial infarction.

Adverse Reactions
See **Amitriptyline hydrochloride.**

Composition and Supply
Capsules (pamoate)   75 mg, 100 mg, 125 mg, and 150 mg
Injection (hydrochloride)   12.5 mg/ml, in 2 ml ampuls
Tablets (hydrochloride)   10 mg, 25 mg, and 50 mg

Legal Status
Prescription

Immu-G®

See **Globulin, immune human serum.**

IMMU-Tetanus®

See **Tetanus immune human globulin.**

Imodium®

See **Loperamide hydrochloride.**

Imuran®

See **Azathioprine.**

Inapsine®

See **Droperidol.**

Inderal®

See **Propranolol hydrochloride.**

Indigo carmine

See **Indigotindisulfonate sodium.**

Indigotindisulfonate sodium (indigo carmine)

Action and Use
Diagnostic used to assess renal function; localizes ureteral orifices during cystoscopy and catheterization.

Dosage and Administration
5 ml IV; 50 to 100 mg IM.

Cautions
Should be protected from light.

Adverse Reactions
None if properly used.

Composition and Supply
Injection   8 mg/ml, in 5 ml vials

Legal Status
Prescription

Indocin®

See **Indomethacin.**

Indocyanine green (Cardio-Green®, CG®)

See DIAGNOSTICS, cardiac output.

Indomethacin (Indocin®)

Action and Use
Nonsteroidal anti-inflammatory, analgesic, and antipyretic agent effective in rheumatoid arthritis, rheumatoid spondylitis, osteoarthritis, and acute gouty arthritis.

Dosage and Administration
50 to 200 mg daily in divided doses, orally, after meals or with food and/or antacids.

Cautions
This is a potent drug with a high incidence of side effects, usually involving the central nervous system and the gastrointestinal tract. It may increase the anticoagulant effect of sodium warfarin and may mask symptoms of infection. Plasma levels are increased if indomethacin is given with probenecid; consequently a lower dose is needed.

Adverse Reactions
Gastrointestinal side effects include ulceration, bleeding, perforation, nausea, vomiting, abdominal pain, and diarrhea. The CNS side effects include headache, occasional confusion, lightheadedness, and vertigo. Rare adverse reactions include hepatic impairment, blood dyscrasias, hypersensitivity, psychological problems, hypotension, hematuria, and alopecia. Renal tests are recommended with prolonged use of indomethacin.

Composition and Supply
Capsules   25 mg and 50 mg

Legal Status
Prescription

Influenza virus vaccine

Action and Use
Used to achieve active immunization against influenza. Includes strains of viruses adjusted to current recommendations of the U.S. Public Health Service.

Dosage and Administration
0.5 ml (500 µl) IM (preferably) or SC.

Cautions

Contraindicated in persons with hypersensitivity to chicken egg and in those with acute respiratory disease. Use with caution in highly allergic persons and in pregnant women.

Adverse Reactions

Local tenderness at the injection site may develop within the first 48 hours, occasionally with swelling and redness. There may be mild fever, chills, and malaise, lasting a few hours, especially in children. Rare side effects include postvaccinal neurological symptoms.

Composition and Supply

Injection   0.5 ml (500 μl) disposable syringes and 2.5 ml and 5 ml vials

Legal Status

Prescription

INH

See **Isoniazid.**

Innovar®

See under **Fentanyl citrate.**

Inpersol®/Dextrose (peritoneal dialysis solution)

See DIALYZING SOLUTIONS.

Insulin

Action and Use

Pancreatic hormone used for replacement therapy in the treatment of diabetes mellitus.

Dosage and Administration

Dosage is individualized to the patient. Insulin is generally given SC, but regular insulin may be given IM or IV if necessary.

Cautions

Keep in a cool place and always examine the label for the expiration date and the number of units in the solution. Use the correct syringe and needle. Use only the form of insulin prescribed; one type should never be substituted for another. An overdose causes hypoglycemia, which can be disastrous if it is severe. The addition of insulin to infusion solutions results in losses of up to 20% of the insulin as a result of its absorption into glass and tubing. Insulin may be potentiated by anabolic steroids, cyclophosphamide, MAO inhibitors, guanethidine monosulfate, and salicylates. The hypoglycemic effect may be antagonized by thyroid therapy, corticosteroids, dextro-thyroxine, phenytoin sodium, and epinephrine.

Adverse Reactions

Hypoglycemia (insulin shock) may result from hyperinsulinism, lack of food, or excessive exercise. Hypoglycemia may cause weakness, diaphoresis, nervousness, anxiety, drowsiness, irritability, fatigue, giddiness, belligerence, "hunger pains," nausea and epigastric distress, cool skin, pallor, palpitations, tremors, headache, blurred vision, diplopia, convulsions, coma, and possibly death. Hyperglycemia or diabetic acidosis (diabetic coma) may occur if too little insulin has been given, or if the administration of insulin is timed incorrectly in relation to eating. Hyperglycemia may result in lethargy, irritability, anorexia, nausea, vomiting, dry skin, flushed face, hyperpnea, tachycardia, drowsiness, abdominal pain, acetone breath, deep respirations, coma, and possibly death. Allergic reactions to insulin include urticaria, redness, itching, angioedema, and possibly anaphylaxis. Edema occasionally develops, characterized by generalized fluid retention; this usually results from the restoration of diabetic control in a patient whose disease has been unsatisfactorily managed over a period of time. (The edema usually subsides in 3 to 5 days after the institution of diuretic therapy.) Lipodystrophy occasionally occurs after repeated injections in the same site (especially after injections of protamine zinc insulin); this can be avoided by the use of deep SC or IM route, or by rotating the site so that no 2-cm area is injected more than once every 3 to 4 weeks.

Composition and Supply

The following preparations are available in 10 ml vials of 40 units/ml, 80 units/ml, and 100 units/ml. *Note:* the vial should be rotated gently between the palms and inverted several times before a dose is withdrawn; do not shake (to avoid foaming).

Rapid (short) acting:
Insulin injection (Regular Iletin®)
    onset   ½ to 1 hour
    peak   2 to 6 hours
    duration   5 to 8 hours
Prompt insulin zinc suspension (Semilente® Iletin®)
    onset   ½ to 1 hour
    peak   3 to 9 hours
    duration   13 to 16 hours

Intermediate acting:
Isophane insulin suspension (NPH Iletin®)
    onset   1 to 2 hours
    peak   7 to 12 hours
    duration   24 to 30 hours

Insulin zinc suspension (Lente® Iletin®)
    onset 1 to 4 hours
    peak 7 to 12 hours
    duration 24 to 30 hours
Globin zinc insulin
    onset 1 to 4 hours
    peak 6 to 16 hours
    duration 16 to 24 hours

Slow (long) acting:
Protamine zinc insulin suspension (PZI) (Protamine, Zinc & Iletin®)
    onset 1 to 8 hours
    peak 12 to 24 hours
    duration 30 to 36 hours
Extended insulin zinc suspension (Ultralente® Iletin®)
    onset 4 to 8 hours
    peak 10 to 30 hours
    duration 34 to 46 hours

Legal Status
Nonprescription

Intal®

See **Cromolyn sodium.**

Intrinsic factor/cyanocobalamin/ferrous fumarate/ascorbic acid
(Falvin®, Trinsicon®)

See HEMATINICS.

Intropin®

See **Dopamine hydrochloride.**

Invert sugar injections 5%, 10%, and 20%

See PARENTERAL ALIMENTATION.

Iodine

Action and Use
Antiseptic-disinfectant.

Dosage and Administration
Apply to affected areas.

Cautions
Do not cover surfaces to which iodine is applied. When used preoperatively, it should be removed from skin with alcohol to prevent possible irritation.

Adverse Reactions
Irritates (stings) abraded skin. Skin burns may occur in hypersensitive patients.

Composition and Supply
Iodine solution   2%
Iodine tincture   2%
Strong iodine solution   7% (Lugol's solution)

Legal Status
Nonprescription

Iodipamide meglumine (Cholografin®)

Action and Use
Contrast medium used in cholangiography and cholescystography.

Dosage and Administration
Injection 52%: 20 ml, IV, slowly over a period of 10 minutes.
Injection 10.3%: 100 ml, IV, over a period of 30 to 45 minutes.

Cautions
Caution should be used in patients with pheochromocytoma, hypertension, and debilitation. See **Diatrizoate meglumine** for further cautions.

Adverse Reactions
See **Diatrizoate meglumine.**

Composition and Supply
Injection   52%, in 20 ml vials
Injection   10.3%, in 100 ml bottles

Legal Status
Prescription

Iodipamide meglumine/diatrizoate meglumine (Sinografin®)

See DIAGNOSTICS, roentgenography.

Iodochlorhydroxyquin (Vioform®)

Action and Use
Local anti-infective.

Dosage and Administration
Apply 2 or 3 times a day.

Cautions
May prove irritating to sensitized skin in rare cases.

Adverse Reactions
May cause stains.

Composition and Supply
Cream and ointment   3%
Cream and ointment   3% with hydrocortisone 0.5%
Cream and ointment   3% with hydrocortisone 1%
Lotion   3% with hydrocortisone 1%

Legal Status
Nonprescription (preparations without hydrocortisone)
Prescription (preparations with hydrocortisone)

Iodoform

See ANTI-INFECTIVES, miscellaneous antiseptic-disinfectants.

Ionamin® (phentermine resin)

See CEREBRAL STIMULANTS, anorectics.

Iopanoic acid (Telepaque®)

Action and Use
Contrast medium used in cholecystography and cholangiography.

Dosage and Administration
3 to 6 g, orally.

Cautions
Iopanoic acid is a potent cholinesterase inhibitor. Use cautiously in patients with renal and hepatic disease. Interferes with BSP and PBI determinations.

Adverse Reactions
Sensitivity may occur in persons who are allergic to iodine. Possible effects include nausea, vomiting, diarrhea, skin reaction, dry throat, dizziness, headache, and dysuria.

Composition and Supply
Tablets   500 mg

Legal Status
Prescription

Iophendylate (Pantopaque®)

See DIAGNOSTICS, roentgenography.

Iothalamate meglumine (Conray®)

Action and Use
Contrast medium.

Dosage and Administration
20 to 50 ml, IV, with dosage adjusted to procedure performed.

Cautions
There is a potential for anaphylaxis. Administer cautiously in patients with renal disease, systemic disease, allergies, and asthma. May interfere with thyroid laboratory tests. See **Diatrizoate meglumine** for further cautions.

Adverse Reactions
See **Diatrizoate meglumine.**

Composition and Supply
Injection   60%, in 20 ml and 30 ml vials

Legal Status
Prescription

Ipecac syrup

Action and Use
Expectorant and emetic.

Dosage and Administration
Emetic: 15 ml; second dose is given after 20 to 30 minutes if needed. *Expectorant:* 1 to 2 ml.

Cautions
If patient does not vomit, dosage should be recovered by gastric lavage. See **Apomorphine hydrochloride.**

Adverse Reactions
Alkaloids of ipecac may be toxic if absorbed.

Composition and Supply
Syrup

Legal Status
Nonprescription

Ipodate (Oragrafin®)

Action and Use
Contrast medium used in oral cholecystography.

Dosage and Administration
3 to 6 g.

Cautions
See **Iopanoic acid.**

Adverse Reactions
See **Iopanoic acid.**

Composition and Supply
Capsules   500 mg (Oragrafin® Sodium)
Packets   3 g (Oragrafin® Calcium)

Legal Status
Prescription

Iron dextran injection (Imferon®)

Action and Use
Hematinic used to correct iron deficiency anemia.

Dosage and Administration
Dosage is individualized and ranges from 100 to 250 mg daily, IM or
IV. Test dose (25 mg) given to rule out sensitivity.

Cautions
It is recommended that iron dextran be given IM (by Z track method).
Not more than 5 ml should be given IV in 2 minutes. Hypersensitivity
and anaphylaxis may occur, especially after IV administration. Use
with caution in patients with liver impairment and in pregnant
women.

Adverse Reactions
Pain may occur at intramuscular site. Local reaction is possible, with
soreness and inflammation. Symptoms that may appear ½ hour to 24
hours after injection include dizziness, syncope, fever, chills, rash,
urticaria, chest pain, backache, generalized body aches, encephalopathy, convulsions, generalized lymphadenopathy, and leukemoid
reactions. Hemosiderosis may occur with an overdose or with prolonged therapy.

Composition and Supply
Injection   elemental iron 50 mg/ml, in 2 ml and 5 ml ampuls
Injection   elemental iron 50 mg/ml with 0.5% phenol, in 10 ml vials
   (*Note:* for IM use only)

Legal Status
Prescription

I-sedrin®

See **Ephedrine sulfate.**

Ismelin®

See **Guanethidine sulfate.**

Iso-Bid®

See **Isosorbide dinitrate.**

Isocarboxazid (Marplan®)

Action and Use
Potent MAO inhibitor with antidepressant activity; its main use is in treatment of patients not responsive to other antidepressants or to ECT.

Dosage and Administration
30 mg initially, followed by 10 to 20 mg daily as maintenance, orally.

Cautions
Contraindicated in patients with congestive heart failure or pheochromocytoma. Concomitant use with tricyclic antidepressants, such as imipramine, has produced serious toxicity; there should be a 2 week period without MAO inhibitors before the patient begins to receive tricyclic antidepressants. A possibly fatal hypertensive crisis may result if isocarboxazid is combined with adrenergic drugs and foods high in tryptophan (broad beans) and tyramine (cheese, beers, wines, pickled herring, chicken livers, and yeast extract). The patient should avoid excessive amounts of caffeine.

Adverse Reactions
The most frequent side effect is postural hypotension with dizziness, weakness, and faintness. Occasional side effects include dry mouth, blurred vision, constipation, anorexia, headache with hypertension, skin reactions, edema, weight gain, euphoria, hyperactivity, confusion, agitation, hallucinations, delirium, muscle twitching, tremors, and convulsions. Rare effects include black tongue, akathisia, ataxia, coma, dysuria, urinary retention, incontinence, delayed ejaculation, impotence, neuritis, and photosensitivity. Side effects of an overdose include hypotension, tachycardia, coma, convulsions, respiratory depression, sluggish reflexes, pyrexia, and diaphoresis.

Composition and Supply
Tablets   10 mg

Legal Status
Prescription

Isoflurophate (Floropryl®)

See MIOTICS.

Isoniazid (INH) (Nydrazid®)

Action and Use
Adjunctive antitubercular agent used in treatment and preventive therapy.

Dosage and Administration
Treatment, in adults: 5 mg/kg, up to 300 mg (single dose) daily, orally or IM.
Treatment, in children: 10 to 30 mg/kg, up to 500 mg (single dose) daily, orally.
Prevention, in adults: 300 mg per day (single dose), orally or IM.
Prevention, in children: 10 mg/kg, up to 300 mg (single dose) daily, orally or IM.

Cautions
Must be administered along with pyridoxine (50 to 100 mg per day) to prevent peripheral neuritis. Use cautiously in patients with pre-existing hepatic disease, renal dysfunction, or convulsive disorders.

Adverse Reactions
Common side effects include nausea and vomiting, constipation, dry mouth, urinary retention in males, headache, insomnia, and orthostatic hypotension. Large doses may produce convulsions. Irritation may result from intramuscular injection.

Composition and Supply
Injection   100 mg/ml, in 10 ml vials
Syrup   50 mg/5 ml
Tablets   100 mg and 300 mg
Tablets   100 mg with pyridoxine 5 mg (Uniad Plus 5™)

Legal Status
Prescription

Isopaque® 280 (metrizoate meglumine/metrizoate/calcium)

See DIAGNOSTICS, roentgenography.

Isopaque® 440 (metrizoate meglumine/metrizoate sodium/metrizoate calcium/metrizoate magnesium)

See DIAGNOSTICS, roentgenography.

Iso-Par® (coparaffinate)

See ANTI-INFECTIVES, LOCAL, fungicides.

Isopropamide iodide (Darbid®)

See ANTICHOLINERGICS.

Isopropamide iodide/prochlorperazine (Combid®)

See ANTICHOLINERGICS.

Isopropyl alcohol

Action and Use
Disinfectant, solvent, and "rubbing compound."

Dosage and Administration
50 to 99%, applied topically.

Cautions
Highly toxic if taken by mouth. Flammable.

Adverse Reactions
Irritating to sensitive areas.

Composition and Supply
Isopropyl alcohol   99%
Isopropyl rubbing alcohol   70%

Legal Status
Nonprescription

Isoproterenol hydrochloride (Isuprel®)

Isoproterenol sulfate (Medihaler-Iso®, Norisodrine®)

Action and Use
Bronchodilator in the treatment of asthma and adjunct in the treatment of shock, cardiac arrest, carotid sinus hypersensitivity, Adams-Stokes syndrome, and ventricular tachycardia and arrhythmias.

Dosage and Administration
Inhalation: administered with a metered aerosol, as directed.
Sublingual: 10 to 20 mg 3 or 4 times a day, with a maximum dose of 60 mg per day.
Injection: diluted solution given by IV infusion according to manufacturer's directions.

Cautions

Injection may be detrimental to myocardial function in patients who are in cardiogenic shock as a result of coronary artery occlusion and myocardial infarction. Use cautiously in patients with heart disease, hyperthyroidism, hypertension, diabetes, or tuberculosis. Should not be used concurrently with epinephrine (serious arrhythmias might result). Hypovolemia should be corrected before treatment with isoproterenol begins (to prevent hypotension). The inhalation preparation should not be used if a precipitate or brownish discoloration is observed. Isoproterenol may be habituating.

Adverse Reactions

The usual dosage may produce transient headache, nervousness, palpitations, tachycardia, hypertension, substernal pain, dizziness, tremors, nausea, vomiting, diaphoresis, and flushing of the face. Severe symptoms may include acute cardiac dilatation, pulmonary edema, and shock. Cardiac arrhythmias can occur. Large or repeated doses may lead to myocardial necrosis or cardiac arrest when the heart is subjected to an increased work load.

Composition and Supply

Injection   1 : 5,000, in 1 ml and 5 ml ampuls (Isuprel®)
Solution, inhalant   0.25%, 0.5%, and 1%
Tablets, sublingual   10 mg and 15 mg (Isuprel®)

Legal Status

Prescription

Isopto®Atropine

See under **Atropine sulfate.**

Isopto® Carbachol

See **Carbachol.**

Isopto® Carpine

See **Pilocarpine hydrochloride.**

Isopto® Tears

See **Hydroxypropyl methylcellulose.**

Isordil®

See **Isosorbide dinitrate.**

Isosorbide dinitrate (Iso-Bid®, Isordil®, Laserdil®, Sorate®, Sorbitrate®)

Action and Use
Coronary vasodilator for the treatment and prevention of angina pectoris.

Dosage and Administration
Sublingual tablets: 5 to 10 mg every 2 or 3 hours.
Tablets: 5 to 30 mg every 4 hours.
Sustained-release capsules and tablets: 1 every 6 to 12 hours.

Cautions
Use cautiously in patients with glaucoma. Tolerance may occur.

Adverse Reactions
See **Nitroglycerin.**

Composition and Supply
Tablets   5 mg, 10 mg, and 20 mg
Tablets, chewable   5 mg and 10 mg
Tablets, sublingual   2.5 mg and 5 mg
Tablets and capsules, sustained-release   40 mg

Legal Status
Prescription

Isovex-100® (ethaverine hydrochloride)

See ANTISPASMODICS; VASODILATORS, PERIPHERAL.

Isoxsuprine hydrochloride (Vasodilan®)

Action and Use
Peripheral and cerebral vasodilator.

Dosage and Administration
5 to 20 mg 3 or 4 times a day, orally; 5 to 10 mg 2 or 3 times a day, IM.

Cautions
Use with caution in patients with hypotension or tachycardia.

Adverse Reactions
Occasional effects include transient hypotension, tachycardia, weakness, dizziness, nervousness, and trembling. Severe rash is a rare effect.

Composition and Supply
Injection   5 mg/ml, in 2 ml ampuls
Tablets   10 mg

Legal Status
Prescription

Isuprel®

See **Isoproterenol hydrochloride.**

Janimine®

See **Imipramine hydrochloride.**

Kafocin® (cephaloglycin)

See ANTIBIOTICS, cephalosporins.

Kanamycin sulfate (Kantrex®)

Action and Use
Broad-spectrum antibiotic, especially useful against gram-negative bacteria.

Dosage and Administration
Intestinal action: in hepatic coma, 8 to 12 g daily in divided doses, orally; in preoperative bowel sterilization, 1 g every hour for 4 hours followed by 1 g every 6 hours for 36 to 72 hours.
Systemic infections: 15 mg/kg per day (maximum 1.5 g) in divided doses every 8 to 10 hours, IM or IV.

Cautions
Kanamycin sulfate is nephrotoxic and ototoxic; the concurrent use of other nephrotoxic and ototoxic drugs should be avoided.

Adverse Reactions
Nausea, vomiting, diarrhea, stomatitis, and proctitis may occur. Less common effects include hypersensitivity (eosinophilia, fever, rash, pruritus, and anaphylaxis), superinfection, paresthesias, nervousness, headache, bulging fontanel, blurred vision, sensory involvement of ninth cranial nerve, and tachycardia. Prolonged therapy or high dosage may damage the kidneys and eighth cranial nerve. Intramuscular injections may result in pain, nodules, and sterile abscesses (rotate injection sites and use deep injection).

Composition and Supply
Capsules   500 mg
Injection   500 mg/2 ml vials; 1 g/3 ml vials
Injection, pediatric   75 mg/2 ml vials

Legal Status
Prescription

Kantrex®

See **Kanamycin sulfate.**

Kanulase® (pepsin/pancreatin/cellulase/glutamic acid/ox bile extract)

See ANTIFLATULENTS; DIGESTANTS.

Kaochlor®

See **Potassium chloride.**

Kaolin/pectin (Kaopectate®)

Action and Use
Adsorbent antidiarrheal.

Dosage and Administration
60 to 120 ml after each bowel movement.

Cautions
Contraindicated in persons who display idiosyncratic reactions.

Adverse Reactions
None.

Composition and Supply
Suspension   kaolin 5.8 g/30 ml and pectin 130 mg/30 ml (Kao-pectate®)
Suspension   kaolin 8.8 g/30 ml and pectin 185 mg/30 ml (Kaopectate Concentrate®)
Suspension   kaolin 5.8 g/30 ml, pectin 130 mg/30 ml, and opium 15 mg/30 ml (Parepectolin®) (*Note:* dosage for Parepectolin® is 15 to 30 ml after each loose bowel movement)

Legal Status
Schedule V (Parepectolin®)
Nonprescription (Kaopectate®, Kaopectate Concentrate®)

Kaolin/pectin/belladonna alkaloids (Donnagel®)

Action and Use
Adsorbent (kaolin, pectin) and antispasmodic (belladonna alkaloids) indicated for diarrhea and acute gastrointestinal upsets.

Dosage and Administration
Diarrhea: 30 ml at once and 15 or 30 ml after each stool.
Other conditions: 15 ml every 3 hours as necessary.

Cautions
Contraindicated in patients with glaucoma and in those with advanced renal or hepatic disease. Administer with care in patients with incipient glaucoma or urinary bladder neck disease obstruction.

Adverse Reactions
Possible but uncommon side effects include blurring of vision, dry mouth, difficult urination, flushing, and dryness of skin.

Composition and Supply
Suspension   kaolin 6 g/30 ml, pectin 142.8 mg/30 ml, hyoscyamine sulfate 104 μg/30 ml, atropine sulfate 19.4 μg, and hyoscine hydrochloride 6.5 μg (Donnagel®)
Suspension   Donnagel® with opium 24 mg/30 ml (Donnagel®-PG)

Legal Status
Nonprescription (Donnagel®)
Prescription (Donnagel®-PG)

Kaon®

See **Potassium gluconate.**

Kaon-Cl® Tabs

See **Potassium chloride oral.**

Kaopectate®

See **Kaolin/pectin.**

Kay Ciel®

See **Potassium chloride oral.**

Kayexalate®

See **Sodium polystyrene sulfonate.**

Keflex®

See **Cephalexin.**

Keflin®Neutral

See **Cephalothin sodium.**

Kefzol® (cefazolin)

See ANTIBIOTICS, cephalosporins.

Kemadrin®

See **Procyclidine hydrochloride.**

Kenacort®

See **Triamcinolone.**

Kenalog®

See **Triamcinolone.**

Keralyt®

See **KERATOLYTICS.**

Ketaject® (ketamine hydrochloride)

See **ANESTHETICS, general.**

Ketalar® (ketamine hydrochloride)

See **ANESTHETICS, general.**

Ketamine hydrochloride (Ketaject®, Ketalar®)

See **ANESTHETICS, general.**

Kinesed® (belladonna alkaloids/phenobarbital/simethicone)

See **ANTICHOLINERGICS.**

K-Lor®

See **Potassium chloride oral.**

K-Lyte®

See **Potassium bicarbonate/potassium citrate.**

Koāte® (antihemophilic factor [human] VIII)

See **HEMOSTATICS.**

Kolyum®

See under **Potassium gluconate.**

Konakion®

See **Phytonadione.**

Konsyl®

See **Psyllium hydrophilic mucilloid.**

Konȳne® (antihemophilic factor [human] IX)

See HEMOSTATICS.

K-Phos® (potassium acid phosphate)

See ELECTROLYTE SOLUTIONS AND WATER-BALANCE AGENTS, acidifying agents.

Kwell®

See **Gamma benzene hexachloride.**

Lactinex®

See *Lactobacillus acidophilus/L. bulgaricus.*

Lactobacillus acidophilus/L. bulgaricus (Lactinex®)

Action and Use
Antidiarrheal; also useful in treatment of fever blisters and canker sores. Acts by helping to restore the normal intestinal flora.

Dosage and Administration
4 tablets or 1 packet of granules 3 or 4 times a day with milk.

Cautions
Should not be used without medical direction for more than 2 days, in patients with high fever, or in children under 3 years of age.

Adverse Reactions
May produce increase in flatus at onset of therapy, but this effect usually subsides with continued therapy.

Composition and Supply
Capsules with sodium carboxymethylcellulose   100 mg (Bacid®)
Tablets and granules

Legal Status
Nonprescription

Lactulose syrup (Cephulac™)

See ELECTROLYTE SOLUTIONS AND WATER-BALANCE AGENTS, ammonia detoxicants.

Lanatoside C (Cedilanid®)

See CARDIACS, cardiac glycosides.

Lanolin (hydrous wool fat)

See EMOLLIENT-PROTECTANTS.

Lanolin, anhydrous

See EMOLLIENT-PROTECTANTS.

Lanoxin®

See **Digoxin.**

Larodopa®

See **Levodopa.**

Larotid®

See **Amoxicillin.**

Lasan® Unguent

See **Anthralin.**

Laserdil®

See **Isosorbide dinitrate.**

Lasix®

See **Furosemide.**

Lassar's paste

See under **Zinc oxide.**

L.C.D.

See under **Coal tar.**

Ledercillin® VK

See **Penicillin V potassium.**

Lederplex® Capsules

See VITAMINS, MULTIPLE, oral.

Leritine®

See **Anileridine.**

Letter®

See **Levothyroxine sodium.**

Leucovorin calcium (citrovorum factor)

Action and Use
Antidote for overdose of folic acid antagonists; also used in the treatment of megaloblastic anemias.

Dosage and Administration
Antidote: dosage in amounts equal to weight of antagonist given, IM.
Megaloblastic anemia: up to a maximum of 1 mg daily, IM.

Cautions
Not to be used in pernicious anemia and other megaloblastic anemias resulting from a deficiency in vitamin B_{12}.

Adverse Reactions
Allergic sensitization may occur.

Composition and Supply
Injection   3 mg/ml, in 1 ml ampuls

Legal Status
Prescription

Leukeran®

See **Chlorambucil.**

Levallorphan tartrate (Lorfan®)

Action and Use
Narcotic antagonist used in counteracting acute narcotic poisoning.

Dosage and Administration
1 mg IV followed, if required, by 500 μg at 10 to 15 minute intervals; the maximum dose is 3 mg. In children, IM or SC route may be used if necessary.

Cautions
Should not be relied on as the sole agent in patients with severe depression. Not effective against respiratory depression resulting from barbiturates, anesthetics, or other nonnarcotic depressants. Should not be used to treat narcotic addicts.

Adverse Reactions
Dysphoria, miosis, lethargy, dizziness, drowsiness, gastric upset, pallor, and perspiration may occur. High doses may produce hallucinations, weird dreams, and disorientation.

Composition and Supply
Injection   1 mg/ml, in 1 ml ampuls and 10 ml vials

Legal Status
Prescription

Levarterenol bitartrate (Levophed®)

Action and Use
Peripheral vasoconstrictor used to restore and maintain blood pressure in all acute hypotensive or shock states.

Dosage and Administration
4 ml of 0.2% solution is added to 1 liter of 5% dextrose solution and given by IV infusion at a rate of flow adjusted to establish and maintain a low normal blood pressure (the usual rate of flow is 0.5 to 1 ml per minute).

Cautions
Except in dire emergencies, hypovolemia should always be corrected as fully as possible before administration of levarterenol. Must be administered carefully to avoid hypertension and cardiac arrhythmias (pressure should be checked every 2 minutes initially, and then every 5 minutes until the desired level is attained, usually 80 to 100 mm Hg systolic). Levarterenol is contraindicated while cyclopropane anesthesia is being used, and it should not be used if the color of the solution is brown. The infusion should be started in a large vein, especially the antecubital vein, to decrease risk of necrosis of overlying skin from prolonged vasoconstriction. Avoid using leg veins in elderly patients or in those with occlusive vascular diseases. Avoid extravasation with resulting blanching, ischemia, sloughing of tissues, necrosis, or even gangrene (caused by vasoconstriction). (*Note:* Local infiltration of the area with phentolamine, an alpha-adrenergic blocking agent that antagonizes the local vasoconstrictor effect of levarterenol, may prevent tissue damage and necrosis. Phentolamine may be added prophylactically to the infusion.)

Adverse Reactions
Tremors, nervous apprehension, palpitation, and precordial distress may be observed. Severe side effects include acute cardiac dilatation, pulmonary edema, respiratory difficulty, bradycardia, and headache. An overdose or a conventional dose in hypersensitive persons (for example, patients with hyperthyroidism) may cause severe hypertension with violent headache, photophobia, stabbing

retrosternal and pharyngeal pain, pallor, intense perspiration, and vomiting.

Composition and Supply
Injection   2 mg/ml (0.2%), in 4 ml ampuls

Legal Status
Prescription

Levodopa (Bendopa®, Dopar®, Larodopa®)

Action and Use
Levodopa, a metabolic precursor of the neurohormone dopamine, is useful in the symptomatic treatment of idiopathic Parkinson's disease, postencephalitic parkinsonism, and symptomatic parkinsonism resulting from carbon monoxide and manganese poisoning.

Dosage and Administration
Dosage is carefully individualized; total daily dosage should not exceed 8 g, orally.

Cautions
Contraindicated in patients receiving adrenergics or MAO inhibitors and in those with narrow-angle glaucoma, suspicious skin lesions, or a history of melanoma. The therapeutic effects are antagonized by pyridoxine. Use cautiously in patients with a history of myocardial infarction, bronchial asthma, emphysema, convulsions, strokes, neuroses, psychoses, or wide-angle glaucoma.

Adverse Reactions
Nausea, vomiting, anorexia, dry mouth, dysphagia, sialorrhea, dizziness, weakness, insomnia, anxiety, and fatigue are relatively common. Adventitious movements are the most frequent serious reactions. Other less frequent serious reactions include cardiac irregularities, orthostatic hypotension, and mental changes. Gastrointestinal bleeding, duodenal ulcers, hypertension, phlebitis, hemolytic anemia, agranulocytosis, and convulsions are rarer effects. Elevations of BUN, SGOT, SGPT, LDH, PBI, and alkaline phosphatase levels have been reported.

Composition and Supply
Capsules   100 mg, 250 mg, and 500 mg
Tablets   100 mg, 250 mg, and 500 mg
Tablets   levodopa with carbidopa
    carbidopa 10 mg with levodopa 100 mg (Sinemet®-10/100)
    carbidopa 25 mg with levodopa 250 mg (Sinemet®-25/250)

Note: carbidopa potentiates levodopa; the maximum dosage should not exceed 8 tablets of Sinemet®-25/250.

Legal Status
Prescription

Levophed®

See **Levarterenol bitartrate.**

Levopropoxyphene napsylate (Novrad®)

See ANTITUSSIVES AND EXPECTORANTS, antitussives.

Levothyroxine sodium (Letter®, Synthroid®)

Action and Use
Thyroid hormone.

Dosage and Administration
The dosage is individualized, starting at low levels. For most patients the final dosage is 100 to 400 μg daily, orally, IM, or IV.

Cautions
Use cautiously in patients with angina pectoris and other cardiovascular disorders. Contraindicated in patients with myocardial infarction and thyrotoxicosis.

Adverse Reactions
Essentially the same as adverse reactions to thyroid.

Composition and Supply
Injection   500 μg
Tablets   25 μg, 50 μg, 100 μg, 150 μg, 200 μg, 300 μg, and
    500 μg

Legal Status
Prescription

Levsin® (hyoscyamine sulfate)

See ANTICHOLINERGICS.

Levugen® (fructose 5% and 10%)

See PARENTERAL ALIMENTATION.

Librax® (clidinium bromide/chlordiazepoxide hydrochloride)

See ANTICHOLINERGICS.

Librium®

See **Chlordiazepoxide hydrochloride.**

Lidex®

See **Fluocinonide.**

Lidocaine hydrochloride (Xylocaine®)

Action and Use
Local anesthetic, antiarrhythmic.

Dosage and Administration
Arrhythmias:
Continuous infusion: Initial bolus of 100 mg is followed by IV infusion given at a rate of 20 to 50 µg per kg per minute. Solutions prepared by adding 1 g of lidocaine to 1 liter of 5% dextrose in water (the preferred diluent).

Intramuscular: The recommended dose is 300 mg delivered in the deltoid muscle, the preferred site. If necessary, an additional injection may be given 60 to 90 minutes later. *Note: Injections should be made with frequent aspirations to avoid possible inadvertent injection into a vein.*

Local anesthesia: used in infiltration, peripheral nerve block, and central neural block techniques.

Cautions
Constant monitoring of electrocardiogram and blood pressure is essential during IM and IV administration; resuscitative drugs and equipment should be available. Use extreme caution in patients with liver disease or congestive heart failure. Contraindicated in patients with Adams-Stokes syndrome or with severe degrees of sinoatrial, atrioventricular, or intraventricular heart block. In sinus bradycardia the elimination of ventricular ectopic beats without prior acceleration of heart rate (by isoproterenol or by electronic pacing) may provoke more frequent and more serious ventricular arrhythmias.

Adverse Reactions
Toxic reactions are similar to those produced by procaine. CNS reactions may include nervousness, dizziness, blurred vision, and tremors, followed by drowsiness, convulsions, unconsciousness, and possibly respiratory arrest. Cardiovascular reactions may include hypotension, myocardial depression, bradycardia, and possibly cardiac arrest.

Composition and Supply
Injection (IM) for cardiac arrhythmias: 100 mg/ml, in 5 ml ampuls
Injection (IV) for cardiac arrhythmias: 5 ml, 100 mg ampuls; 5 ml, 100 mg prefilled syringes; and 1 and 2 g vials
Injection 0.5%: 2 ml, 30 ml, and 50 ml vials
Injection 1%: 2 ml, 5 ml, and 30 ml ampuls; 20 ml, 30 ml, 50 ml, and 100 ml vials; and 5 ml prefilled syringes
Injection 1.5%: 20 ml ampuls

Injection 2%: 2 ml and 10 ml ampuls; and 20 ml and 50 ml vials
Injection 5% with dextrose: 2 ml ampuls
Injection 0.5% with epinephrine 1 : 200,000: 50 ml vials
Injection 1% with epinephrine 1 : 200,000: 30 ml ampuls
Injection 1% with epinephrine 1 : 100,000: 20 ml and 50 ml vials
Injection 2% with epinephrine 1 : 200,000: 20 ml ampuls and 20 ml
vials
Injection 2% with epinephrine 1 : 100,000: 20 ml and 50 ml vials

Legal Status
Prescription

Limbitrol®

See under **Chlordiazepoxide hydrochloride.**

Lincocin®

See **Lincomycin hydrochloride.**

Lincomycin hydrochloride (Lincocin®)

Action and Use
Antibiotic effective against most common gram-positive pathogens.

Dosage and Administration
500 mg every 6 to 8 hours, orally; 600 mg to 1.2 g, daily, IM; 600 mg
every 8 to 12 hours, IV.

Cautions
Can cause severe, possibly fatal colitis. Use cautiously in patients with
gastrointestinal, kidney, liver, or endocrine disease and in those with
a history of asthma or pronounced allergies.

Adverse Reactions
Oral preparations may cause glossitis, stomatitis, nausea, vomiting,
and diarrhea. Superinfections are common. Other side effects include
pruritus, rash, urticaria, vaginitis, angioedema, anaphylaxis, photosensitivity, and cardiopulmonary arrest. Hypotension, leukopenia,
agranulocytosis, and purpura are possible after parenteral administration. Abnormal results from liver function tests occur rarely.

Composition and Supply
Capsules   250 mg and 500 mg
Injection   300 mg/ml, in 2 ml vials
Syrup   250 mg/5 ml

Legal Status
Prescription

Lioresal® (baclofen)

See SKELETAL MUSCLE RELAXANTS.

Liothyronine sodium (Cytomel®)

Action and Use
Thyroid replacement.

Dosage and Administration
25 µg per day initially, then increased by increments to a maintenance dose as determined by the response.

Cautions
Use cautiously in patients with angina pectoris or other cardiovascular disorders. Contraindicated in patients with myocardial infarction or thyrotoxicosis. In rare instances, liothyronine sodium may precipitate a hyperthyroid state.

Adverse Reactions
Essentially the same as the adverse reactions for thyroid.

Composition and Supply
Tablets   5 µg, 25 µg, and 50 µg

Legal Status
Prescription

Liotrix® (Euthroid®, Thyrolar®)

See THYROID PREPARATIONS.

Lipase/amylase/protease/hemicellulase/bile constituents (Festal®)

See ANTIFLATULENTS.

Lipo-Hepin®

See **Heparin sodium injection.**

Lipo-Lutin®

See **Progesterone.**

Liquaemin®

See **Heparin sodium injection.**

Liquamar® (phenprocoumon)

See ANTICOAGULANTS.

Lithane®

See **Lithium carbonate.**

Lithium carbonate (Eskalith®, Lithane®, Lithonate®, Lithotabs™)

Action and Use
Used for the control of manic episodes in patients with manic depressive psychoses.

Dosage and Administration
Dosage is individualized, ranging from 300 to 600 mg 3 times a day, orally.

Cautions
Lithium carbonate is a highly toxic drug with a low margin of safety. Serum lithium levels should not exceed 2 mEq/L during the acute treatment phase or 1.5 mEq/L during maintenance. Restricted sodium diets may potentiate lithium toxicity. Contraindicated in patients with significant cardiovascular disease, renal disease, or brain damage.

Adverse Reactions
Nausea, thirst, and transient tremors are common. Occasional side effects include exophthalmos, leukocytosis, dermatitis, nephrogenic diabetes insipidus (with polydipsia), and polyuria. Nontoxic goiter is a rare side effect.

Composition and Supply
Capsules   300 mg
Tablets   300 mg

Legal Status
Prescription

Lithonate®

See **Lithium carbonate.**

Lithotabs™

See **Lithium carbonate.**

Locorten® (flumethasone pivalate)

See CORTICOSTEROIDS.

Loestrin®

See under **Norethindrone.**

Lomidine® (pentamidine)

See ANTIPROTOZOALS, antitrypanosomals.

Lomotil®

See **Diphenoxylate hydrochloride/atropine sulfate.**

Lomustine (CCNU) (Cee Nu®)

Action and Use
Antineoplastic indicated as a palliative in brain tumors and Hodgkin's disease.

Dosage and Administration
130 mg per square meter of body surface area every 6 weeks as a single dose.

Cautions
Bone marrow depression may occur; consequently weekly blood studies are necessary.

Adverse Reactions
Nausea, vomiting, stomatitis, anemia, or alopecia may occur.

Composition and Supply
Dose pack   2 capsules each of strengths 10 mg, 40 mg, and 100 mg

Legal Status
Prescription

Lo/Ovral® (norgestrel/ethinyl estradiol)

See CONTRACEPTIVES, ORAL.

Loperamide hydrochloride (Imodium®)

Action and Use
Antidiarrheal.

Dosage and Administration
4 mg initially followed by 2 mg after each unformed stool, up to 16 mg daily.

Cautions
Not to be used in acute diarrhea associated with organisms that penetrate intestinal mucosa. Not recommended in children under the age of 12. Should be discontinued if improvement is not observed in 48 hours.

Adverse Reactions
Possible effects include abdominal pain or discomfort, constipation, drowsiness or dizziness, dry mouth, nausea and vomiting, skin rash, and tiredness.

Composition and Supply
Capsules   2 mg

Legal Status
Prescription

Lorazepam (Ativan®)

See PSYCHOTROPICS, tranquilizers.

Lorelco® (probucol)

See ANTILIPEMICS.

Lorfan®

See **Levallorphan tartrate.**

Loridine®

See **Cephaloridine.**

Lorophyn® (phenylmercuric acetate)

See CONTRACEPTIVES, TOPICAL.

Loroxide® (benzoyl peroxide preparation)

See KERATOLYTICS.

Lotrimin® (clotrimazole)

See ANTI-INFECTIVES, LOCAL, fungicides.

Lotusate® (talbutal)

See SEDATIVE-HYPNOTICS, barbiturates.

Lowila® Cake

See **Sodium lauryl sulfoacetate.**

Loxapine succinate (Daxolin®, Loxitane®)

See PSYCHOTROPICS, antipsychotics.

Loxitane® (loxapine succinate)

See PSYCHOTROPICS, antipsychotics.

Lugol's solution

See under **Iodine.**

Luminal®

See **Phenobarbital.**

Luride®

See **Sodium fluoride.**

Lypressin (Diapid®)

See PITUITARY HORMONES.

Lysodren®

See **Mitotane.**

Maalox®

See **Magnesium hydroxide/aluminum hydroxide.**

Maalox® Plus

See under **Magnesium hydroxide/aluminum hydroxide.**

Macrodantin®

See **Nitrofurantoin.**

Macrodex® (dextran 70)

See ELECTROLYTE SOLUTIONS AND WATER-BALANCE AGENTS, plasma extenders.

Mafenide acetate cream (Sulfamylon®)

Action and Use
Topical anti-infective used in the treatment of second- and third-degree burns.

Dosage and Administration
Applied topically.

Cautions
Use with caution in patients who are hypersensitive or have allergies to sulfonamides, and in those with pulmonary or adrenal dysfunction.

Adverse Reactions
May cause burning when first applied. Eschar separation is delayed. Absorption may result in acidosis and respiratory embarrassment.

Composition and Supply
Cream   0.5%

Legal Status
Prescription

Magaldrate (Riopan®)

Action and Use
Antacid, low in sodium content (700 μg for each 400 mg).

Dosage and Administration
800 mg 4 times a day, between meals and at bedtime, orally.

Cautions
Contraindicated in patients with kidney failure.

Adverse Reactions
Rare.

Composition and Supply
Suspension   400 mg/5 ml
Tablets, regular and chewable   400 mg

Legal Status
Nonprescription

Magnesia magma

See **Magnesia, milk of.**

Magnesia, milk of (magnesia magma, magnesium hydroxide)

Action and Use
Antacid and laxative.

Dosage and Administration
Antacid: 5 to 10 ml, orally.
Laxative: 15 to 30 ml, orally.

Cautions
Increases absorption of sodium warfarin. Neurological, neuromuscular, and cardiovascular impairment may result in a patient with renal insufficiency. Contraindicated in patients with nausea, vomiting, or abdominal pain.

Adverse Reactions
Diarrhea and possibly slight acid rebound may occur.

Composition and Supply
Suspension 8% magnesium hydroxide

Legal Status
Nonprescription

Magnesium citrate solution (citrate of magnesia)

Action and Use
Cathartic.

Dosage and Administration
200 to 300 ml, orally.

Cautions
Contraindicated in patients with nausea, vomiting, abdominal pain, or kidney failure.

Adverse Reactions
Some distention may occur.

Composition and Supply
Solution (carbonated and flavored)

Legal Status
Nonprescription

Magnesium hydroxide

See **Magnesia, milk of.**

Magnesium hydroxide/aluminum hydroxide (Aludrox®, Creamalin®, Maalox®)

Action and Use
Antacid.

Dosage and Administration
Suspension: 10 to 20 ml 4 times a day after meals and at bedtime.
Tablets (No. 1): 2 to 4 after meals and at bedtime, well chewed or swallowed with water.
Tablets (No. 2): 1 or 2 after meals and at bedtime, well chewed.

Cautions
Not to be used with any form of tetracycline. Contraindicated in kidney failure.

Adverse Reactions
None.

Composition and Supply
Suspension   27 mEq/10 ml
Suspension with simethicone   magnesium hydroxide 200 mg/5 ml, aluminum hydroxide 225 mg/5 ml, and simethicone 25 mg/5 ml (Maalox® Plus)
Tablets   17 mEq/2 tablets (No. 1) and 18 mEq/tablet (No. 2)
Tablets with simethicone   magnesium hydroxide 200 mg/5 ml, aluminum hydroxide 200 mg/5 ml, and simethicone 25 mg/5 L (Maalox® Plus)

Legal Status
Nonprescription

Magnesium hydroxide/aluminum hydroxide/calcium carbonate
(Camalox®)

See ANTACIDS.

Magnesium hydroxide/aluminum hydroxide/simethicone
(Mylanta®)

Action and Use
Antacid and antiflatulent.

Dosage and Administration
Suspension: 5 or 10 ml 4 times a day between meals and at bedtime.
Tablets: 1 or 2 tablets (well chewed) 4 times a day between meals and at bedtime.

Cautions
See **Magnesium hydroxide/aluminum hydroxide.**

Adverse Reactions
None.

Composition and Supply
Suspension   aluminum hydroxide 200 mg/5 ml, magnesium hydroxide 200 mg/5 ml, and simethicone 20 mg/5 ml
Tablets   each tablet provides the same dosage as 5 ml of suspension
Suspension   aluminum hydroxide 400 mg/5 ml, magnesium hydroxide 400 mg/5 ml, and simethicone 30 mg/5 ml (Mylanta®-II)
Tablets   aluminum hydroxide 400 mg/5 ml, magnesium hydroxide 400 mg/5 ml, and simethicone 30 mg/5 ml (Mylanta®-II)

Legal Status
Nonprescription

Magnesium sulfate (Epsom salt)

Action and Use
Cathartic; solution used as a soak or compress for relief of inflammatory conditions.

Dosage and Administration
Cathartic: 15 g in glass of ice water as needed.
Topical: 25 to 50% aqueous solution.

Cautions
Contraindicated in patients with nausea, vomiting, abdominal pain, or kidney failure.

Adverse Reactions
Has a disagreeable taste.

Composition and Supply
Crystals and powder

Legal Status
Nonprescription

Magnesium sulfate injection

Action and Use
Anticonvulsant used for the prevention and control of seizures in preeclampsia and eclampsia. Magnesium ion supplement in hyperalimentation management of uterine tetany.

Dosage and Administration
Dosage is individualized and adjusted carefully to the patient's needs. The total daily dose should not exceed 30 to 40 g, IM (sometimes administered IV).

Cautions
The patient should not be left alone during the administration of this agent, because respiratory depression or cardiac arrest is possible. Serum magnesium levels should be monitored closely. Administer cautiously in patients with impaired renal function. Contraindicated in patients with heart block or myocardial damage.

Adverse Reactions
CNS depression may occur.

Composition and Supply
Injection   10%, 25%, and 50%

Legal Status
Prescription

Mandelamine®

See **Methenamine mandelate.**

Mannitol injection (Osmitrol®)

Action and Use
Osmotic diuretic; diagnostic agent used to determine glomerular filtration rate.

Dosage and Administration
Diuresis: dosage is individualized, administered by IV infusion.
Diagnosis: 280 ml of 7.2% solution (100 ml of 20% solution diluted with 180 ml of sodium chloride injection), infused at a rate of 20 ml per minute.

Cautions
Contraindicated in patients with anuria, pulmonary congestion, pulmonary edema, congestive heart disease, marked dehydration, or intracranial hemorrhage. There should be a filter on the infusion set when 20% mannitol is being administered.

Adverse Reactions
Common side effects include headache, nausea, circulatory overload, and hyponatremia. Occasional side effects include vomiting, fever, chills, mild chest pain, fluid and electrolyte imbalance, thirst, urinary retention, and rhinitis. Convulsions are a rare side effect.

Composition and Supply
Injection   5% and 10%, in 1,000 ml containers
Injection   15% and 20%, in 500 ml containers

Legal Status
Prescription

Maolate® (chlorphenesin carbamate)

See SKELETAL MUSCLE RELAXANTS.

Marax® (theophylline/ephedrine/hydroxyzine)

See ANTIASTHMATICS, xanthine preparations.

Marcaine®

See **Bupivacaine hydrochloride.**

Marezine®

See **Cyclizine hydrochloride.**

Marplan®

See **Isocarboxazid.**

Matulane®

See **Procarbazine hydrochloride.**

Maxidex®

See under **Dexamethasone.**

Mazindol (Sanorex®)

See CEREBRAL STIMULANTS, anorectics.

M-B Tabs

See **Methylene blue.**

Measles, mumps, and rubella virus vaccine, live (M-M-R)

See BIOLOGICALS, vaccines.

Measles virus vaccine, live attenuated (Attenuvax®)

Action and Use
Vaccine used to achieve active immunization against measles.

Dosage and Administration
0.5 ml SC, preferably into the outer aspect of the upper arm.

Cautions
Contraindications include active infection; concomitant use of corticosteroids, antineoplastic agents, or radiotherapy; pregnancy; malignancies involving bone marrow or lymphatic system; gamma globulin deficiency; and sensitivity to eggs, chicken, chicken feathers, or neomycin. Delay the administration of the vaccine for 12 weeks if the patient received a transfusion of whole blood or if more than 0.01 ml per pound of body weight of immune serum globulin was administered within preceding 6 weeks. Measles vaccine should be administered no less than 4 weeks after use of live attenuated poliomyelitis virus vaccine or smallpox vaccine. Schedule a tuberculin test before giving the vaccine to avoid the possibility of a false-negative response.

Adverse Reactions
Moderate fever may occur 7 to 10 days after vaccination. Generally, fever, rash, or both, appear between the fifth and twelfth days. A reaction at the injection site is possible in children who have been vaccinated with killed measles vaccine.

Composition and Supply
Injection   single-dose vials, with disposable syringes containing diluent (*Note:* keep vials in dark place at 2° to 8°C; discard reconstituted vaccine if not used within 8 hours)

Legal Status
Prescription

Mebaral®

See **Mephobarbital.**

Mebendazole (Vermox®)

Action and Use
Anthelmintic indicated for the treatment of *Trichuris trichiura* (whipworm), *Enterobius vermicularis* (pinworm), *Ascaris lumbricoides* (roundworm), and *Necator americanus* (American hookworm), in single or mixed infestations.

Dosage and Administration
Pinworm: 1 tablet, orally, 1 time.
Other indications: 1 tablet, orally, morning and evening, on 3 consecutive days.
Note: If patient is not cured three weeks after treatment, a second course of treatment is advised.

Cautions
Contraindicated in pregnant women and in children under 2 years of age. Relative benefit and risk should be considered.

Adverse Reactions
Possible abdominal pain and diarrhea in patients with massive infestation.

Composition and Supply
Tablets   100 mg

Legal Status
Prescription

329

Mechlorethamine hydrochloride (nitrogen mustard) (Mustargen®)

Action and Use
Antineoplastic.

Dosage and Administration
400 μg/kg, not to exceed 8 to 10 mg daily, IV.

Cautions
This is a highly toxic agent, especially to the bone marrow. It should not come into contact with skin or mucous membranes. Contraindicated in patients with infectious granuloma.

Adverse Reactions
The most common side effects include nausea, vomiting, diarrhea, amenorrhea, fever, tinnitus, deafness, metallic taste, headache, and alopecia. Local reactions to extravasation into subcutaneous tissue result in a severe, brawny, tender induration that may persist for a long time; in severe extravasation, a slough may result. (*Note:* the drug may be neutralized by injecting sodium thiosulfate 1% into the infiltrated tissue.) Thrombophlebitis and thrombosis rarely occur if the drug is injected into the tubing during the course of an IV infusion.

Composition and Supply
Vials   10 mg

Legal Status
Prescription

Meclizine hydrochloride (Antivert®, Bonine®)

Action and Use
Antiemetic used in the prevention and treatment of motion sickness; it also controls vertigo.

Dosage and Administration
25 to 100 mg daily in divided doses, orally.

Cautions
Drowsiness may occur. There may be additive effects when this drug is given with other CNS depressants. Contraindicated in pregnant women.

Adverse Reactions
Dry mouth and blurred vision are possible adverse reactions.

Composition and Supply
Tablets   12.5 mg and 25 mg

Legal Status
Prescription

Medihaler-Epi® (epinephrine bitartrate)

See ADRENERGICS; ANTIASTHMATICS, adrenergics.

Medihaler-Iso®

See **Isoproterenol sulfate.**

Medrol®

See **Methylprednisolone.**

Medroxyprogesterone acetate (Amen®, Depo-Provera®, Provera®)

Action and Use
Progestogen used in the treatment of amenorrhea, dysmenorrhea, functional uterine bleeding, and threatened abortion.

Dosage and Administration
2.5 to 30 mg daily, orally; 50 to 100 mg, IM.

Cautions
Contraindicated in patients with cancer of the breast and genitals, liver disease, kidney disease, or a history of thrombophlebitis or pulmonary embolism.

Adverse Reactions
Hypertension may occur in susceptible individuals. There may be dizziness or fatigue. When this drug is combined with estrogens, glucose tolerance may be decreased. Discontinue if a sudden alteration of vision occurs. See **Progesterone** for further cautions.

Composition and Supply
Injection   100 mg/ml, in 5 ml vials; and 400 mg/ml, in 2.5 ml and 10 ml vials (Depo-Provera®)
Tablets   2.5 mg and 10 mg (Provera®)
Tablets   10 mg (Amen®)

Legal Status
Prescription

Mefenamic acid (Ponstel®)

See ANALGESICS, nonnarcotic.

Megace®

See **Megestrol acetate.**

Megestrol acetate (Megace®)

Action and Use
Antineoplastic used to treat carcinoma of the breast and endometrium.

Dosage and Administration
Breast carcinoma: 160 mg daily in 4 divided doses, orally.
Endometrial carcinoma: 40 to 320 mg daily in divided doses, orally.

Cautions
Not recommended for use in other types of neoplastic disease. Use with caution in patients with a history of thrombophlebitis.

Adverse Reactions
No untoward effects have been reported.

Composition and Supply
Tablets   20 mg and 40 mg

Legal Status
Prescription

Mellaril®

See **Thioridazine hydrochloride.**

Melphalan (Alkeran®)

Action and Use
Nitrogen mustard antineoplastic used to treat multiple myeloma.

Dosage and Administration
6 mg daily, orally.

Cautions
This is a toxic drug, especially to bone marrow.

Adverse Reactions
Similar to adverse reactions to mechlorethamine hydrochloride (see).

Composition and Supply
Tablets   2 mg

Legal Status
Prescription

Menadiol sodium diphosphate (vitamin K) (Synkayvite®)

Action and Use
Synthetic water-soluble derivative of menadione (vitamin K_3) used in the treatment of hypoprothrombinemia resulting from poor absorption of vitamin K or the administration of salicylates.

Dosage and Administration
5 to 10 mg daily, orally; 6 to 75 mg, SC, IM, or IV, depending on the condition being treated.

Cautions
This agent does not counteract the anticoagulant action of heparin and may cause temporary resistance to prothrombin-depressing anticoagulants. It can induce hemolysis in patients with a deficiency of glucose-6-phosphate dehydrogenase in their red cells. Should be used with caution in patients with liver impairment. Contraindicated during last the few weeks of pregnancy. Check prothrombin time during the course of therapy.

Adverse Reactions
Large doses may cause decreased BSP excretion and prolongation of prothrombin time. In infants (especially premature babies), an excessive dose may produce hyperbilirubinemia, which may lead to kernicterus, brain damage, and possibly death.

Composition and Supply
Injection   5 mg/ml, in 1 ml ampuls; 10 mg/ml, in 1 ml ampuls; and
    75 mg/2 ml, in 2 ml ampuls
Tablets   5 mg

Legal Status
Prescription

Menest™

See **Estrogens, esterified.**

Menotropins (Pergonal®)

See GONADOTROPICS.

Menthol preparations (Derma Medicone®, Rhulicream®, Solarcaine®)

See ANTIPRURITICS, topical preparations.

Mepenzolate bromide (Cantil®)

See ANTICHOLINERGICS.

Mepenzolate bromide/phenobarbital (Cantil®-PHB)

See ANTIDIARRHEALS.

Meperidine hydrochloride (Demerol®)

Action and Use
Narcotic analgesic.

Dosage and Administration
50 to 150 mg every 3 to 4 hours, orally, SC, or IM.

Cautions
Meperidine hydrochloride is addicting, and may cause respiratory depression. It potentiates CNS depressants and MAO inhibitors. Blood pressure and respiration should be checked before administration. Solutions are physically incompatible with barbiturates.

Adverse Reactions
Pain at the injection site is possible; rotate the site to avoid local tissue irritation. Common systemic adverse responses include dizziness, lightheadedness, syncope, orthostatic hypotension, tachycardia, nausea, vomiting, and weakness. Other symptoms include diaphoresis, flushing, dry mouth, headache, euphoria, visual disturbances, disorientation, and possibly agitation. Uterine contractions are decreased. With overdose, meperidine may appear in the milk of nursing mothers. Toxicity produces dilated pupils, confusion, incoordination, tremors, convulsions, gradual coma, shock, respiratory depression, and possibly cardiac arrest.

Composition and Supply
Injection   50 mg/ml, 75 mg/ml, and 100 mg/ml, in ampuls, vials, and disposable syringes
Syrup   50 mg/5 ml
Tablets   50 mg and 100 mg

Legal Status
Schedule II

Mephenytoin (Mesantoin®)

Action and Use
Anticonvulsant.

Dosage and Administration
Dosage is adjusted to individual requirements; maintenance dose is 200 to 800 mg daily, in divided doses, orally.

Cautions
Mephenytoin should be used only after safer anticonvulsants have been given an adequate trial and have failed.

Adverse Reactions
Similar to adverse reactions to phenytoin sodium (see).

Composition and Supply
Tablets   100 mg

Legal Status
Prescription

Mephobarbital (Mebaral®)

Action and Use
Long-acting barbiturate used as a sedative and anticonvulsant.

Dosage and Administration
Epilepsy: 400 to 600 mg daily in divided doses, orally.
Sedative: 32 to 100 mg 3 or 4 times a day, orally.

Cautions
Drowsiness may occur. Potentiates other CNS depressants. Mephobarbital is habituating. Use cautiously if the patient is receiving phenytoin sodium. See **Phenobarbital** for further cautions.

Adverse Reactions
See **Phenobarbital.**

Composition and Supply
Tablets   30 mg, 50 mg, 100 mg, and 200 mg

Legal Status
Schedule IV

Mephyton®

See **Phytonadione.**

Mepivacaine hydrochloride (Carbocaine®)

Action and Use
Local anesthetic used for infiltration, nerve block, and caudal or other epidural blocks.

Dosage and Administration
5 to 7 mg/kg; the total dose should not exceed 1 g in any 24 hour period.

Cautions
Resuscitative equipment and drugs should be immediately available when any local anesthetic is used. Use cautiously in patients with allergies. High doses can cause cardiovascular depression.

Adverse Reactions
Adverse reactions are similar to those of lidocaine. Possible symptoms include excitation, depression, nervousness, dizziness, blurred vision, tremors, drowsiness, convulsions, unconsciousness, respiratory arrest, depression of myocardium, hypotension, cutaneous lesions, edema, and possibly anaphylactoid reactions.

Composition and Supply
Injection   1%, in 30 ml and 50 ml vials
Injection   1.5%, in 30 ml vials
Injection   2%, in 20 ml and 50 ml vials
Injection   3%, in 20 ml vials

Legal Status
Prescription

Meprednisone (Betapar®)

See CORTICOSTEROIDS.

Meprobamate (Equanil®, Miltown®)

Action and Use
Tranquilizer.

Dosage and Administration
400 mg 3 or 4 times a day, orally.

Cautions
Drowsiness may occur. Prolonged use can lead to addiction. May lower tolerance to alcohol. Contraindicated in patients with porphyria.

Adverse Reactions
Possible side effects include slurred speech, weakness, paresthesias, visual accommodation impairment, euphoria, overstimulation, diarrhea, arrhythmias, hypotensive crisis, skin eruptions, peripheral edema, fever, adenopathy, and syncope. Rare effects include hyperpyrexia, chills, angioneurotic edema, bronchospasm, oliguria, anuria, anaphylaxis, stomatitis, and proctitis. The effects of an overdose may

involve drowsiness, stupor, ataxia, coma, shock, and vasomotor and respiratory collapse.

Composition and Supply
Suspension, oral   200 mg/5 ml
Tablets   200 mg and 400 mg

Legal Status
Schedule IV

Mercaptomerin sodium (Thiomerin®)

Action and Use
Mercurial diuretic (reserved for use in patients who are resistant to other diuretics).

Dosage and Administration
Dosage is adjusted to the patient, ranging from 125 to 250 mg daily, SC or IM.

Cautions
Contraindicated in patients with renal insufficiency, ulcerative colitis, dehydration, or hypersensitivity to mercury. Store ready-to-use solution in refrigerator (but freezing should be avoided). Protect solution from light; do not use if a color or precipitate develops.

Adverse Reactions
Rather common side effects include hypotension, arrhythmias, cyanosis, and dyspnea. Other possible effects include: stomatitis, gingivitis, increased salivation, nausea, vomiting, diarrhea, hypochloremic alkalosis, cramps, lethargy, circulatory collapse, oliguria, azotemia, albuminuria, hematuria, thrombocytopenia, and agranulocytosis (the patient should be observed for sore throat and bleeding). Rare side effects include flushing, fever, chills, skin eruptions, and pruritus. Local irritation may occur at the injection site.

Composition and Supply
Injection   125 mg/ml, in 2 ml and 10 ml vials

Legal Status
Prescription

Mercaptopurine (6-MP) (Purinethol®)

Action and Use
Antineoplastic useful in the treatment of acute leukemia.

Dosage and Administration
Dosage is individualized; the usual initial dose is 2.5 mg/kg, orally.

Cautions
Mercaptopurine is highly toxic, especially to bone marrow.

Adverse Reactions
The principal toxic effect is bone marrow depression 4 to 6 weeks after dosage. A weekly blood examination is recommended; discontinue the drug at the first evidence of bone marrow depression. Other adverse reactions include nausea, vomiting, anorexia, diarrhea, and bloody stools. Large doses may result in stomatitis, mucosal ulcerations, jaundice, biliary stasis, and possibly liver damage. Skin eruptions occasionally develop.

Composition and Supply
Tablets 50 mg

Legal Status
Prescription

Mercocresols (Mercresin®)

See ANTI-INFECTIVES, LOCAL, miscellaneous antiseptic-disinfectants.

Mercresin® (mercocresols)

See ANTI-INFECTIVES, LOCAL, miscellaneous antiseptic-disinfectants.

Mercuric oxide, yellow

See ANTI-INFECTIVES, LOCAL, miscellaneous antiseptic-disinfectants.

Merethoxylline procaine (Dicurin®)

See DIURETICS.

Merthiolate® (thimerosal)

See ANTI-INFECTIVES, LOCAL, miscellaneous antiseptic-disinfectants.

Meruvax®

See **Rubella virus vaccine, live.**

Mesantoin®

See **Mephenytoin.**

Mesoridazine (Serentil®)

See PSYCHOTROPICS, antipsychotics.

Mestinon®

See **Pyridostigmine bromide.**

Metamucil®

See **Psyllium hydrophilic mucilloid.**

Metandren®

See **Methyltestosterone.**

Metaprel®

See **Metaproterenol sulfate.**

Metaproterenol sulfate (Alupent®, Metaprel®)

Action and Use
Bronchodilator.

Dosage and Administration
Oral: 20 mg 3 or 4 times a day.
Inhalation: dosage should not exceed 12 inhalations at 3- to 4-hour
intervals.

Cautions
Use cautiously in patients with hypertension, hyperthyroidism, diabetes, or cardiac problems. Avoid concomitant use with other adrenergic agents. Response to reserpine and guanethidine sulfate may be
diminished.

Adverse Reactions
Similar to adverse reactions to isoproterenol (see). The most common
side effects include tachycardia, hypertension, palpitations, nervousness, tremors, nausea, and vomiting. A bad taste may occur with
inhalants.

Composition and Supply
Inhalants   1.5%
Tablets   20 mg

Metaraminol bitartrate (Aramine®)

Action and Use
Vasopressor useful in shock and other hypotensive conditions.

Dosage and Administration
500 μg to 5 mg, IV; 2 to 10 mg, IM or SC.

Cautions
Monitor closely to avoid rapidly induced hypertension. Use cautiously in digitalized patients and those with hyperthyroidism, hypertension, heart disease, cirrhosis, and diabetes. Should not be used with halogenated anesthetics. In hypovolemic shock, blood volume should be corrected prior to metaraminol administration. Only normal saline or 5% dextrose injection should be used as diluent. Incompatible with phenytoin, methicillin, thiopental, warfarin, invert sugar solutions, protein hydrolysates, Ringer's injection, lactated Ringer's injection, and Solu-Cortef®.

Adverse Reactions
Headache, tachycardia, hypertension, dizziness, nervousness, reflex bradycardia, and occasionally sinus arrhythmia may occur.

Composition and Supply
Injection   10 mg/ml, in 1 ml ampuls and 10 ml vials

Legal Status
Prescription

Metaxalone (Skelaxin®)

See SKELETAL MUSCLE RELAXANTS.

Methacycline hydrochloride (Rondomycin®)

See ANTIBIOTICS, tetracyclines.

Methadone hydrochloride (Dolophine®)

Action and Use
Narcotic analgesic for severe pain and for treatment of narcotic addiction.

Dosage and Administration

When used as an analgesic, the dosage is 2.5 to 10 mg every 3 or 4 hours, orally, IM, or SC. (*Note:* for information about the use of methadone in detoxification treatment, the reader should consult the relevant literature and federal regulations.)

Cautions

An addicting drug, with the toxic potential of other narcotics. It produces slightly more severe respiratory depression than morphine does. Parenteral doses larger than 10 mg should not be given.

Adverse Reactions

Similar to adverse reactions to morphine, with less euphoria and no constipation. Addiction develops more slowly and withdrawal symptoms are less severe than with morphine.

Composition and Supply

Injection   10 mg/ml, in 1 ml ampuls and 20 ml vials
Tablets   5 mg and 10 mg

Legal Status

Schedule II

Methamphetamine hydrochloride (Fetamin®)

See CEREBRAL STIMULANTS, anorectic.

Methandrostenolone (Dianabol®)

See ANDROGENS.

Methantheline bromide (Banthīne®)

See ANTICHOLINERGICS.

Methapyrilene fumarate (Histadyl® Fumarate)

See ANTIHISTAMINES.

Methapyrilene hydrochloride (Histadyl®)

See ANTIHISTAMINES.

Methaqualone (Parest®, Quāālude®, Sopor®)

See SEDATIVE-HYPNOTICS, nonbarbiturates.

Metharbital (Gemonil®)

See ANTICONVULSANTS.

Methazolamide (Neptazane®)

See CARBONIC ANHYDRASE INHIBITORS.

Methdilazine hydrochloride (Tacaryl®)

See ANTIPRURITICS, systemic preparations.

Methenamine hippurate (Hiprex®, Urex®)
Methenamine mandelate (Mandelamine®)

Action and Use
Urinary tract antibacterial.

Dosage and Administration
1 g 4 times a day, orally.

Cautions
For therapy to be effective, the urine must have a pH of at least 5.5, and the urine should be monitored. Contraindicated in patients with renal or hepatic insufficiency.

Adverse Reactions
Hypersensitivity and gastric distress may occur; this can be minimized by administering the drug after meals or in enteric-coated form.

Composition and Supply
Tablets   1 g (Hiprex®, Urex®)
Tablets   250 mg, 500 mg, and 1 g (Mandelamine®)

Legal Status
Prescription

Methenamine mandelate/phenazopyridine hydrochloride (Azo-Mandelamine®)

See URINARY ANTISEPTICS.

Methenamine mandelate/phenazopyridine hydrochloride/belladonna alkaloids/phenobarbital (Donnasep®)

See URINARY ANTISEPTICS.

Methergine®

See **Methylergonovine maleate.**

Methicillin sodium (Celbenin®, Staphcillin®)

Action and Use
Antibiotic used in the treatment of staphylococcal infections caused by penicillinase-producing organisms.

Dosage and Administration
1 g every 4 or 6 hours, IM; 1 g every 6 hours using sodium chloride injection at the rate of 10 ml per minute, IV.

Cautions
Penicillin type allergies are possible. Bone marrow depression is also possible. See **Penicillin G potassium** for further cautions.

Adverse Reactions
See **Penicillin G potassium.**

Composition and Supply
Injection   1 g, 4 g, and 6 g vials
Injection   1 g, 2 g, 4 g, and 6 g piggyback bottles

Legal Status
Prescription

Methimazole (Tapazole®)

Action and Use
Antithyroid agent.

Dosage and Administration
5 to 20 mg 3 times a day, orally.

Cautions
See **Propylthiouracil.**

Adverse Reactions
See **Propylthiouracil.**

Composition and Supply
Tablets   5 mg and 10 mg

Legal Status
Prescription

Methionine (Pedameth®, Uracid®, Uranap®)

Action and Use
Methionine effects an ammonia-free urine and is indicated in control of odor in incontinent adults and in the management of diaper rash in infants.

Dosage and Administration
Odor control in adults: 200 mg, orally, 3 times daily with meals.
Diaper rash: 200 mg daily, added to evening formula or orange juice.

Cautions
Contraindicated in patients with a history of liver disease.

Adverse Reactions
Prolonged excessive doses may result in subnormal weight gain. Adequate protein intake should be assured during long periods of methionine therapy.

Composition and Supply
Capsules   200 mg
Liquid (Pedameth®)   75 mg/5 ml

Legal Status
Prescription

Methixene hydrochloride (Trest®)

See ANTICHOLINERGICS.

Methocarbamol (Robaxin®)

Action and Use
Skeletal muscle relaxant.

Dosage and Administration
1 to 1.5 g 4 times a day, orally; 300 mg to 3 g, IV.

Cautions
May cause color interference in certain screening tests for 5-HIAA and VMA. Safety has not been established in pregnant women and in children below the age of 12 years.

Adverse Reactions
Headache, lightheadedness, dizziness, drowsiness, and nausea may occur. There may also be allergic reactions, such as urticaria, pruritus, rash, and conjunctivitis.

Composition and Supply
Injection   100 mg/ml
Tablets   500 mg and 750 mg
Tablets   400 mg with aspirin 325 mg (Robaxisal®)

Legal Status
Prescription

Methohexital sodium (Brevital®)

Action and Use
Ultrashort-acting barbiturate anesthetic agent.

Dosage and Administration
Dosage is individualized according to the patient's response; the usual range is 5 to 12 ml of a 1% solution (50 to 120 mg), IV.

Cautions
Incompatible with acid solutions, such as atropine sulfate and succinylcholine chloride, and with silicone materials. See **Thiopental sodium** for further cautions.

Adverse Reactions
See **Thiopental sodium.**

Composition and Supply
Injection   500 mg, 2.5 g, and 5 g ampuls

Legal Status
Prescription

Methotrexate

Action and Use
Antineoplastic used to treat acute lymphocytic leukemia, gestational choriocarcinoma, and advanced stages of lymphosarcoma. Also useful in the control of refractory psoriasis.

Dosage and Administration
Dosage is individualized to the patient; administered orally, IM, IV, or intrathecally.

Cautions
Methotrexate is highly toxic (with a low therapeutic index), especially to the bone marrow and gastrointestinal tract. Toxicity may be increased with the concomitant use of salicylates, sulfonamides, phenytoin sodium, tetracycline, or chloramphenicol.

Adverse Reactions
Common side effects include nausea, vomiting, diarrhea, gastrointestinal ulcers, stomatitis, photosensitivity, bone marrow depression (the patient should be observed for infection and bleeding), and alopecia. Methotrexate may be hepatotoxic, especially at high dosage or with prolonged treatment. Other possible adverse reactions include malaise, fatigue, chills, fever, aggravated psoriasis, defective oogenesis or spermatogenesis, abortion, fetal defects, rash, pruritus, urticaria, depigmentation, acne, furunculosis, telangiectasia, headache, drowsi-

ness, blurred vision, aphasia, hemiparesis, paresis, convulsions, pneumonitis, metabolic changes (precipitating diabetes), and osteoporosis.

Composition and Supply
Injection 25 mg/ml, in 2 ml ampuls
Tablets 2.5 mg

Legal Status
Prescription

Methoxamine hydrochloride (Vasoxyl®)

See ADRENERGICS.

Methoxsalen (Oxsoralen®)

See ANTIPSORIATICS; EMOLLIENT-PROTECTANTS.

Methoxyflurane (Penthrane®)

See ANESTHETICS, general.

Methscopolamine bromide (Pamine®)

See ANTICHOLINERGICS.

Methsuximide (Celontin®)

Action and Use
Anticonvulsant used in the treatment of petit mal seizures refractory to other drugs.

Dosage and Administration
300 mg to 1.2 g per day, orally; the optimum dosage is determined by trial.

Cautions
There is a risk of possibly fatal fatal blood dyscrasias. Periodic blood counts are essential. Use cautiously in patients with liver or renal disease. Gastric irritation may occur. There may be CNS depression.

Adverse Reactions
Similar to adverse reactions to phenytoin sodium (see). In addition, anorexia is possible, and occasional dream-like states occur.

Composition and Supply
Capsules 150 mg and 300 mg

Legal Status
Prescription

Methychlothiazide (Enduron®)

See ANTIHYPERTENSIVES, diuretics.

Methylbenzethonium chloride (Dalidyne®)

See MOUTHWASHES.

Methyldopa (Aldomet®)

Action and Use
Antihypertensive.

Dosage and Administration
250 mg 2 or 3 times a day for 2 days, then adjusted to maintenance of 500 mg to 2 g daily in divided doses, orally; 250 mg to 1 g (maximum) at 6 hour intervals, IV.

Cautions
Methyldopa is contraindicated in patients with hepatic disease or pheochromocytoma. May cause false-positive Coombs' test results, hemolytic anemia, and liver disorders.

Adverse Reactions
Depression and sedation (larger doses should be taken at night) occur frequently. Occasional side effects include orthostatic hypotension, altered results in liver function tests, leukopenia, hemolytic anemia, thrombocytopenia, bradycardia, headache, dry mouth, sore or black tongue, nasal congestion, nausea, vomiting, diarrhea, constipation, edema, allergic reactions, pancytopenia, and positive results on tests for lupus erythematosus and rheumatoid factor. Other side effects include gynecomastia, impotence, decreased libido, lactation, extrapyramidal signs, nightmares, depression, skin eruptions, increased BUN levels, and angina type pains. Rarely, the patient's urine may darken upon exposure to air.

Composition and Supply
Injection (as methyldopate hydrochloride)   50 mg/ml, in 5 ml ampuls
Tablets   125 mg, 250 mg, and 500 mg
Tablets   250 mg with hydrochlorothiazide 15 mg (Aldoril®-15)
Tablets   250 mg with hydrochlorothiazide 25 mg (Aldoril®-25)

Legal Status
Prescription

Methylene blue (Urolene Blue®, M-B Tabs)

Action and Use
Mild antiseptic (of limited value) for urinary tract infections. Also used by injection for management of methemoglobinemia and as a diagnostic agent for outlining body cavities.

Dosage and Administration
Urinary antiseptic: 120 to 300 mg every 4 hours, orally.
Methemoglobinemia: 1 to 1.5 mg/kg, IV.

Cautions
Contraindicated in patients with renal insufficiency and in those allergic to methylene blue.

Adverse Reactions
Occasional side effects include nausea, vomiting, and diarrhea. Urine becomes blue-green in color. Large intravenous doses may cause nausea, abdominal and precordial pain, headache, diaphoresis, dizziness, and confusion.

Composition and Supply
Injection   1%
Tablets   65 mg, 120 mg, and 300 mg

Legal Status
Prescription

Methylergonovine maleate (Methergine®)

Action and Use
Oxytocic used to prevent or control postpartum hemorrhage.

Dosage and Administration
200 µg 3 or 4 times a day, orally; 200 µg (may be repeated in 2 or 4 hours), IM or IV.

Cautions
Contraindicated in pregnant women. Must be used cautiously in presence of sepsis or impaired renal or hepatic function. Use sparingly with vasopressors to avoid hypertensive reactions.

Adverse Reactions
See **Ergonovine maleate.**

Composition and Supply
Injection   200 µg/ml, in 1 ml ampuls
Tablets   200 µg

Legal Status
Prescription

Methylphenidate hydrochloride (Ritalin®)

Action and Use
Cerebral stimulant. Adjunctive therapy to other medical measures in minimal brain dysfunction in children. Methylphenidate is also effective in narcolepsy, mild depression, and apathetic or withdrawn senile behavior.

Dosage and Administration
Adults: 10 mg 2 or 3 times a day, orally.
Children: 5 mg per day, initially, gradually increased by increments of 5 to 10 mg per week. Daily recommended dosage not to exceed 60 mg.

Cautions
Habit-forming. May lower convulsive threshold in patients with history of seizures. Use cautiously in patients with hypertension. Contraindicated in patients with marked anxiety or glaucoma. Methylphenidate should not be used in children under 6 years of age nor should it be used for severe depression or in the prevention or treatment of normal fatigue states.

Adverse Reactions
The most common side effects are nervousness and insomnia. Less common effects include hypersensitivity with rash, urticaria, fever, dermatitis, arthralgia, vasculitis, anorexia, weight loss, drowsiness, dizziness, headache, dyskinesia, hypertension or hypotension, tachycardia, anemia, leukopenia, and thrombocytopenia. Other reported reactions include vomiting, tremors, euphoria, twitching, hallucinations, hyperpyrexia, psychosis, convulsions, palpitations, hypertension, diaphoresis, mydriasis, dryness of mucous membranes, and coma.

Composition and Supply
Tablets   5 mg, 10 mg, and 20 mg

Legal Status
Schedule II

Methylprednisolone (Medrol®)

Action and Use
Glucocorticoid.

Dosage and Administration
Oral: Initial dose is 4 to 96 mg per day, depending on disease being treated.
Intravenous (Solu-Medrol®): For shock, 250 mg every 4 to 6 hours (according to Melby); for other conditions, 10 to 40 mg.
Intramuscular, intra-articular, and intralesional (Depo-Medrol®): Dosage is highly individualized; range, 4 to 80 mg.

Cautions
Essentially the same as the cautions for cortisone acetate (see).

Adverse Reactions
Similar to adverse reactions to cortisone acetate (see), except that methylprednisolone causes less sodium and water retention.

Composition and Supply
Capsules, sustained release   4 mg
Injection (as sodium succinate salt)   40 mg, 125 mg, and 1,000 mg vials (Solu-Medrol®)
Injection (as acetate salt)   20 mg/ml, 40 mg/ml, and 80 mg/ml ampuls and vials (Depo-Medrol®)
Tablets   2 mg, 4 mg, and 16 mg

Legal Status
Prescription

Methyl salicylate (wintergreen oil)

Action and Use
Counterirritant.

Dosage and Administration
Applied topically.

Cautions
Irritant poison when taken by mouth, except as a flavoring agent. Excessive use may produce salicylism. Should not be used on denuded or irritated skin.

Adverse Reactions
Causes burning when applied to sensitive areas.

Composition and Supply
Liniment and ointment   10%

Legal Status
Nonprescription

Methyltestosterone (Android®, Metandren®, Oreton® Methyl, Testred®)

Action and Use
Androgen.

Dosage and Administration
Dosage must be strictly individualized according to use. Range, 15 to 50 mg daily, in divided doses, orally or buccally.

Cautions
Same as cautions for fluoxymesterone (see).

Adverse Reactions
Essentially the same as adverse reactions to fluoxymesterone (see).

Composition and Supply
Capsules   10 mg
Tablets   5 mg, 10 mg, and 25 mg
Tablets, buccal   5 mg, 10 mg, and 25 mg

Legal Status
Prescription

Methyprylon (Noludar®)

Action and Use
Hypnotic and sedative.

Dosage and Administration
Hypnotic: 200 to 400 mg, orally.
Sedative: 50 to 100 mg 3 or 4 times a day, orally.

Cautions
Methyprylon is habit-forming and is a potent CNS depressant. Should be used cautiously in patients with hepatic or renal disease. Total daily dose should not exceed 400 mg.

Adverse Reactions
Possible adverse effects include nausea, vomiting, constipation, diarrhea, morning drowsiness, dizziness, headache, rash, and pruritus. The effects of an overdose include miosis, somnolence, coma, respiratory distress, and hypotension.

Composition and Supply
Capsules   300 mg
Tablets   50 mg and 200 mg

Legal Status
Schedule III

Methysergide maleate (Sansert®)

Action and Use
Used for prophylaxis of vascular headache.

Dosage and Administration
4 to 8 mg in divided doses daily, orally.

Cautions
Should be used cautiously in patients suspected of having heart problems, psychic disturbances, and hallucinations. Contraindicated in patients with renal or hepatic disease, hypertension, infectious diseases, peptic ulcer, coronary artery disease, collagen or fibrotic disorders, peripheral vascular disease, pulmonary disease, cellulitis of lower extremities, and pregnancy. The patient should be warned that coolness of extremities should be reported immediately.

Adverse Reactions
The most common symptoms include nausea, vomiting, diarrhea, heartburn, cramps, anorexia, insomnia, mild euphoria, nervousness, weakness, ataxia, and lightheadedness. Other side effects include drowsiness, dizziness, hyperesthesia, dissociation and hallucinations, skin reactions, peripheral edema, weight gain, neutropenia, eosinophilia, arthralgia, and myalgia.

Composition and Supply
Tablets   2 mg

Legal Status
Prescription

Meticortelone®

See **Prednisolone.**

Meticorten®

See **Prednisone.**

Meti-Derm®

See under **Prednisolone.**

Metimyd® (prednisolone/sodium sulfacetamide

See CORTICOSTEROIDS.

Metocurine iodide (Metubine®)

See SKELETAL MUSCLE RELAXANTS.

Metolazone (Zaroxolyn®)

See DIURETICS.

Metopirone®

See **Metyrapone.**

Metrazol®

See **Pentylenetetrazole.**

Metreton®

See under **Prednisolone.**

Metrizoate preparations (Isopaque® 280, Isopaque® 440)

See DIAGNOSTICS, roentgenography.

Metronidazole (Flagyl®)

Action and Use
Antiprotozoal used to treat trichomoniasis and amebiasis.

Dosage and Administration
Trichomoniasis: In women, the dosage is 250 mg 3 times a day, orally, or 250 mg twice a day, orally, with 500 mg intravaginally each night. In men the dosage is 250 mg twice a day, orally.
Acute amebiasis: 750 mg 3 times a day for 5 to 10 days, orally.
Amebic liver abscess: 500 to 750 mg 3 times a day for 5 to 10 days, orally.

Cautions
Contraindicated in patients with blood dyscrasias or CNS disease, or in women in the first trimester of pregnancy. Should not be used with alcoholic beverages. The course of therapy should not exceed 10 days; a second course may be given after 4 to 6 weeks.

Adverse Reactions
The most common side effects include metallic taste, anorexia, and nausea. Occasional side effects include headache, vomiting, diarrhea, glossitis and stomatitis (resulting from overgrowth of *Candida*), and neutropenia. Rare side effects include dizziness, vertigo, incoordination, ataxia, paresthesias, irritability, depression, urticaria, flushing, pruritus, dysuria, cystitis, and dryness of the mouth, vagina, and vulva. A high dose may color urine deep reddish brown. Concomitant

use of alcoholic beverages may cause gastrointestinal discomfort, headache, and flushing.

Composition and Supply
Tablets   250 mg

Legal Status
Prescription

Metubine® (metocurine iodide)

See SKELETAL MUSCLE RELAXANTS.

Metyrapone (Metopirone®)

Action and Use
Drug used in diagnostic testing of hypothalamic and pituitary function.

Dosage and Administration
750 mg every 4 hours for 6 doses, orally; 30 mg/kg over a 4 hour period, IV infusion.

Cautions
Patients with poorly functioning adrenals may develop acute adrenal insufficiency.

Adverse Reactions
Nausea, rash, dizziness, headache, and sedation may occur. Thrombophlebitis is an occasional side effect after intravenous injection.

Composition and Supply
Injection (as tartrate)   100 mg/ml, in 10 ml ampuls (*Note:* 100 mg metyrapone tartrate is equivalent to 43.8 mg metyrapone base)
Tablets   250 mg

Legal Status
Prescription

MicaTin®

See **Miconazole nitrate.**

Miconazole nitrate (MicaTin®, Monistat®)

Action and Use
Antifungal used in the local treatment of tinea pedis, tinea cruris, tinea corporis, and vulvovaginal candidiasis.

Dosage and Administration
Applied topically or intravaginally.

Cautions
Should not come in contact with the eyes.

Adverse Reactions
Occasional side effects include initial vulvovaginal itching or burning with vaginal preparations. Urticaria and skin rash are other possible side effects.

Composition and Supply
Cream, topical   2%
Cream, vaginal   2%

Legal Status
Prescription

Microfibrillar collagen hemostat (Avitene®)

See HEMOSTATICS.

Microstix®-Candida

See DIAGNOSTICS, vaginal candidiasis.

Microstix®-3

See DIAGNOSTICS, urine (bacteriuria).

Midicel® (sulfamethoxypyridazine)

See SULFONAMIDES.

Migral®

See under **Ergotamine tartrate.**

Milontin®

See **Phensuximide.**

Miltown®

See **Meprobamate.**

Mineral oil (liquid petrolatum)

Action and Use
Lubricant laxative.

Dosage and Administration
Liquid: 15 to 30 ml at bedtime.
Emulsion: 30 ml at bedtime.

Cautions
May prevent absorption of fat-soluble vitamins in food. Lipid pneumonia may result if the drops coating the pharynx gain access to the trachea. Indiscriminate use should be discouraged, especially in elderly, debilitated, or dysphagic persons.

Adverse Reactions
When mineral oil is used in large doses, it tends to seep from the rectum, which may interfere with healing of postoperative wounds of the anus and perineum and may also cause pruritus ani.

Composition and Supply
Liquid
Emulsion (Agoral®) with or without phenolphthalein

Legal Status
Nonprescription

Minipress®

See **Prazosin hydrochloride.**

Minocin®

See **Minocycline hydrochloride.**

Minocycline hydrochloride (Minocin®, Vectrin®)

Action and Use
Tetracycline antibiotic.

Dosage and Administration
200 mg initially, followed by 100 mg every 12 hours, orally or IV.

Cautions
Parenteral therapy is indicated only when the oral route is not adequate or is not tolerated (see **Tetracycline hydrochloride).**

Adverse Reactions
See **Tetracycline hydrochloride.**

Composition and Supply
Capsules   50 mg and 100 mg
Injection   100 mg vials
Syrup   50 mg/5 ml
Tablets   100 mg

Legal Status
Prescription

Mintezol®

See **Thiabendazole.**

Miochol®

See **Acetylcholine chloride.**

Miradon® (anisindione)

See ANTICOAGULANTS.

Mithracin®

See **Mithramycin.**

Mithramycin (Mithracin®)

Action and Use
Antineoplastic used in the management of hypercalcemia associated with neoplasms and in the treatment of testicular tumors.

Dosage and Administration
25 to 30 µg/kg daily for 8 to 10 days, IV.

Cautions
Mithramycin has a low therapeutic index and is highly toxic to bone marrow and the gastrointestinal tract; it may interfere with liver function tests. Daily doses should not exceed 30 µg/kg, and a course of therapy of more than 10 days is not recommended.

Adverse Reactions
The most important toxic response is bone marrow depression, with infection and bleeding. Common side effects include nausea, vomiting, anorexia, diarrhea, stomatitis, hypocalcemia, and hypokalemia. Less frequent responses include fever, malaise, weakness, lethargy, phlebitis, facial flush, and skin rash. There may be renal and liver toxicity, and periodic tests of kidney and liver function are recommended. Warn the patient that headache, depression, and drowsiness may occur.

Composition and Supply
Injection   2.5 mg vials

Legal Status
Prescription

Mitomycin (Mutamycin®)

See ANTINEOPLASTICS, antibiotics.

Mitotane (Lysodren®)

Action and Use
Antineoplastic.

Dosage and Administration
2 to 16 g daily, orally.

Cautions
May cause adrenal insufficiency. Use with caution in patients with liver disease. There are many other side effects, including those involving the CNS and the gastrointestinal tract.

Adverse Reactions
The most frequent side effects include nausea, vomiting, anorexia, diarrhea, dermatitis, depression, lethargy, somnolence, vertigo, and tremors. Less common side effects include visual blurring, diplopia, lens opacity, toxic retinopathy, hematuria, hemorrhagic cystitis, albuminuria, hypertension, orthostatic hypotension, flushing, generalized aching, hyperpyrexia, and lowered PBI. Discontinue the drug immediately if shock or severe trauma occurs, since adrenal suppression is its prime action. Steroid metabolism is altered, which may cause insufficiency and the need for cortisone replacement.

Composition and Supply
Tablets   500 mg

Legal Status
Prescription

6-MP

See **Mercaptopurine.**

M-M-R® (measles, mumps, and rubella virus vaccine, live)

See BIOLOGICALS, vaccines.

Moban® (molindone hydrochloride)

See PSYCHOTROPICS, antipsychotics.

Modane® (danthron)

See CATHARTICS.

Moderil® (rescinnamine)

See ANTIHYPERTENSIVES, nondiuretic.

Molindone hydrochloride (Moban®)

See PSYCHOTROPICS, antipsychotics.

Mol-Iron® Panhemic™ Chronosule®

See under **Ferrous sulfate.**

Monistat®

See **Miconazole nitrate.**

Monocaine® (butethamine hydrochloride)

See ANESTHETICS, local.

Monospot™

See DIAGNOSTICS, mononucleosis.

Morphine sulfate

Action and Use
Potent narcotic analgesic.

Dosage and Administration
10 to 15 mg every 4 hours, orally, SC, IM, or IV.

Cautions
Morphine sulfate is addicting and causes respiratory depression. If the rate of respiration is below 10 to 12 per minute, withhold the drug and consult a physician. Check rate of respiration 20 to 30 minutes after oral administration and 10 minutes after parenteral administration. Use carefully in patients with toxic psychosis, liver or kidney dysfunction, hypotension, prostatic hypertrophy, convulsive disorders, myxedema, Addison's disease, head injury, and acute alcoholism; in pregnant women; and in elderly and debilitated persons.

Adverse Reactions
The most common side effects include constipation, anorexia, and respiratory depression. Other adverse responses include difficulty in voiding, nausea and vomiting, postural hypotension, diaphoresis, drowsiness, euphoria, pruritus, decreased body temperature, and urticaria. With large doses, the T wave of the ECG may be depressed or inverted, which may interfere with the interpretation of the ECG in patients with suspected myocardial infarction.

Composition and Supply

Injection   10 mg/ml in 1 ml ampuls; 15 mg/ml in 1 ml ampuls and 20 ml vials

Injection   15 mg/ml with atropine 400 μg/ml, 20 ml and 30 ml vials

Tablets   10 mg and 15 mg

Legal Status

Schedule II

Morrhuate sodium

See SCLEROSING AGENTS.

Motrin®

See **Ibuprofen.**

Mucomyst®

See **Acetylcysteine.**

Mudrane®-GG (aminophylline/guaifenesin/ephedrine/phenobarbital)

See ANTIASTHMATICS, xanthine preparations.

Multicebrin® Tablets

See VITAMINS, MULTIPLE, oral.

Mumps immune globulin (Hyparotin®)

See BIOLOGICALS, immune serums.

Mumps skin test antigen

See DIAGNOSTICS, mumps.

Mumpsvax®

See **Mumps virus vaccine, live.**

Mumps virus vaccine, live (Mumpsvax®)

Action and Use

Used to achieve active immunity against mumps.

Dosage and Administration

0.5 ml (500 μl) reconstituted vaccine (5,000 TCID$_{50}$), SC into upper arm.

Cautions

Postpone immunization in the presence of active infection. Contraindicated in pregnant women; in patients with gamma globulin deficiency, leukemia, or other malignancies; in those receiving ACTH or corticosteroids (except in replacement therapy), irradiation, or antineoplastics; and in persons with sensitivity to eggs, chicken, chicken feathers, or neomycin. Store the vaccine at 2° to 8° C and protect from light. Discard reconstituted vaccine if it is not used within 8 hours.

Adverse Reactions
Rare side effects include allergic reactions, purpura, encephalitis, and fever (usually 39° C).

Composition and Supply
Injection   5,000 TCID$_{50}$ vials with 0.7 ml (700 μl) of diluent

Legal Status
Prescription

Mustargen®

See **Mechlorethamine hydrochloride.**

Mutamycin® (mitomycin)

See ANTINEOPLASTICS, antibiotics.

M.V.I.®

See VITAMINS, MULTIPLE, parenteral.

Myambutal®

See **Ethambutol hydrochloride.**

Mycifradin®

See **Neomycin sulfate.**

Mycolog® (nystatin/neomycin sulfate/gramicidin/triamcinolone acetonide)

See ANTI-INFECTIVES, LOCAL, fungicides.

Mycostatin®

See **Nystatin.**

Mydriacyl®

See **Tropicamide.**

Mylanta®

See **Magnesium hydroxide/aluminum hydroxide/simethicone.**

Mylanta®-II

See **Magnesium hydroxide/aluminum hydroxide/simethicone.**

Myleran®

See **Busulfan.**

Mylicon®

See **Simethicone.**

Myochrysine®

See **Gold sodium thiomalate.**

Mysoline®

See **Primidone.**

Mysteclin-F® (tetracycline/amphotericin B)

See ANTIBIOTICS, tetracyclines.

Mytelase®

See **Ambenonium chloride.**

Nafcillin sodium (Unipen®)

Action and Use
Antibiotic used in the treatment of infections caused by penicillinase-producing staphylococci.

Dosage and Administration
250 mg to 1 g every 4 to 6 hours, orally; 500 mg every 4 to 6 hours, IM; or 500 mg to 1 g every 4 hours, IV.

Cautions
Use with caution in patients who may have penicillin type allergy. Periodic renal function assessments should be made. See **Penicillin G potassium** for further cautions.

Adverse Reactions
See **Penicillin G potassium.**

Composition and Supply
Capsules   250 mg
Injection   500 mg, 1 g, and 2 g vials
Solution, oral   250 mg/5 ml
Tablets   500 mg

Legal Status
Prescription

Nalfon®

See **Fenoprofen calcium**.

Nalidixic acid (NegGram®)

Action and Use
Urinary tract anti-infective used primarily against gram-negative organisms.

Dosage and Administration
500 mg to 1 g 4 times a day, orally.

Cautions
Use cautiously in patients with hepatic or renal disease. Contraindicated in patients with epilepsy and in those being treated with nitrofurantoin.

Adverse Reactions
Occasional side effects include nausea, vomiting, diarrhea, and abdominal pain. Infrequent side effects include pruritus, urticaria, photosensitivity, eosinophilia, fever, rash, headache, malaise, drowsiness, vertigo, visual disturbances, myalgia, and asthenia. Increased intracranial pressure with bulging fontanel and headache may occasionally develop in infants and children. Rare side effects include cholestasis, leukopenia, thrombocytopenia, hemolytic anemia, paresthesia, and metabolic acidosis; renal and liver studies are recommended with prolonged therapy. Convulsions may occur in children given high doses, or in patients with cardiovascular insufficiency, parkinsonism, or epilepsy. False-positive results may occur in urine glucose tests with Benedict's solution or Clinitest® tablets.

Composition and Supply
Tablets   250 mg and 500 mg

Legal Status
Prescription

Nalline®

See **Nalorphine hydrochloride.**

Nalorphine hydrochloride (Nalline®)

Action and Use
Antidote for narcotic respiratory depression.

Dosage and Administration
Neonates: 200 to 500 μg (maximum) SC, IM, or IV.
Adults: 5 to 10 mg for up to 3 doses, SC, IM, or IV.

Cautions
Ineffective against depression produced by barbiturates or general anesthetics. Contraindicated in patients addicted to narcotics and in patients with mild narcotic-induced respiratory depression.

Adverse Reactions
See **Levallorphan tartrate.**

Composition and Supply
Injection, adult   5 mg/ml, in 1 ml and 2 ml ampuls and 10 ml vials
Injection, neonatal   200 μg/ml, in 1 ml ampuls

Legal Status
Schedule III

Naloxone hydrochloride (Narcan®)

Action and Use
Narcotic antagonist used to treat narcotic depression, including respiratory depression, caused by natural and synthetic narcotics, propoxyphene, and pentazocine. It is the drug of choice when the nature of the depressant drug is unknown.

Dosage and Administration
Adults: 400 μg IV, IM, or SC, repeated every 2 to 3 minutes if needed.
Neonates: 10 μg/kg, IV, IM, or SC, repeated every 2 to 3 minutes if needed.

Cautions
Use with caution in patients who may be addicted to narcotics.

Adverse Reactions
After the administration of naloxone to a person who has taken a narcotic overdose, respirations will increase and the depression will lighten. Withdrawal syndrome may be precipitated. Nausea and vomiting may occur.

Composition and Supply
Adults   400 μg/ml, in 1 ml ampuls
Neonatal   20 μg/ml, in 2 ml ampuls

Legal Status
Prescription

Nandrolone decanoate (Deca-Durabolin®)

See ANDROGENS.

Nandrolone phenpropionate (Durabolin®)

See ANDROGENS.

Naphazoline hydrochloride (Privine®)

Action and Use
Nasal and ophthalmic vasoconstrictor.

Dosage and Administration
Eye: instill 1 or 2 drops once or twice a day.
Nose: apply 3 or 4 drops or 2 or 3 sprays 3 or 4 times a day.

Cautions
Contraindicated in patients with narrow-angle glaucoma. Excessive use may lead to drowsiness, local mucous membrane irritation, and rebound congestion. Use with caution in patients with hypertension, cardiac irregularities, hyperglycemia, or hyperthyroidism, and in those receiving MAO inhibitors (since a hypertensive crisis might result).

Adverse Reactions
Pupillary dilatation with increased intraocular pressure may occur. Systemic adrenergic effects may be caused by absorption. An overdose depresses the central nervous system.

Composition and Supply
Solution, nasal   0.05%
Solution, ophthalmic   0.1%
Spray, nasal   0.05%

Legal Status
Nonprescription

Naphuride® (suramin)

See ANTIPROTOZOALS, antitrypanosomals.

Naprosyn®

See **Naproxen.**

Naproxen (Naprosyn®)

Action and Use
Nonsteroidal anti-inflammatory agent used to relieve rheumatoid arthritis.

Dosage and Administration
250 mg twice daily (morning and evening), orally; daily doses higher than 750 mg are not recommended.

Cautions
See **Fenoprofen calcium.**

Adverse Reactions
See **Fenoprofen calcium.**

Composition and Supply
Tablets   250 mg

Legal Status
Prescription

Naqua® (trichlormethiazide)

See DIURETICS.

Narcan®

See **Naloxone hydrochloride.**

Nardil®

See **Phenelzine sulfate.**

Naturetin®

See **Bendroflumethiazide.**

Navane®

See **Thiothixene hydrochloride.**

Nebcin®

See **Tobramycin sulfate.**

Nebs®

See **Acetaminophen.**

NegGram®

See **Nalidixic acid.**

Nembutal®

See **Pentobarbital.**

Neo-Betalin® 12 (hydroxocobalamin)

See HEMATINICS; VITAMINS, water-soluble.

Neobiotic®

See **Neomycin sulfate.**

Neo-Cortef® (neomycin sulfate/hydrocortisone acetate)

See ANTI-INFECTIVES, LOCAL, antibiotics.

Neomycin palmitate/trypsin/chymotrypsin (Biozyme®)

See DEBRIDEMENT ENZYMES.

Neomycin sulfate (Mycifradin®, Neobiotic®)

Action and Use
Broad-spectrum antibiotic for topical use; also used as a preoperative intestinal antiseptic and as a urinary antiseptic for hospital cases in which no other antimicrobial agent is effective.

Dosage and Administration
Applied topically as a solution or ointment; 500 mg to 1 g, orally; or 15 mg/kg per day divided in 4 equally spread doses, IM.

Cautions
Neomycin sulfate is nephrotoxic and ototoxic. Allergic manifestations may occur and possibly superinfection from nonsusceptible organisms.

Adverse Reactions
Topical applications occasionally cause rash and fever. Oral preparations may produce intestinal malabsorption and mild diarrhea. Systemic toxicity (following parenteral use) involves damage to the kidney and the eighth cranial nerve.

Composition and Supply
Injection   500 mg vials
Suspension, oral   125 mg/5 ml
Tablets   500 mg
Topical preparations   creams, ointments, or solutions, containing neomycin alone or combined with other topical antibiotics and/or corticosteroids (several combinations are listed in Section 1 under anti-infectives, local, antibiotics)

Legal Status
Prescription

Neomycin sulfate/hydrocortisone acetate (Neo-Cortef®)

See ANTI-INFECTIVES, LOCAL, antibiotics.

Neosporin®

See under **Polymyxin B sulfate.**

Neosporin® Aerosol

See under **Polymyxin B sulfate.**

Neosporin-G® Cream

See under **Polymyxin B sulfate.**

Neosporin® G.U. Irrigant

See **Polymyxin B sulfate.**

Neosporin® Ointment

See under **Polymyxin B sulfate.**

Neosporin® Ointment Ophthalmic

See under **Polymyxin B sulfate.**

Neosporin® Solution Ophthalmic

See under **Polymyxin B sulfate.**

Neostigmine (Prostigmin®)

Action and Use
Cholinergic used to treat urinary retention, bowel ileus, megacolon, myasthenia gravis, and tubocurarine poisoning.

Dosage and Administration
Dosage is individualized to the patient and condition being treated. The usual dosage is in the range of 15 to 30 mg 3 times a day, orally; or 250 µg to 1.0 mg 3 or 4 times a day, SC or IM.

Cautions
Cholinergic crisis is possible; keep atropine at hand.

Adverse Reactions
Adverse reactions are more pronounced than those from bethanechol chloride (see).

Composition and Supply
Injection (as methylsulfate)   1 : 4,000, in 1 ml ampuls; 1 : 2,000, in
   1 ml ampuls; and 1 : 1,000, in 5 ml and 10 ml vials
Tablets (as bromide)   15 mg

Legal Status
Prescription

Neo-Synalar®

See under **Fluocinolone acetonide.**

Neo-Synephrine®

See **Phenylephrine hydrochloride.**

Neptazane® (methazolamide)

See CARBONIC ANHYDRASE INHIBITORS.

Nesacaine® (chloroprocaine hydrochloride)

See ANESTHETICS, local.

Niac®

See under **Niacin.**

Niacin (nicotinic acid)

Niacinamide (nicotinamide)

Action and Use
Niacin, a B-complex vitamin, is converted in the body to niacinamide,
the active metabolite. Both compounds may be used in the treatment
and prophylaxis of pellagra, but niacinamide is preferred because of
its lack of side effects. Niacin is used chiefly as a vasodilator and
antilipemic.

Dosage and Administration
Niacin: 50 to 500 mg in divided doses, orally or parenterally.
Niacinamide: 500 mg in divided doses, orally.

Cautions
Liver impairment is possible with large doses. Use with caution in
patients with a history of glaucoma, severe diabetes, peptic ulcer, or
impaired gallbladder or liver function.

Adverse Reactions
Therapeutic dose of nicotinic acid may produce superficial vasodilatation for 2 hours (seen as flushing), accompanied by pruritus and burning. Occasional side effects (for both compounds) include gastric distress, skin rash, and allergies.

Composition and Supply
Nicotinic acid
Capsules   25 mg, 50 mg, and 100 mg
Capsules, sustained-release   300 mg (Niac®)
Elixir   50 mg/5 ml (Nicotinex®)
Injection   10 mg/ml, in 10 ml vials
Injection   50 mg/ml, in 10 ml vials
Injection   100 mg/ml, in 10 ml vials
Tablets   25 mg, 50 mg, and 100 mg

Niacinamide
Capsules   50 mg
Injection   50 mg/2 ml, in 2 ml ampuls and 10 ml vials
Tablets   25 mg, 50 mg, and 100 mg

Legal Status
Prescription (injection)
Nonprescription (oral preparations)

Niclosamide (Yomesan®)

See ANTHELMINTICS, tapeworm.

Nicotinamide

See **Niacinamide.**

Nicotinex®

See under **Niacin.**

Nicotinic acid

See **Niacin.**

Nicotinyl alcohol (Roniacol®)

Action and Use
Vasodilator used in treating peripheral vascular diseases.

Dosage and Administration
50 to 100 mg 3 to 4 times a day, orally.

Cautions
Contraindicated in those who are hypersensitive to this agent.

Adverse Reactions
Occasional and transient side effects include flushing, gastric disturbances, and minor skin rashes and allergies.

Composition and Supply
Elixir   50 mg/5 ml
Tablets   50 mg
Tablets, sustained-release   150 mg

Legal Status
Prescription

Nikethamide (Coramine®)

See RESPIRATORY STIMULANTS.

Nilstat®

See **Nystatin.**

Nipride®

See **Sodium nitroprusside.**

Niridazole (Ambilhar®)

See ANTHELMINTICS, schistosomiasis.

Nisentil®

See **Alphaprodine hydrochloride.**

Nitro-Bid®

See **Nitroglycerin.**

Nitrofurantoin (Cyantin®, Furadantin®, Macrodantin®)

Action and Use
Urinary tract antibacterial.

Dosage and Administration
50 to 100 mg 4 times a day, orally. May be given with food or milk to minimize gastric upset.

Cautions
Hemolytic anemia, possibly linked with glucose-6-phosphate dehydrogenase deficiency, may occur. Contraindicated in patients with anuria, oliguria, or significant impairment of renal function. Discon-

tinue use if there is any sign of hemolysis. Peripheral neuropathy may occur with nitrofurantoin therapy.

Adverse Reactions
The most common side effects include nausea, vomiting, and diarrhea. Occasional side effects include headache, dizziness, drowsiness, muscular aches, and nystagmus. Sensitization may occur, with urticaria, rash, chills, fever, angioedema, leukopenia, anaphylaxis, drug fever, arthralgia, and granulocytopenia. Prolonged treatment may produce interstitial pulmonary fibrosis. Rare side effects include liver damage, transient alopecia, and superinfections.

Composition and Supply
Capsules (macrocrystals)   50 mg and 100 mg (Macrodantin®)
Suspension   25 mg/5 ml
Tablets   50 mg and 100 mg

Legal Status
Prescription

Nitrofurazone (Furacin®)

Action and Use
Local anti-infective for adjunctive therapy of second- and third-degree burns (when bacterial resistance is a problem), and in skin grafting (when bacterial contamination may cause rejection).

Dosage and Administration
Applied topically.

Cautions
Contraindicated in cases of prior sensitization.

Adverse Reactions
Sensitization develops occasionally.

Composition and Supply
Cream   0.2%
Dressing, soluble   0.2%
Powder   0.2%
Solution   0.2%

Legal Status
Prescription

Nitrogen mustard

See **Mechlorethamine hydrochloride.**

Nitroglycerin (glyceryl trinitrate) (Nitro-Bid®, Nitroglyn®, Nitrol®, Nitrong®, Nitrospan®, Nitrostat®)

Action and Use
Vasodilator used in the treatment of angina pectoris.

Dosage and Administration
Oral: 1 capsule 2 or 3 times daily.
Sublingual: 400 to 600 µg every 2 or 3 hours, as needed.
Topical: applied every 2 or 3 hours.

Cautions
Oral forms (capsules) are not intended for immediate relief of angina attacks. Tolerance develops, and the dose must be increased. Consult the physician if the patient's chest pain is not relieved in 15 to 20 minutes after 1 or more tablets. Nitroglycerin is unstable and should be kept cool and dry, in a tightly closed container.

Adverse Reactions
Common side effects include reflex tachycardia, headache, nausea, vomiting, flushing, vertigo, postural hypotension with weakness, dizziness, and faintness (the patient should use caution on rising); alcohol may intensify these effects. There may occasionally be increased intraocular pressure (use with caution in patients with glaucoma). Sensitivity to the hypotensive effect is a contraindication, since it may lead to collapse (nitrate syncope). Effects of an overdose include flushing, headache, tachycardia, and dizziness.

Composition and Supply
Capsules, sustained-release   2.5 mg and 6.5 mg
Ointment   2%
Tablets, sublingual   150 µg, 300 µg, 400 µg, and 600 µg

Legal Status
Prescription

Nitroglyn®

See **Nitroglycerin.**

Nitrol®

See **Nitroglycerin.**

Nitrong®

See **Nitroglycerin.**

Nitrospan®

See **Nitroglycerin.**

Nitrostat®

See **Nitroglycerin.**

Nitrous oxide

See ANESTHETICS, general.

N-Multistix™

See DIAGNOSTICS, urine (protein, glucose, ketones, bilirubin, blood, urobilinogen, nitrite, pH).

Noctec®

See **Chloral hydrate.**

Noludar®

See **Methyprylon.**

Nolvadex® (tamoxifen citrate)

See ANTINEOPLASTICS, antimetabolites.

Nonoxynol 9 (Conceptrol®, Ortho-Creme®, Semicid®)

See CONTRACEPTIVES, TOPICAL.

Nonylphenoxypolyoxyethylene ethanol (Because®)

See CONTRACEPTIVES, TOPICAL.

Norethindrone (Norlutate®, Norlutin®)

Action and Use
Progestogen; in combination used as an oral contraceptive.

Dosage and Administration
5 to 40 mg daily, orally, depending on condition being treated.

Cautions
See **Progesterone.**

Adverse Reactions
See **Progesterone.**

Composition and Supply
Norethindrone:
Tablets   5 mg (Norlutin®)

Norethindrone acetate:
Tablets   5 mg (Norlutate®)

Contraceptive combinations:
Tablets   norethindrone 10 mg with mestranol 60 μg (Norinyl®, Ortho-Novum®)
Tablets   norethindrone 2 mg with mestranol 100 μg (Norinyl®, Ortho-Novum®)
Tablets   norethindrone acetate 1 mg and 2.5 mg with ethinyl estradiol 50 μg (Norlestrin®)
Tablets   norethindrone acetate 1 mg and 1.5 mg with ethinyl estradiol 20 μg and 30 μg (Loestrin®)

Legal Status
Prescription

Norethynodrel/mestranol (Enovid-E®)

See CONTRACEPTIVES, ORAL.

Norflex®

See **Orphenadrine citrate.**

Norgesic®

See under **Orphenadrine citrate.**

Norgestrel/ethinyl estradiol (Lo/Ovral®)

See CONTRACEPTIVES, ORAL.

Norinyl®

See under **Norethindrone.**

Norisodrine®

See **Isoproterenol sulfate.**

Norlestrin®

See under **Norethindrone.**

Norlutate®

See **Norethindrone.**

Norlutin®

See **Norethindrone.**

Nolvadex® (tamoxifen citrate)

See ANTINEOPLASTICS, antimetabolites.

Norpace®

See **Disopyramide phosphate.**

Norpramin®

See **Desipramine hydrochloride.**

Nortriptyline hydrochloride (Aventyl®)

Action and Use
Antidepressant.

Dosage and Administration
Dosage is adjusted to the individual, and ranges from 20 to 100 mg daily, orally.

Cautions
Concomitant use with MAO inhibitors is contraindicated. The action of adrenergic drugs may be potentiated. Use cautiously in patients with cardiovascular disorders or a history of epilepsy or hypotensive states.

Adverse Reactions
See **Amitriptyline hydrochloride.**

Composition and Supply
Capsules   10 mg and 25 mg
Solution, oral   10 mg/5 ml

Legal Status
Prescription

Novafed®

See **Pseudoephedrine hydrochloride.**

Novafed® A Capsules

See COUGH-COLD PREPARATIONS, common cold preparations.

Novahistine® (phenylpropanolamine hydrochloride/chlorpheniramine maleate)

See NASAL DECONGESTANTS.

Novahistine® Preparations

See COUGH-COLD PREPARATIONS, cough preparations.

Novocain®

See **Procaine hydrochloride.**

Novrad® (levopropoxyphene napsylate)

See ANTITUSSIVES AND EXPECTORANTS, antitussives.

Numorphan® (oxymorphone hydrochloride)

See ANALGESICS, narcotic.

Nupercainal®

See **Dibucaine.**

Nupercaine®

See **Dibucaine hydrochloride.**

Nursoy®

See INFANT FORMULAS.

Nydrazid®

See **Isoniazid.**

Nylidrin hydrochloride (Arlidin®)

Action and Use
Adrenergic vasodilator used to treat peripheral vascular disease and circulatory disturbances of the inner ear.

Dosage and Administration
3 to 12 mg 3 or 4 times a day, orally.

Cautions
Use cautiously in patients with myocardial lesions, thyrotoxicosis, or angina pectoris.

Adverse Reactions
Possible side effects include nervousness, palpitations, weakness, dizziness, nausea, and vomiting.

Composition and Supply
Injection   5 mg/ml, in 1 ml ampuls and 10 ml vials
Tablets   6 mg and 12 mg

Nystatin (Mycostatin®, Nilstat®)

Action and Use
Antifungal antibiotic used in the treatment of candidiasis.

Dosage and Administration
500,000 to 1,000,000 units 3 times a day, orally; applied topically as an ointment, cream, or powder, or vaginally as a suppository.

Cautions
Hypersensitivity may occur. High oral doses are likely to produce gastrointestinal disturbances.

Adverse Reactions
Occasional side effects include nausea, vomiting, and diarrhea, especially with large oral doses. Urticaria and hypersensitivity have been reported following topical application.

Composition and Supply
Cream   100,000 units/g
Ointment   100,000 units/g
Powder   100,000 units/g
Suppositories, vaginal   100,000 units/g
Suspension, oral   100,000 units/ml
Tablets, oral   500,000 units
Tablets, vaginal   100,000 units

Legal Status
Prescription

Nystatin/neomycin sulfate/gramicidin/triamcinolone acetonide
(Mycolog®)

See ANTI-INFECTIVES, LOCAL, fungicides.

Oatmeal, colloidal (Aveeno®)

Action and Use
Demulcent and antipruritic.

Dosage and Administration
1 cup (premixed with 4 cups cold tap water) to a tubful of lukewarm water and use as a soaking bath for 30 minutes.

Cautions
None.

Adverse Reactions
None.

Composition and Supply
Powdered oatmeal   500 mg boxes

Legal Status
Nonprescription

Ogen®

See **Piperazine estrone sulfate.**

Olive oil

See EMOLLIENT-PROTECTANTS.

Omnipen®

See **Ampicillin.**

Oncovin®

See **Vincristine sulfate.**

Ophthaine®

See **Proparacaine hydrochloride.**

Opium alkaloids (Pantopon®)

Action and Use
Narcotic recommended for relief of severe pain.

Dosage and Administration
5 to 20 mg, given only IM or SC.

Cautions
Same as cautions for morphine sulfate (see).

Adverse Reactions
Same as adverse reactions to morphine sulfate (see).

Composition and Supply
Injection   hydrochlorides of opium alkaloids, 20 mg/ml, in 1 ml
   ampuls

Legal Status
Schedule II

Opium, camphorated tincture of

See **Paregoric.**

Opium, deodorized tincture of (DTO)

Action and Use
Antidiarrheal.

Dosage and Administration
0.6 ml (600 µl) 4 times a day, orally.

Cautions
Habit-forming; 25 times the strength of paregoric.

Adverse Reactions
See **Morphine sulfate.**

Composition and Supply
Tincture   morphine, 10 mg/ml

Legal Status
Schedule II

Opium/belladonna suppositories

See ANALGESICS, narcotic.

Optimyd®

See under **Prednisolone.**

Oragrafin®

See **Ipodate.**

Oretic®

See **Hydrochlorothiazide.**

Oreton® Methyl

See **Methyltestosterone.**

Oreton® Propionate

See under **Testosterone propionate.**

Orimune®

See **Poliovirus vaccine, live oral.**

Orinase®

See **Tolbutamide.**

Orinase® Diagnostic (tolbutamide sodium)

See DIAGNOSTICS, diabetes mellitus.

Oriodide® (sodium iodide I 131)

See ANTITHYROIDS; ANTINEOPLASTICS, radioisotopes.

Ornade® Spansule® Capsules

See COUGH-COLD PREPARATIONS, common cold preparations.

Orphenadrine citrate (Norflex®)
Orphenadrine hydrochloride (Disipal®)

Action and Use
Central-acting muscle relaxant for use in patients with parkinsonism or with acute, painful musculoskeletal conditions.

Dosage and Administration
150 to 400 mg daily, orally.

Cautions
Contraindicated in patients with glaucoma, cardiospasm, intestinal obstruction, urinary retention, or myasthenia gravis.

Adverse Reactions
Side effects mainly result from the drug's mild anticholinergic action, which may cause dryness of mouth, tachycardia, palpitation, urinary hesitancy, urinary retention, blurred vision, dilatation of the pupil, increased occular tension, weakness, nausea, vomiting, headache, dizziness, constipation, drowsiness, hypersensitivity reactions, pruritus, and rarely urticaria.

Composition and Supply
Tablets   50 mg and 100 mg
Tablets   25 mg with APC (Norgesic®)

Legal Status
Prescription

Ortho-Creme® (nonoxynol 9)

See CONTRACEPTIVES, TOPICAL.

Ortho-Novum®

See under **Norethindrone.**

Osmitrol®

See **Mannitol.**

Osmoglyn®

See under **Glycerin.**

Otic Domeboro® Solution (acetic acid/aluminum acetate)

See ANTI-INFECTIVES, LOCAL, miscellaneous antiseptic-disinfectants.

Otrivin®

See **Xylometazoline hydrochloride.**

Ouabain (G-strophanthin)

Action and Use
Cardiotonic glycoside.

Dosage and Administration
The digitalizing dose is 1 mg in divided doses, IV (slowly).

Cautions
Administer cautiously in patients who have received other cardiotonic glycosides within the past 3 weeks. See **Digitalis** for further cautions.

Adverse Reactions
See **Digitalis.**

Composition and Supply
Injection   250 μg/ml, in 2 ml ampuls

Legal Status
Prescription

Ovulen® (ethynodiol diacetate/mestranol)

See CONTRACEPTIVES, ORAL.

Oxacillin sodium (Bactocill®, Prostaphlin®)

Action and Use
Antibiotic useful against penicillinase-producing organisms.

Dosage and Administration
250 to 500 mg every 4 to 6 hours, orally; 250 mg to 1 g (or more) every 4 to 6 hours, IM or IV.

Cautions
Use with caution in patients who may be allergic to penicillin.

Adverse Reactions
See **Penicillin G potassium.**

Composition and Supply
Capsules   250 mg and 500 mg
Injection   1 g, 2 g and 4 g vials

Legal Status
Prescription

Oxalid®

See **Oxyphenbutazone.**

Oxazepam (Serax®)

Action and Use
Tranquilizer.

Dosage and Administration
10 to 30 mg 3 or 4 times a day, orally.

Cautions
Oxazepam is a CNS depressant; administer cautiously to patients taking other depressant drugs. Contraindicated in patients with psychoses.

Adverse Reactions
Occasionally, skin eruptions, edema, slurred speech, tremor, and altered libido may result. See **Chlordiazepoxide hydrochloride** for further cautions.

Composition and Supply
Capsules   10 mg, 15 mg, and 30 mg

Legal Status
Schedule IV

Ox bile extract (bile salts)

Action and Use
A choleretic and digestant that promotes absorption of fat.

Dosage and Administration
325 to 750 mg 2 or 3 times a day, orally.

Cautions
Tablets should not be chewed.

Adverse Reactions
Diarrhea may result.

Composition and Supply
Tablets   325 mg

Legal Status
Prescription

Oxolinic acid (Utibid®)

Action and Use
Antibacterial agent indicated for the treatment of initial or recurrent nonobstructive urinary tract infections caused by susceptible gram-negative organisms, including *Escherichia coli, Enterobacter aerogenes, Proteus* species, and *Klebsiella* species.

Dosage and Administration
1 tablet twice daily for 2 weeks.

Cautions
Contraindicated in infants, nursing mothers, and in persons with a history of convulsive disorders. Oxolinic acid has CNS stimulant potential, especially in elderly patients, and should be used cautiously in patients with severely impaired renal function.

Adverse Reactions
The most frequent reactions include insomnia, dizziness, nausea, nervousness, and headache; less frequent reactions include restlessness, weakness, itching, constipation, diarrhea, abdominal cramps, anorexia, and vomiting.

Composition and Supply
Tablets   750 mg

Legal Status
Prescription

Oxsoralen® (methoxsalen)

See ANTIPSORIATICS; EMOLLIENT-PROTECTANTS.

Oxtriphylline (Choledyl®)

Action and Use
Xanthine bronchodilator used to treat acute asthma and broncho-spasm associated with bronchitis or emphysema.

Dosage and Administration
200 to 400 mg 4 times a day, orally.

Cautions
Concurrent use with other xanthine preparations may lead to adverse reactions, especially CNS stimulation in children. See **Aminophylline** for further cautions.

Adverse Reactions
Better absorbed from gastrointestinal tract and less irritating to gas-tric mucosa than aminophylline (see).

Composition and Supply
Tablets   100 mg and 200 mg

Legal Status
Prescription

Oxtryphylline/guaifenesin (Brondecon®)

See ANTIASTHMATICS, xanthine preparations.

Oxybenzone/dioxybenzone (Solbar®)

See EMOLLIENT-PROTECTANTS.

Oxybutynin chloride (Ditropan®)

See ANTISPASMODICS.

Oxycodone hydrochloride/acetaminophen (Percocet™-5, Tylox™)

See ANALGESICS, narcotic.

Oxycodone/APC (Percodan®)

Action and Use
Narcotic analgesic used for moderate pain.

Dosage and Administration
1 or 2 tablets every 6 hours, orally.

Cautions
Oxycodone compound is habit-forming; it is more potent and more likely to produce dependency than codeine. Should not be adminis-

tered to children. Use with caution in patients with head injury, acute abdominal conditions, peptic ulcer, coagulation abnormalities, hepatic or renal impairment, hypothyroidism, Addison's disease, prostatic hypertrophy, and urethral stricture, and in elderly or debilitated persons.

Adverse Reactions
Similar to but more pronounced than adverse reactions to codeine (see).

Composition and Supply
Tablets   oxycodone 4.88 mg with APC (Percodan®)
Tablets   oxycodone 2.44 mg with APC (Percodan®-Demi)

Legal Status
Schedule II

Oxymetazoline hydrochloride (Afrin®)

Action and Use
Nasal decongestant.

Dosage and Administration
2 to 4 drops or 2 or 3 sprays twice a day, morning and evening.

Cautions
Use cautiously in patients with coronary heart disease, hypertension, hyperthyroidism, or diabetes, and in those being treated with MAO inhibitors (to avoid a hypertensive crisis).

Adverse Reactions
Mild and transitory burning, stinging, and dryness of the nasal mucosa may occur. Other possible side effects include sneezing, headache, lightheadedness, insomnia, and palpitations. Rebound congestion may occur with prolonged or excessive use.

Composition and Supply
Solution   0.05%

Legal Status
Nonprescription

Oxymetholone (Anadrol®-50)

See ANDROGENS.

Oxymorphone hydrochloride (Numorphan®)

See ANALGESICS, narcotic.

Oxyphenbutazone (Oxalid®, Tandearil®)

Action and Use
Potent anti-inflammatory analgesic.

Dosage and Administration
300 to 600 mg daily in divided doses, orally, after meals.

Cautions
Contraindicated in children younger than 14 years old, in senile patients, and in patients with gastrointestinal disease, blood dyscrasias, hypertension, thyroid disease, systemic edema, or renal, hepatic, or cardiac dysfunction. Not to be used in conjunction with other potent chemotherapeutic agents in long-term anticoagulant therapy. Use cautiously in women in the first trimester of pregnancy and in nursing mothers. May potentiate the action of insulin, sulfonylureas, and sulfonamides. Periodic blood examinations are recommended.

Adverse Reactions
Common side effects include fever, sore throat, mouth lesions, and other symptoms of blood dyscrasias. Other possible responses include dyspepsia, epigastric pain, black or tarry stools (or other evidence of intestinal ulcer or hemorrhage), allergic reactions, skin eruptions, kidney dysfunction, fluid and electrolyte disturbances, hypertension, confusion, and blurred vision. The patient should be advised to report any unusual symptoms immediately.

Composition and Supply
Tablets   100 mg

Legal Status
Prescription

Oxyphencyclimine hydrochloride (Daricon®)
See CHOLINERGICS.

Oxyquinoline sulfate (Triva® Combination)
See ANTIPROTOZOALS, antitrichomonials.

Oxytetracycline (Terramycin®)

Action and Use
Broad-spectrum antibiotic.

Dosage and Administration
250 to 500 mg every 6 to 12 hours, orally, IM, or IV.

Cautions

Use cautiously in patients with renal impairment. Do not administer concurrently with food or milk. Patients being treated with oxytetracycline should not be given antacids. See **Tetracycline hydrochloride** for further cautions.

Adverse Reactions
See **Tetracycline hydrochloride.**

Composition and Supply
Capsules (oxytetracycline hydrochloride)   250 mg
Suspension, oral (calcium oxytetracycline)   125 mg/5 ml
Injection   250 mg and 500 mg vials
Injection   50 mg/ml and 62.5 mg/ml, in 2 ml ampuls

Legal Status
Prescription

Oxytetracycline hydrochloride/sulfamethizole/ phenazopyridine hydrochloride (Urobiotic®)

See URINARY ANTISEPTICS.

Oxytocin (Pitocin®, Syntocinon®)

Action and Use
Oxytocic used to control postpartum hemorrhage and to induce labor.

Dosage and Administration
The dosage is individualized; administered by buccal, intranasal, SC, IM, or IV route.

Cautions

Oxytocin is a potent drug; it should be administered by only one route at a time. Contraindicated in patients with a history of uterine surgery (including cesarean section), or when the uterus is overdistended. Oxytocin may produce coronary vasoconstriction, myocardial ischemia, and hypotension during anesthesia.

Adverse Reactions

Possible side effects include nausea and vomiting, anaphylactic reaction, premature ventricular contractions, pelvic hematoma, hypotension, anxiety, dyspnea, chest pain, cyanosis, and flushing. Occasionally severe uterine contractions occur as a result of excessive dosage or hypersensitivity, which may lead to a ruptured uterus, cardiac and/or respiratory fetal distress, or fetal death. Prolonged infusion may rarely lead to water intoxication (with convulsions and coma) and increased blood loss (following hypofibrinogenemia or afibrinogenemia).

Composition and Supply
Injection   10 units/ml, in 0.5 ml and 1 ml ampuls
Solution, nasal spray   40 units/ml (Syntocinon® Nasal Spray)
Tablets, buccal   200 units (Pitocin® Citrate, Buccal)

Legal Status
Prescription

Pabanol™ (para-aminobenzoic acid ointment)

See EMOLLIENT-PROTECTANTS.

Pagitane® (cycrimine hydrochloride)

See ANTIPARKINSONICS.

Pamine® (methscopolamine bromide)

See ANTICHOLINERGICS.

Pamisyl®

See **Aminosalicylic acid.**

Panafil® (papain/urea/chlorophyll derivatives)

See DEBRIDEMENT ENZYMES.

Pancreatin (Viokase®)

See DIGESTANTS.

Pancrelipase (Cotazym®, Ilozyme®)

Action and Use
Pancreatic enzymes (lipase, protease, and amylase) used in replacement therapy.

Dosage and Administration
1 to 3 capsules or tablets (or 1 or 2 packets) just before each meal or snack.

Cautions
Avoid inhalation of the powder. Use with caution in patients who are allergic to pork protein.

Adverse Reactions
Temporary indigestion may result unless the proper balance between fat, protein, and starch is maintained.

Composition and Supply
Capsules   300 mg

Legal Status
Prescription

Pancuronium bromide (Pavulon®)

Action and Use
Skeletal muscle relaxant.

Dosage and Administration
The dosage is individualized and carefully adjusted, ranging from 40 to 100 μg/kg, IV.

Cautions
There is a danger of respiratory paralysis. Not recommended for use in children under 10 years of age. The intensity of blockade and the duration of action are increased by potent volatile inhalation anesthetics.

Adverse Reactions
Hypersensitivity may occur. The patient may complain of muscle soreness caused by the initial contractions that often occur prior to the onset of paralysis. Occasional side effects include bradycardia, tachycardia, hypertension, hypotension, cardiac arrest, increased intraocular pressure, and excessive salivation. Large doses injected quickly may produce hypotension, circulatory collapse, and occasionally bronchospasm. Respiratory depression, hypoxia, and death are possible.

Composition and Supply
Injection   1 mg/ml, in 10 ml vials
Injection   2 mg/ml, in 2 ml and 5 ml ampuls

Legal Status
Prescription

Panheprin®

See **Heparin sodium injection.**

Panmycin®

See **Tetracycline hydrochloride.**

Pantopaque® (iophendylate)

See DIAGNOSTICS, roentgenography.

Pantopon®

See **Opium alkaloids.**

Pantothenic acid

See VITAMINS, water-soluble, vitamin B complex.

Panwarfin®

See **Sodium warfarin.**

Papain/urea/chlorophyll derivatives (Panafil®)

See DEBRIDEMENT ENZYMES.

Papaverine hydrochloride (Cerespan®, Pavabid®, Pavakey®, Vasospan®)

Action and Use
Antispasmodic and peripheral vasodilator.

Dosage and Administration
100 to 300 mg 3 to 5 times a day, orally; 30 to 120 mg, SC, IM, or IV, repeated every 3 hours if needed.

Cautions
May be potentiated by CNS depressants. Use cautiously in patients with glaucoma. Injections must be given slowly to avoid serious side effects.

Adverse Reactions
Large intravenous doses may cause arrhythmias. Rare side effects include nausea, diarrhea, anorexia, constipation, malaise, drowsiness, vertigo, headache, diaphoresis, and rash.

Composition and Supply
Capsules, long-acting 150 mg and 300 mg (Pavabid® Plateau CAPS®)
Injection 30 mg/ml, in 1 ml and 2 ml ampuls
Tablets 30 mg, 60 mg, 100 mg, and 200 mg

Legal Status
Prescription

Para-aminobenzoic acid ointment (Pabanol®, PreSun®)

See EMOLLIENT-PROTECTANTS.

Para-diisobutylphenoxypolyethoxyethanol (Preceptin®)

See CONTRACEPTIVES, TOPICAL.

Paradione®

See **Paramethadione.**

Paraflex® (chlorzoxazone)

See SKELETAL MUSCLE RELAXANTS.

Paraldehyde

Action and Use
Sedative and hypnotic used to treat delirium tremens and alcohol withdrawal.

Dosage and Administration
4 to 15 ml, orally; 10 to 20 ml, rectally; 3 to 5 ml, IM; or 3 to 5 ml (well diluted in saline), IV.

Cautions
Use cautiously in patients with hepatitis. IV injection may cause circulatory collapse or pulmonary edema (the risk is diminished by injecting the drug slowly). Contraindicated in patients with liver disease, bronchitis, or pneumonia. Keep liquid in a tightly sealed, amber-colored glass container to avoid decomposition. Discolored parenteral preparations should not be used.

Adverse Reactions
Nausea, vomiting, and gastric distress may occur. Paraldehyde has an unpleasant taste and imparts a pungent odor to the breath; it is irritating to the mucous membranes. Pain may occur on injection if more than 5 ml is given.

Composition and Supply
Capsules   1 g
Injection   2 ml, 5 ml, and 10 ml ampuls
Liquid, oral   100%
Solution   30 ml
Suppositories   1.5 g

Legal Status
Schedule IV

Paramethadione (Paradione®)

Action and Use
Anticonvulsant indicated for the management of petit mal seizures.

Dosage and Administration
900 mg to 2.4 g daily, orally.

Cautions
Drowsiness occurs frequently. Blood dyscrasias may occur. Use with caution in pregnant women, since there is a potential for birth defects. See **Trimethadione** for further cautions.

Adverse Reactions
Similar to adverse reactions to trimethadione, except that there is a lower incidence of photophobia and rash.

Composition and Supply
Capsules   150 mg and 300 mg
Solution, oral   300 mg/ml, in 50 ml vials

Legal Status
Prescription

Paramethasone acetate (Haldrone®)

See CORTICOSTEROIDS.

Parathyroid injection

Action and Use
Hormone replacement used to treat parathyroid tetany.

Dosage and Administration
The initial dose is 100 to 300 units, followed by 20 to 40 units every 12 hours as a maintenance dose, SC, IM, or IV.

Cautions
Frequent serum calcium determinations should be made in patients being treated with parathyroid injections. It should not be given to patients whose blood levels of the hormone are already above normal. Skin tests should be made before IV injection, and desensitization should be employed if the tests are positive. Use cautiously in patients with renal or cardiac disease.

Adverse Reactions
Anorexia, vomiting, diarrhea, and weakness may occur with overdosage.

Composition and Supply
Injection   100 units/ml, in 1 ml and 5 ml vials

Legal Status
Prescription

Paredrine® (hydroxyamphetamine hydrobromide)

See MYDRIATICS.

Paregoric (camphorated tincture of opium)

Action and Use
Antidiarrheal.

Dosage and Administration
5 to 10 ml 1 to 4 times a day, orally.

Cautions
Paregoric is habit-forming.

Adverse Reactions
Constipation and other morphine-like effects in excessive dosage.

Composition and Supply
Tincture   morphine 400 µg/ml

Legal Status
Schedule III

Parenogen® (fibrinogen, human)

See HEMOSTATICS.

Parenteral hyperalimentation kit (amino acids–dextrose) (Aminosol® Kit, FreAmine® Kit, Polynute® Kit)

See PARENTERAL ALIMENTATION.

Parepectolin®

See under **Kaolin/pectin.**

Parest® (methaqualone)

See SEDATIVE-HYPNOTICS, nonbarbiturates.

Pargyline hydrochloride (Eutonyl®)

Action and Use
Antihypertensive (MAO inhibitor).

Dosage and Administration
25 to 75 mg daily, orally.

Cautions
Use extreme caution in patients concurrently being treated with catecholamine-releasing antihypertensives, antidepressants, adrenergic agents, CNS depressants or stimulants, or anesthetic agents. Contraindicated in patients with renal failure, pheochromocytoma, paranoid schizophrenia, or hypothyroidism. See **Isocarboxazid** for further cautions.

Adverse Reactions
See **Isocarboxazid.**

Composition and Supply
Tablets   10 mg, 25 mg, and 50 mg
Tablets   25 mg with methyclothiazide 5 mg (Eutron®)

Legal Status
Prescription

Parnate® (tranylcypromine)

See PSYCHOTROPICS, MAO inhibitors.

Paromomycin sulfate (Humatin®)

Action and Use
Antibiotic used to treat enteric bacterial infections, amebiasis, and hepatic coma, and to achieve bowel sterilization.

Dosage and Administration
25 to 100 mg/kg daily in 4 divided doses, orally.

Cautions
Contraindicated in patients with intestinal obstruction.

Adverse Reactions
Possible side effects include vomiting, nausea, diarrhea, abdominal cramps, headache, and skin rash.

Composition and Supply
Capsules   250 mg
Syrup   125 mg/5 ml

Legal Status
Prescription

Parsidol®

See **Ethopropazine hydrochloride.**

PAS

See **Aminosalicylic acid.**

Pascorbic®

See under **Aminosalicylic acid.**

Pathocil®

See **Dicloxacillin sodium.**

Pavabid®

See **Papaverine hydrochloride.**

Pavakey®

See **Papaverine hydrochloride.**

Paveril® (dioxyline phosphate)

See ANTISPASMODICS.

Pavulon®

See **Pancuronium bromide.**

Pedameth®

See **Methionine.**

Pediaflor®

See **Sodium fluoride.**

Pedialyte® (electrolyte solution, oral)

See ELECTROLYTE SOLUTIONS AND WATER-BALANCE AGENTS, replacement solutions.

Pediamycin®

See **Erythromycin ethylsuccinate.**

Peganone® (ethotoin)

See ANTICONVULSANTS.

Pemoline (Cylert®)

See CEREBRAL STIMULANTS.

Penbritin®

See **Ampicillin.**

Penicillamine (Cuprimine®)

Action and Use
Chelating agent that removes excess copper and mercury; used principally in Wilson's disease.

Dosage and Administration
250 mg 4 times a day, orally; the dosage may be increased to 4 to 5 g daily, if needed.

Cautions
Contraindicated in patients who are hypersensitive to the drug.

Adverse Reactions
Rash and blood dyscrasias are occasional side effects. Renal damage may rarely develop.

Composition and Supply
Capsules   250 mg

Legal Status
Prescription

Penicillin G benzathine (Bicillin®, Bicillin® L-A)

Action and Use
Antibiotic, particularly useful in the treatment of syphilis (see p. 11).

Dosage and Administration
Depending on condition, 200,000 to 600,000 units every 4 to 6 hours, orally, or 600,000 to 2.4 million units, IM.

Cautions
Sensitivity reactions may occur. Shake multiple-dose vials vigorously before use. See **Penicillin G potassium** for further cautions.

Adverse Reactions
See **Penicillin G potassium.**

Composition and Supply
Suspension, oral   150,000 units/5 ml and 300,000 units/5 ml
   (Bicillin®)

Suspension, injectable   300,000 units/ml, 600,000 units/ml, and 1.2 million units/ml (Bicillin® L-A)

Legal Status
Prescription

Penicillin G benzathine/penicillin G procaine (Bicillin® C-R, Bicillin® C-R 900/300)

Action and Use
Antibiotic (see p. 11).

Dosage and Administration
The dosage is 600,000 to 2.4 million units, individualized to the patient and condition being treated, deep IM.

Cautions
Sensitivity may occur. Should not be used in the treatment of venereal diseases. Shake multiple-dose vials vigorously before use. See **Penicillin G potassium** for further cautions.

Adverse Reactions
See **Penicillin G potassium.**

Composition and Supply
Cartridges   450,000 units penicillin G benzathine and 150,000 units penicillin G procaine per ml
Cartridges and syringes   300,000 units penicillin G benzathine and 300,000 units penicillin G procaine per ml
Vials   150,000 units penicillin G benzathine and 150,000 units penicillin G procaine per ml

Legal Status
Prescription

Penicillin G potassium injection

Penicillin G potassium oral (Pentids®, Pfizerpen G®)

Action and Use
Antibiotic (see p. 11).

Dosage and Administration
400,000 to 80 million units per day (individualized to the patient and the condition being treated), orally or IV drip.

Cautions
Use with caution in patients who may be allergic to penicillin; anaphylaxis may occur. Patients should remain close to medical facilities for at least 30 minutes after injection.

Adverse Reactions
Relatively nontoxic. There is a small percentage of allergic responses, including dermatitis, urticaria, erythema, pruritus, asthma, local reaction at injection site, fever, eosinophilia, nephritis, and polyarthritis. Anaphylaxis is possible, especially when the drug is administered by the parenteral route. Superinfections may occur. Nausea, vomiting, diarrhea, and dehydration may limit drug excretion and raise the blood level to a toxic range. Irritation, pain, and inflammation may occur at the injection site with some preparations. Phlebitis or thrombophlebitis may occasionally develop with intravenous administration of some preparations.

Composition and Supply
Injection   1 million unit, 5 million unit, and 20 million unit vials (*Note:* dilute with sterile water for injection, isotonic sodium chloride injection, or dextrose injection, depending on the route of administration)
Syrup (prepared from Pentids® "400" powder)
Tablets   400,000 units and 800,000 units

Legal Status
Prescription

Penicillin G procaine (Crysticillin®, Duracillin® A.S., Wycillin®)

Action and Use
Antibiotic (see p. 11).

Dosage and Administration
300,000 to 2.4 million units, IM.

Cautions
Penicillin allergy and possibly anaphylaxis may occur. Procaine hypersensitivity is also possible. See **Penicillin G potassium** for further cautions.

Adverse Reactions
See **Penicillin G potassium.**

Composition and Supply
Injection   300,000 units/ml and 600,000 units/ml, in ampuls, vials, and disposable syringes

399

Legal Status
Prescription

Penicillin G sodium

Action and Use
Antibiotic (see p. 11).

Dosage and Administration
See **Penicillin G potassium.**

Cautions
See **Penicillin G potassium.**

Adverse Reactions
See **Penicillin G potassium.**

Composition and Supply
Injection   1 million unit and 5 million unit vials

Legal Status
Prescription

Penicillin V potassium (Compocillin®-VK, Ledercillin® VK, Pen-Vee® K, SK-Penicillin VK™, V-Cillin® K, Veetids®)

Action and Use
Antibiotic (see p. 11).

Dosage and Administration
200,000 to 800,000 units every 6 to 8 hours, orally.

Cautions
See **Penicillin G potassium.**

Adverse Reactions
See **Penicillin G potassium.**

Composition and Supply
Suspension   125 mg/5 ml and 250 mg/5 ml (200,000 units/125 mg)
Tablets   125 mg, 250 mg, and 500 mg (200,000 units/125 mg)

Legal Status
Prescription

Pensin®

See **Ampicillin.**

Pentaerythritol tetranitrate (Pentritol®, Peritrate®)

Action and Use
Coronary vasodilator.

Dosage and Administration
The initial dose is 10 to 20 mg 4 times a day, orally, titrated upward to 40 mg 4 times a day ½ hour before or 1 hour after meals and at bedtime.

Cautions
Use carefully in patients with glaucoma.

Adverse Reactions
See **Nitroglycerin.**

Composition and Supply
Tablets   10 mg and 20 mg
Tablets   10 mg and 20 mg with phenobarbital 15 mg
Tablets, long-acting   30 mg (Pentritol®) and 80 mg (Peritrate® SA)
  (*Note:* the dosage is 1 tablet twice daily)
Tablets, long-acting   80 mg with phenobarbital 45 mg (Peritrate®
  with phenobarbital SA) (*Note:* the dosage is 1 tablet twice daily)

Legal Status
Prescription

Pentamidine (Lomidine®)

See ANTIPROTOZOALS, antitrypanosomals.

Pentazocine (Talwin®)

Action and Use
Nonnarcotic analgesic used to relieve moderate to severe pain.

Dosage and Administration
50 to 100 mg every 3 or 4 hours, orally; or 30 to 60 mg every 3 or 4 hours, SC, IM, or IV.

Cautions
Use cautiously in patients being treated with other depressant drugs, and in those with renal and hepatic malfunction, intracranial pressure, respiratory depression, liver disease, kidney disease, myocardial infarction, or seizures. Pentazocine weakly antagonizes the analgesic effect of morphine and other narcotics; it can produce dependency in abusers.

Adverse Reactions
The most common side effects include sedation, diaphoresis, nausea, dizziness, and lightheadedness. Other possible symptoms include euphoria, vomiting, constipation, diarrhea, dry mouth, weakness, headache, syncope, and blurred vision. High doses produce marked respiratory depression associated with hypertension and tachycardia.

Composition and Supply
Injection (as lactate)   30 mg and 60 mg ampuls
Tablets (as hydrochloride)   50 mg
Tablets (Caplets®)   12.5 mg with aspirin 325 mg (Talwin® Compound) (*Note:* the dosage is 2 Caplets® 3 or 4 times a day)

Legal Status
Prescription

Penthrane® (methoxyflurane)

See ANESTHETICS, general.

Pentids®

See **Penicillin G potassium.**

Pentobarbital (Nembutal®)

Action and Use
Barbiturate—sedative, hypnotic.

Dosage and Administration
Sedation: 15 to 40 mg 3 or 4 times a day, orally.
Sleep: 60 to 120 mg at bedtime, orally.
IV use: 100 to 500 mg (cautiously).

Cautions
Use cautiously in patients being treated with other CNS depressants. Pentobarbital is habit-forming. See **Amobarbital** for further cautions.

Adverse Reactions
See **Amobarbital.**

Composition and Supply
Capsules (as sodium salt)   30 mg, 50 mg, and 100 mg
Elixir   18.2 mg/5 ml
Injection (as sodium salt)   50 mg/ml
Suppositories, rectal   15 mg, 30 mg, 60 mg, 120 mg, and 200 mg
Tablets, long-acting   100 mg (Nembutal®, Gradumet®)

Legal Status
Schedule II (except suppositories Schedule III)

Pentothal®

See **Thiopental sodium.**

Pentritol®

See **Pentaerythritol tetranitrate.**

Pentylenetetrazole (Metrazol®)

Action and Use
CNS, respiratory, and circulatory stimulant.

Dosage and Administration
100 to 300 mg 3 times a day, orally; or 100 to 500 mg, IV, repeated as necessary.

Cautions
Use with caution in treating patients with low convulsive threshold and in those with focal brain lesion.

Adverse Reactions
Relatively safe in recommended dosage. Symptoms of toxicity include convulsions, exhaustion, and depression of vital centers.

Composition and Supply
Injection   100 mg/ml, in 1 ml and 3 ml ampuls
Liquid   100 mg/5 ml
Tablets   100 mg

Legal Status
Prescription

Pen-Vee® (penicillin V)

See ANTIBIOTICS, penicillins.

Pen-Vee® K

See **Penicillin V potassium.**

Peppermint spirit

See DIGESTANTS.

Pepsin

See DIGESTANTS.

Pepsin/pancreatin/bile salts (Entozyme®)
See DIGESTANTS.

Pepsin/pancreatin/bile salts/belladonna alkaloids/phenobarbital (Donnazyme®)
See DIGESTANTS.

Pepsin/pancreatin/cellulase/glutamic acid/ox bile extract (Kanulase®)
See ANTIFLATULENTS; DIGESTANTS.

Pepto-Bismol® (bismuth subsalicylate)
See ANTIDIARRHEALS.

Percocet™-5 (oxycodone hydrochloride/acetaminophen)
See ANALGESICS, narcotic.

Percodan®
See **Oxycodone/APC.**

Percorten®
See **Desoxycorticosterone acetate.**

Percorten® Pivalate
See **Desoxycorticosterone pivalate.**

Pergonal® (menotropins)
See GONADOTROPICS.

Periactin®
See **Cyproheptadine hydrochloride.**

Peri-Colace® (dioctyl sodium sulfosuccinate/casanthranol)
See CATHARTICS.

Peridial®/Dextrose 1.5% (peritoneal dialysis solution)
See DIALYZING SOLUTIONS.

Peridial®/Dextrose 4.25% (peritoneal dialysis solution)
See DIALYZING SOLUTIONS.

Peristim® Forte (casanthranol)

See CATHARTICS.

Peritoneal dialysis solution (Inpersol®/Dextrose, Peridial®/Dextrose)

See DIALYZING SOLUTIONS.

Peritrate®

See **Pentaerythritol tetranitrate.**

Permitil®

See **Fluphenazine.**

Perphenazine (Trilafon®)

Action and Use
Tranquilizer and antiemetic.

Dosage and Administration
Dosage is individualized to the patient and condition; the usual range is 4 to 64 mg daily, orally or IM.

Cautions
Perphenazine may elevate serum PBI. There are numerous side effects of the phenothiazine group of tranquilizers. See **Chlorpromazine** for further cautions.

Adverse Reactions
Possible side effects include blurred vision, sedation, ataxia, extrapyramidal effects, dry mouth, constipation, antiemesis, dermatitis, hypotension, blood dyscrasias, and jaundice.

Composition and Supply
Concentrate   16 mg/5 ml
Injection   5 mg/ml, in 1 ml ampuls and 10 ml vials
Tablets   2 mg, 4 mg, 8 mg, and 16 mg

Legal Status
Prescription

Perphenazine/amitriptyline hydrochloride (Etrafon®, Triavil®)

Action and Use
Tranquilizer-antidepressant combination used to treat patients with depression and moderate anxiety.

Dosage and Administration
Initial dosage is usually 1 tablet (of the 2-25 or 4-25 combination) 3 or 4 times a day.

Cautions
See **Perphenazine; Amitriptyline hydrochloride.**

Adverse Reactions
See **Perphenazine; Amitriptyline hydrochloride.**

Composition and Supply
Tablets   perphenazine 2 mg with amitriptyline hydrochloride 10 mg
(Etrafon® 2-10, Triavil® 2-10)
Tablets   perphenazine 4 mg with amitriptyline hydrochloride 10 mg
(Etrafon®-A, Triavil® 4-10)
Tablets   perphenazine 2 mg with amitriptyline hydrochloride 25 mg
(Etrafon®, Triavil® 2-25)
Tablets   perphenazine 4 mg with amitriptyline hydrochloride 25 mg
(Etrafon® Forte, Triavil® 4-25)

Legal Status
Prescription

Persadox® (benzoyl peroxide preparation)

See KERATOLYTICS.

Persa-Gel® (benzoyl peroxide preparation)

See KERATOLYTICS.

Persantine®

See **Dipyridamole.**

Pertofrane®

See **Desipramine hydrochloride.**

Pertussis immune human globulin (Hypertussis®)

See BIOLOGICALS, immune serums–antitoxins.

Petrolatum (petroleum jelly)

Action and Use
Protectant, emollient, lubricant, and ointment base.

Dosage and Administration
Applied topically.

Cautions
Should not be used for wounds, serious burns, or cuts.

Adverse Reactions
None with proper use.

Composition and Supply
Petrolatum, NF (yellow petrolatum)
Petrolatum, hydrophilic, USP (white petrolatum plus cholesterol, stearyl alcohol, and white wax)
Petrolatum, white, USP
Petroleum jelly, pure (Vaseline®)

Legal Status
Nonprescription

Petrolatum, liquid

See **Mineral oil.**

Pfizer-E®

See **Erythromycin stearate.**

Pfizerpen-G®

See **Penicillin G potassium.**

Phazyme® (simethicone/pancreatin)

See **ANTIFLATULENTS.**

Phelantin® (phenobarbital/phenytoin sodium/methamphetamine hydrochloride)

See **ANTICONVULSANTS.**

Phenacemide (Phenurone®)

See **ANTICONVULSANTS.**

Phenaphen®

See **Acetaminophen.**

Phenazopyridine hydrochloride (Pyridium®)

Action and Use
Urinary tract local anesthetic.

Dosage and Administration
100 to 200 mg 3 times a day, orally before meals.

Cautions

Contraindicated in patients with severe hepatitis, uremia, and chronic glomerular nephritis. The patient should be told that phenazopyridine imparts a reddish orange color to the urine.

Adverse Reactions

Occasional gastrointestinal disturbances and sensitivity may result.

Composition and Supply

Tablets   100 mg and 200 mg

Legal Status

Prescription

Phenelzine sulfate (Nardil®)

Action and Use

Antidepressant (MAO inhibitor).

Dosage and Administration

15 to 45 mg daily, orally.

Cautions

Contraindicated in patients with impaired renal or hepatic function, epilepsy, degenerative heart disease, hyperthyroidism, or pheochromocytoma. The patient should avoid adrenergic drugs and foods high in tryptamine and tyramine (namely, cheeses, beer, wine, chicken liver, yeast, and pickled herring).

Adverse Reactions

Common side effects include dizziness, constipation, dry mouth, postural hypotension, drowsiness, weakness, fatigue, gastrointestinal disturbances, tremors, and twitching. Uncommon and severe reactions include reversible jaundice, ataxia, coma, respiratory depression, leukopenia, manic reaction, convulsions, and precipitation of schizophrenia.

Composition and Supply

Tablets   15 mg

Legal Status

Prescription

Phenergan®

See **Promethazine hydrochloride.**

Phenergan® Expectorant

See COUGH-COLD PREPARATIONS, cough preparations.

Phenergan® VC Expectorant

See COUGH-COLD PREPARATIONS, cough preparations.

Phenistix®

See DIAGNOSTICS, urine (phenylketonuria).

Phenmetrazine hydrochloride (Preludin®)

Action and Use
Anorectic.

Dosage and Administration
12.5 mg to 25 mg 2 to 3 times a day, orally.

Cautions
Contraindicated in patients with hypertension, hyperthyroidism, or angina pectoris.

Adverse Reactions
Similar to but less pronounced than those of dextroamphetamine sulfate (see).

Composition and Supply
Tablets   25 mg
Tablets, long-acting   75 mg

Legal Status
Schedule II

Phenobarbital (Luminal®)

Action and Use
A barbiturate used as a sedative, hypnotic, and anticonvulsant.

Dosage and Administration
Sedative: 15 to 30 mg 2 to 4 times a day, orally.
Hypnotic: 100 to 300 mg, orally.
Anticonvulsant (control): 50 to 120 mg a day, orally.
Status epilepticus: 300 to 600 mg, IM or SC.

409

Cautions
Contraindicated in patients with nephritis. Use with caution in patients with pulmonary disease and in those who are aged or debilitated. Phenobarbital is habit-forming.

Adverse Reactions
Adverse reactions are infrequent with doses under 200 mg. Occasional side effects include drowsiness, vertigo, headache, nausea, vomiting, emotional disturbances, allergic reaction, and nightmares. More severe reactions include delirium, stupor, and ataxia.

Composition and Supply
Elixir   20 mg/5 ml
Injection (as sodium salt)   65 mg/ml and 130 mg/ml
Tablets 15 mg, 30 mg, and 100 mg

Legal Status
Schedule III

Phenobarbital/phenytoin sodium/methamphetamine hydrochloride (Phelantin®)

See ANTICONVULSANTS.

Phenolated calamine lotion

See under **Calamine lotion.**

Phenolsulfonphthalein (PSP)

Action and Use
Diagnostic agent used to assess kidney function (in normal individuals no less than 25% of the injected dose is excreted in 15 minutes; within 30 minutes 50 to 65% is usually excreted).

Dosage and Administration
6 mg, IV.

Cautions
False-positive results may occur in patients with gout and in those receiving acidic drugs. Avoid the concurrent administration of drugs that discolor urine.

Adverse Reactions
There are occasional allergic responses.

Composition and Supply
6 mg/ml, in 1 ml ampuls

Legal Status
Prescription

Phenoxybenzamine hydrochloride (Dibenzyline®)

Action and Use
Used in the treatment of vasospastic peripheral vascular disorders and in the control of pheochromocytoma.

Dosage and Administration
10 to 60 mg daily, orally.

Cautions
Use with caution in patients with cerebral arteriosclerosis or renal damage.

Adverse Reactions
Relatively common side effects include tachycardia, orthostatic hypotension (the patient should use caution upon rising), dizziness, weakness, and faintness; the latter may subside, but may reappear under conditions that promote vasodilatation, such as exercise, eating a large meal, or consuming alcohol. Stroke or myocardial infarction may occur in patients with severe cerebral or coronary atherosclerosis or congestive heart failure. Kidney failure is possible in patients with renal damage. Occasional side effects include nausea, vomiting (especially with large doses taken on an empty stomach), nasal congestion, bronchoconstriction, miosis, impotence. The effects of an overdose include hypotension, tachycardia, and shock.

Composition and Supply
Capsules   10 mg

Legal Status
Prescription

Phenprocoumon (Liquamar®)

See ANTICOAGULANTS.

Phensuximide (Milontin®)

Action and Use
Anticonvulsant used to control petit mal epilepsy.

Dosage and Administration
Dosage is adjusted to individual needs; the usual dose is 500 mg to 1 g 2 or 3 times a day, orally.

Cautions
Drowsiness is a frequent side effect. Cases of systemic lupus erythematosus and fatal blood dyscrasias have been reported. Use with caution in patients with hepatic or renal disease and in pregnant women.

Adverse Reactions
Frequent side effects include nausea, vomiting, anorexia, drowsiness, dizziness, and headache. Other possible side effects include skin eruptions, renal damage, blood dyscrasias, alopecia, and muscular weakness.

Composition and Supply
Capsules   250 mg and 500 mg
Suspension   300 mg per 5 ml

Legal Status
Prescription

Phentermine resin (Ionamin®)

See CEREBRAL STIMULANTS, anorectics.

Phentolamine (Regitine®)

Action and Use
Alpha-adrenergic blocking agent used in the diagnosis of pheochromocytoma, in the treatment of hypertensive crises, and in the prevention and treatment of dermal sloughing following intravenous administration or extravasation of norepinephrine.

Dosage and Administration
50 mg 4 to 6 times a day, orally; or 1 to 5 mg, IM or IV.

Cautions
Contraindicated in patients with myocardial infarction, coronary insufficiency, angina, a history of myocardial infection, or other evidence of coronary artery disease.

Adverse Reactions
Side effects include orthostatic hypotension, tachycardia, weakness, dizziness (the patient should use caution when rising), anginal pain (especially with parenteral doses), nausea, vomiting, diarrhea, flushing, chilliness, and apprehension. The effects of an overdose include severe hypotension and shock.

Composition and Supply
Tablets (as hydrochloride)   50 mg
Injection (as mesylate)   5 mg ampuls

Legal Status
Prescription

Phenurone® (phenacemide)

See ANTICONVULSANTS.

Phenylbutazone (Azolid®, Butazolidin®)

Action and Use
Anti-inflammatory analgesic.

Dosage and Administration
200 to 600 mg daily in divided doses, orally.

Cautions
Avoid indiscriminate use in patients with minor musculoskeletal conditions. The incidence of side effects is high; phenylbutazone should be administered to selected patients under close medical supervision.

Adverse Reactions
Similar to adverse reactions to oxyphenbutazone (see), which is its active metabolite.

Composition and Supply
Capsules   100 mg with dried aluminum hydroxide gel 100 mg and
    magnesium trisilicate 150 mg (Azolid-A®, Butazolidin® Alka)
Tablets   100 mg

Legal Status
Prescription

Phenylephrine hydrochloride (Neo-Synephrine®)

Action and Use
Antihypertensive, mydriatic, and ophthalmic and nasal vasoconstrictor.

Dosage and Administration
Antihypertensive: 1 to 10 mg, SC or IM.
Mydriatic: 1 or 2 drops of solution preceded by 1 drop of a local anesthetic.
Ophthalmic vasoconstrictor: 1 or 2 drops of ophthalmic solution once or twice a day.
Nasal vasoconstrictor: 2 to 3 drops (or 2 to 3 sprays) of nasal preparation every 4 hours.

Cautions
Use with caution in patients with diabetes, hyperthyroidism, hypertension, coronary disease, arteriosclerosis, or narrow-angle glaucoma. May cause serious arrhythmias if used with halogenated anesthetics. MAO inhibitors are potentiated. Increased intraocular pressure may occur in patients who are also being treated with long-term corticosteroid therapy. Should not be used in patients who are being treated with phenytoin sodium.

Adverse Reactions
Similar to the adverse reactions to epinephrine (see), but less common and less severe. Overuse of nasal preparations can cause rebound congestion. Systemic absorption can cause nervousness, palpitations, and hypertension.

Composition and Supply
Drops and spray, nasal   0.125%, 0.25%, 0.5%, and 1%
Injection   10 mg/ml, in 1 ml ampuls
Solution, ophthalmic   2.5% and 10%

Legal Status
Prescription (injection and ophthalmic solution)
Nonprescription (nasal preparations)

Phenylephrine hydrochloride/isoetharine mesylate (Bronkometer®)

See ADRENERGICS; ANTIASTHMATICS, adrenergics.

Phenylmercuric acetate (Lorophyn®)

See CONTRACEPTIVES, TOPICAL.

Phenylpropanolamine hydrochloride

See NASAL DECONGESTANTS.

Phenylpropanolamine hydrochloride/chlorpheniramine maleate
(Novahistine®, Triaminicin®)

See NASAL DECONGESTANTS.

Phenytoin sodium (Dilantin®)

Action and Use
Anticonvulsant used to control grand mal seizures and to prevent seizures during neurosurgery.

Dosage and Administration
The dosage is adjusted to individual requirements. The usual oral dose is 6 to 7 mg/kg daily (300 to 600 mg per day); the usual IV dose is

150 to 250 mg initially, followed by 100 to 150 mg 30 minutes later, if needed (slowly).

Cautions
Side effects are numerous and can be serious. Contraindicated in patients with sinus bradycardia, sinoatrial block, atrioventricular block, or Adams-Stokes syndrome. IV administration should not exceed 50 mg per minute. Neonatal hemorrhage and birth defects may be associated with the use of phenytoin and other anticonvulsants during pregnancy. Abrupt withdrawal may precipitate status epilepticus.

Adverse Reactions
The most common side effects include apathy, insomnia, transient nervousness, tremors, hirsutism, and gingival hyperplasia. Occasional side effects include nausea, vomiting, constipation, anorexia, skin rash, fever, pancytopenia, and lymphadenopathy. Rare side effects include inhibition of antidiuretic hormone and insulin, osteomalacia, polyarthropathy, hepatitis, lupus erythematosus, and periarteritis nodosa. IV administration at an excessive rate may cause cardiovascular collapse or CNS depression. The injection should be followed with saline to avoid local venous irritation. Continuous infusion should be avoided.

Composition and Supply
Capsules   100 mg
Injection   50 mg/ml (*Note:* it is not recommended that phenytoin be added to IV infusions, because precipitation may result)
Suspension   30 mg/5 ml and 125 mg/5 ml
Tablets   50 mg

Legal Status
Prescription

pHisoDerm® (entsulfon sodium)

See DETERGENTS.

pHisoHex®

See **Hexachlorophene detergent.**

Phosphaljel® (aluminum phosphate)

See ANTACIDS.

Phospholine Iodide®

See **Echothiophate iodide.**

Phosphotope® (sodium phosphate P 32)

See ANTINEOPLASTICS, radioisotopes.

Phthalylsulfathiazole (Sulfathalidine®)

Action and Use
Sulfonamide used in the treatment of ulcerative colitis and in the suppression of intestinal bacteria prior to bowel surgery.

Dosage and Administration
50 to 125 mg/kg, orally or rectally; the dose should not exceed 8 g.

Cautions
Contraindicated in patients with an allergy or sensitivity to sulfonamides.

Adverse Reactions
See **Sulfisoxazole.**

Composition and Supply
Tablets   500 mg

Legal Status
Prescription

Physostigmine salicylate (eserine) (Antilirium®)

Action and Use
Cholinergic (anticholinesterase) agent used as a miotic and as an antidote to anticholinergic poisons (e.g., belladonna preparations, atropine) and tricyclic antidepressants.

Dosage and Administration
Antidote in poisoning: 1 to 4 mg, IM or IV.
Miotic: the ointment is applied at bedtime, and the solution is used during the day.

Cautions
Should not be used in patients with asthma, gangrene, diabetes, cardiovascular disease, or mechanical obstruction of the intestines or urogenital tract, and in those being treated with depolarizing skeletal muscle relaxants (e.g., decamethonium, succinylcholine). An overdose can cause cholinergic crisis. Use only clear, colorless solutions.

Adverse Reactions
The more common adverse reactions are typical cholinergic effects—miosis, excessive sweating, nausea, vomiting, and slow heart. Hypersensitivity may occur.

Composition and Supply
Injection   1 mg/ml, in 2 ml ampuls
Ointment, ophthalmic   0.25%
Solution, ophthalmic   0.25%

Legal Status
Prescription

Phytonadione (Vitamin K₁) (AquaMEPHYTON®, Konakion®, Mephyton®)

Action and Use
Vitamin K preparation of choice used in the prevention and treatment of hypoprothrombinemia.

Dosage and Administration
Dosage is individualized to the patient and condition being treated; the dosage ranges from 500 μg to 25 mg daily, administered orally, SC, IM, or IV.

Cautions
IV use may cause severe reactions (resembling hypersensitivity and anaphylaxis) and should be restricted to those patients in whom other routes are not feasible and for whom the serious risk involved is justified. The anticoagulant action of heparin is not counteracted. An overdose may produce thrombosis. Use with caution in patients with liver impairment. Temporary resistance to prothrombin-depressing anticoagulants may result. Check prothrombin time during therapy.

Adverse Reactions
Rapid IV administration may produce flushing, dizziness, weak and rapid pulse, sweating, brief hypotension, dyspnea, and cyanosis. SC or IM administration may result in pain at the injection site. Allergic sensitivity and anaphylaxis may occur.

Composition and Supply
Injection   1 mg and 10 mg ampuls
Tablets   5 mg

Legal Status
Prescription

Pilocar®

See **Pilocarpine hydrochloride.**

Pilocarpine hydrochloride (Isopto® Carpine, Pilocar®)

Action and Use
Miotic used in the management of glaucoma and in the neutralization of mydriatics.

Dosage and Administration
1 to 2 drops in conjunctival sac several times daily as required.

Cautions
Pulmonary edema may occur in patients with lung disease. Asthmatic attack may be precipitated. The solution should be protected from light.

Adverse Reactions
Cholinergic effects are possible adverse reactions.

Composition and Supply
Solution, ophthalmic (as hydrochloride or nitrate)   0.5%, 1%, 2%, 4%, and 6%

Legal Status
Prescription

Pipenzolate bromide (Piptal®)

See ANTICHOLINERGICS.

Piperacetazine (Quide®)

See PSYCHOTROPICS, antipsychotics.

Piperazine citrate (Antepar®)

Action and Use
Anthelmintic used for pinworm and roundworm.

Dosage and Administration
50 mg/kg daily, orally; the maximum adult dose is 3.5 g.

Cautions
Contraindicated in patients with hepatic or renal dysfunction, convulsive disorders, hypertension, or hypersensitivity reactions to piperazine and its salts. Use with caution in patients with malnutrition or anemia.

Adverse Reactions
Occasional side effects include nausea, vomiting, diarrhea, and abdominal cramps. Large doses may produce urticaria, muscular weakness, and blurred vision. Discontinue the medication if there

are CNS reactions or major gastrointestinal or hypersensitivity reactions.

Composition and Supply
Syrup   500 mg/5 ml
Tablets   250 mg and 500 mg

Legal Status
Prescription

Piperazine estrone sulfate (Ogen®)

Action and Use
Estrogen.

Dosage and Administration
Dosage is individualized to patient, administered orally.

Cautions
See **Estradiol benzoate.**

Adverse Reactions
See **Estradiol benzoate.**

Composition and Supply
Tablets   625 µg, 1.25 mg, and 2.5 mg

Legal Status
Prescription

Pipobroman (Vercyte®)

See ANTINEOPLASTICS, alkylating agents.

Piptal® (pipenzolate bromide)

See ANTICHOLINERGICS.

Pitocin®

See **Oxytocin.**

Pitocin® Citrate, Buccal

See under **Oxytocin.**

Pitressin®

See **Vasopressin.**

Placidyl®

See **Ethchlorvynol.**

Plaquenil®

See **Hydroxychloroquine sulfate.**

Plasma protein fraction, human (Plasmanate®, Plasmatein®)

See ELECTROLYTE SOLUTIONS AND WATER-BALANCE AGENTS, plasma extenders.

Plasmanate® (plasma protein fraction, human)

See ELECTROLYTE SOLUTIONS AND WATER-BALANCE AGENTS, plasma extenders.

Plasmatein® (plasma protein fraction, human)

See ELECTROLYTE SOLUTIONS AND WATER-BALANCE AGENTS, plasma extenders.

Plexonal® (barbital/butalbital/phenobarbital/dihydroergotamine/scopolamine)

See SEDATIVE-HYPNOTICS, barbiturates.

Pneumococcal vaccine, polyvalent (Pneumorax®)

See BIOLOGICALS, vaccines.

Pneumovax® (pneumococcal vaccine, polyvalent)

See BIOLOGICALS, vaccines.

Podophyllum resin

Action and Use
Keratolytic used in the treatment of venereal warts.

Dosage and Administration
Applied topically; the treated area should be washed ½ to 1 hour after application.

Cautions
Podophyllum resin is cytotoxic and caustic; the surrounding area of the patient's skin should be protected. It is highly poisonous if taken internally.

Adverse Reactions
Exposure to dust may cause conjunctivitis and keratitis. Prolonged topical use may result in the absorption of toxic amounts, which may result in renal insufficiency, coma, and death.

Composition and Supply
Powder   used as 25% suspension in compound benzoin tincture

Legal Status
Prescription

Polaramine® (dexchlorpheniramine maleate)

See ANTIHISTAMINES.

Poliovirus vaccine, live oral (Diplovax®, Orimune®)

Action and Use
Vaccine used to prevent poliomyelitis caused by poliovirus types 1, 2, and 3.

Dosage and Administration
Administered orally in doses of 0.5 ml (500 μl). Primary immunization involves the following schedules:
Infants: The first dose is given at 6 to 12 weeks of age; the second dose 8 weeks later; and the third dose 8 to 12 months after the second dose.
Children and adolescents (through high school age): 2 doses are given 8 weeks apart; and the third dose is given 8 to 12 months after second dose.
Adults: 2 doses are given no less than 6 weeks and preferably 8 weeks apart.

Cautions
Under no circumstances is the vaccine to be given parenterally. Contraindicated during acute illness and in situations having a suppressive effect on immune responses (namely, in steroid, antineoplastic, or radiation therapy and in patients with leukemia, lymphogenous disease, or dysgammaglobulinemia).

Adverse Reactions
There are occasional minor complaints (by the patient), probably not related to the vaccine.

Composition and Supply
0.5 ml (500 μl) dose (single disposable pipette)
2-drop dose (10 dose and 100 dose vials with dropper)

Legal Status
Prescription

Poloxamer iodine (Prepodyne®)

See ANTI-INFECTIVES, LOCAL, miscellaneous.

Polycillin®

See **Ampicillin.**

Polycin®

See under **Polymyxin B sulfate.**

Polycitra® (sodium citrate/potassium citrate)

See ELECTROLYTE SOLUTIONS AND WATER-BALANCE AGENTS, alkalizing agents.

Polyestradiol phosphate (Estradurin®)

See ANTINEOPLASTICS, steroids, estrogens.

Polymyxin B sulfate (Aerosporin®)

Action and Use
Antibiotic effective against susceptible strains of *Pseudomonas aeruginosa* and other common gram-negative bacteria.

Dosage and Administration
Administered topically and by IV infusion (25,000 to 30,000 units/kg/day).

Cautions
Polymyxin B sulfate is nephrotoxic and neurotoxic systemically; parenteral use should be restricted to infections that do not yield to less toxic agents.

Adverse Reactions
Nausea, vomiting, and diarrhea may occur with large doses. Other side effects include superinfection; nephrotoxic effects, with hematuria, albuminuria, casts, azotemia, oliguria, and increased BUN (periodic tests of renal function are recommended); and neurotoxic effects, with flushing, slurred speech, irritability, drowsiness, paresthesias, weakness, ataxia, blurred vision, and rarely respiratory paralysis. The intrathecal injection of more than 5 mg may produce signs of meningeal irritation, headache, fever, and increased cells and protein in the spinal fluid.

Composition and Supply
Polymyxin B sulfate sterile powder   500,000 unit vials
Polymyxin B sulfate/bacitracin (Polycin®, Polysporin®*)
Polymyxin B sulfate/neomycin sulfate (Neosporin® G.U. Irrigant)

Polymyxin B sulfate/neomycin sulfate/bacitracin (Neosporin® Aerosol*, Neosporin® Ointment*, Neosporin® Ointment Ophthalmic)

Polymyxin B sulfate/neomycin sulfate/bacitracin/hydrocortisone acetate (Cortisporin® Ointment*, Cortisporin® Ointment Ophthalmic*)

Polymyxin B sulfate/neomycin sulfate/gramicidin (Neosporin®-G Cream*, Neosporin® Solution Ophthalmic)

Polymyxin B sulfate/neomycin sulfate/hydrocortisone acetate (Cortisporin® Ophthalmic Suspension*, Corticosporin® Otic Solution*)

Legal Status
Prescription (except for products marked with asterisks, which are nonprescription)

Polynute Kit® (parenteral hyperalimentation kit [amino acids–dextrose])

See PARENTERAL ALIMENTATION.

Polyoxyethylene nonyl phenol/sodium edetate/sodium dioctyl sulfosuccinate (Vagisec®)

See ANTIPROTOZOALS, antitrichomonials.

Polysporin®

See under **Polymyxin B sulfate.**

Polythiazide (Renese®)

See DIURETICS.

Pondimin® (fenfluramine hydrochloride)

See CEREBRAL STIMULANTS, anorectics.

Ponstel® (mefenamic acid)

See ANALGESICS, nonnarcotic.

Pontocaine®

See **Tetracaine hydrochloride.**

Potassic saline injection, lactated (Darrow's solution)

See ELECTROLYTE SOLUTIONS AND WATER-BALANCE AGENTS, replacement solutions.

Potassium acid phosphate (K-Phos®)

See ELECTROLYTE SOLUTIONS AND WATER-BALANCE AGENTS, acidifying agents.

Potassium bicarbonate/potassium citrate (K-Lyte®)

Action and Use
K-Lyte® is an oral potassium supplement for therapy or prophylaxis of potassium deficiency.

Dosage and Administration
1 tablet completely dissolved in 3 to 4 ounces of cold water 2 to 4 times daily, depending upon the patient's requirements. To minimize adverse reactions the solution should be taken with meals and sipped slowly over a 5 to 10 minute period.

Cautions
Contraindicated in impaired renal function (with oliguria and azotemia), hyperkalemia, and Addison's disease. To prevent the development of hyperkalemia dosage must be carefully adjusted to the needs of the individual patient.

Adverse Reactions
The usual adverse reactions include abdominal discomfort, nausea, vomiting, and diarrhea.

Composition and Supply
Tablets, effervescent   each tablet in solution supplies 25 mEq of potassium as bicarbonate and citrate

Legal Status
Prescription

Potassium chloride injection

Potassium chloride oral (Kaochlor®, Kaon-Cl Tabs®, Kay Ciel®, K-Lor®, Slow-K®)

Action and Use
Potassium replacement.

Dosage and Administration
Oral forms: 10 to 100 mEq (K$^+$) daily, depending on need.
Injection: diluted and given as required IV.

Cautions
Oral use may cause small bowel ulcerations (liquid preparations should be diluted to minimize this effect). IV use may cause cardiotoxicity. The concentration of the infusion fluid should not exceed 40 mEq/L. Contraindicated in patients with severe renal impairment, untreated Addison's disease, adynamia episodica hereditaria, acute dehydration, heat cramps, and hyperkalemia from any cause.

Adverse Reactions
Possible nausea, vomiting, abdominal discomfort; the effects of potassium intoxication resulting from overdosage include paresthesias, flaccid paralysis, listlessness, confusion, weakness, hypotension, cardiac arrhythmias, and heart block.

Composition and Supply
Injection   20 mEq, 30 mEq, and 40 mEq, in 10 ml, 15 ml, and 20 ml vials (*Note:* these must be diluted)
Liquid, flavored (with sugar or sugar-free)   20 mEq/15 ml and 40 mEq/15 ml
Powder packets, flavored   15 mEq and 20 mEq
Tablets, controlled-release   6.67 mEq (500 mg) (Kaon-Cl Tabs®)
Tablets, slow-release   8 mEq (600 mg) (Slow-K®)

Legal Status
Prescription

Potassium gluconate (Kaon®)

Action and Use
Potassium supplement.

Dosage and Administration
40 to 80 mEq (K⁺) a day, orally.

Cautions
Small bowel ulceration may occur. Liquid preparations must be diluted. See **Potassium chloride** for further cautions.

Adverse Reactions
See **Potassium chloride.**

Composition and Supply
Elixir   20 mEq/15 ml
Liquid and powder with potassium chloride (Kolyum®)   20 mEq/15 ml
Tablets   5 mEq

425

Legal Status
Prescription

Potassium iodide solution (SSKI)

Action and Use
Expectorant. (*Note:* SSKI stands for saturated solution of potassium chloride.)

Dosage and Administration
300 to 600 mg (0.3 to 0.6 ml) is administered with water every 2 hours until desired effect is achieved.

Cautions
Contraindicated in patients with tuberculosis and inflammatory conditions of the respiratory system.

Adverse Reactions
Large doses may produce nausea and vomiting. Prolonged use may produce symptoms of iodism, including coryza, pain in region of frontal sinus, and skin eruptions.

Composition and Supply
Solution, saturated   1 g/ml

Legal Status
Prescription

Potassium permanganate

Action and Use
Local anti-infective; oxidizing antidote.

Dosage and Administration
1 : 25,000 to 1 : 1,000, topically; 1 : 10,000, gastric lavage.

Cautions
The crystals and tablets are poisonous and explosive. Solutions must be freshly prepared, and crystals or tablets must be completely dissolved.

Adverse Reactions
Solutions stronger than 1 : 5,000 may be irritating to tissues. A brown stain is produced on the skin and dressings.

Composition and Supply
Tablets (for preparing solutions)   60 mg, 120 mg, 200 mg, and 300 mg

Legal Status
Prescription

Povan®

See **Pyrvinium pamoate.**

Povidone-iodine (Betadine®)

Action and Use
Water-soluble (nonstinging, nonstaining) iodine complex with the broad-range antimicrobial activity of regular iodine.

Dosage and Administration
Applied topically as directed by manufacturer.

Cautions
Should not be used near or in the eyes.

Adverse Reactions
Povidone-iodine is relatively nonirritating. Its use should be discontinued if redness, swelling, or other signs of irritation develop. It turns blue or black on contact with starch or starched linen.

Composition and Supply
Antiseptic gauze pad
Solution
Solution swabsticks
Aerosol spray
Surgical scrub
Douche
Vaginal gel
Skin cleanser

Legal Status
Nonprescription

Pralidoxime chloride (Protopam®)

Action and Use
Cholinesterase reactivator used as an antidote (in conjunction with atropine) in the treatment of poisoning caused by pesticides and chemicals of the organophosphate class (with anticholinesterase activity) and in the control of overdosage of anticholinesterase drugs.

Dosage and Administration
1 to 2 g by slow IV infusion (over 15 to 30 minutes) every hour until muscle weakness has been relieved. Oral doses of 1 to 3 g may be given every 5 hours, as a follow-up to IV therapy in severe cases, especially

after the ingestion of poison. (*Note:* if IV administration is not feasible, IM or SC injection should be used.)

Cautions
Repeated prophylactic use in workers who are exposed to phosphate ester insecticides is not recommended. Use with caution in patients with myasthenia gravis, because myasthenic crisis may occur. This drug should only be used in hospitalized patients.

Adverse Reactions
Large doses or rapid IV injection (more than 500 mg/minute) can produce weakness, diplopia, blurred vision, drowsiness, headache, dizziness, nausea, tachycardia, and hyperventilation.

Composition and Supply
Injection   1 g vials
Tablets   500 mg

Legal Status
Prescription

Pramoxine hydrochloride (Tronothane®)

Action and Use
Surface anesthetic.

Dosage and Administration
Applied topically.

Cautions
Pramoxine hydrochloride should not be used in the eye, nose, or throat; should not be used for gastroscopy or bronchoscopy; should not be injected; and should not be applied over extensive areas of skin.

Adverse Reactions
Toxicity is low, but allergic reactions are possible. Stinging sometimes occurs on initial application. Discontinue use if redness, irritation, swelling, or pain persists or increases.

Composition and Supply
Cream, jelly, lotion, and solution   1%

Legal Status
Prescription

Prazepam (Verstran®)

See PSYCHOTROPICS, tranquilizers, minor.

Prazosin hydrochloride (Minipress®)

Action and Use
Antihypertensive of mild to moderate action, used as the initial agent or in conjunction with diuretics and/or other antihypertensives.

Dosage and Administration
1 mg 3 times a day, slowly increased to a total daily dose of 20 mg in divided doses, orally. When other drugs are added, the dosage of prazosin hydrochloride should be reduced to 1 or 2 mg 3 times a day, and retitration should be carried out.

Cautions
Syncope with sudden loss of consciousness may occur. Patients should always be started at 1 mg 3 times a day.

Adverse Reactions
The most common reactions include transient dizziness, headache, drowsiness, lack of energy, weakness, palpitations, and nausea. Rarer side effects include gastrointestinal complaints, edema, dyspnea, tachycardia, rash, pruritus, urinary frequency, impotence, blurred vision, tinnitus, dry mouth, nasal congestion, and diaphoresis.

Composition and Supply
Capsules   1 mg, 2 mg, and 5 mg

Legal Status
Prescription

Preceptin® (para-diisobutylphenoxypolyethoxyethanol)

See CONTRACEPTIVES, TOPICAL.

Prednisolone (Delta-Cortef®, Hydeltra®, Meticortelone®)

Action and Use
Corticosteroid (glucocorticoid).

Dosage and Administration
5 to 200 mg daily, depending on the patient and condition being treated, orally, IM, or IV; or 0.5%, topically.

Cautions
Similar in nature to cautions for cortisone acetate (see).

Adverse Reactions
Similar in nature to adverse reactions to cortisone acetate (see), except that there is less electrolyte disturbance.

Composition and Supply

Cream   0.5% (Meti-Derm®)

Injection (as sodium succinate)   50 mg vials (for IV use) (Meti-cortelone® Soluble Sterile Powder)

Injection (as acetate)   25 mg/ml, in 5 ml vials (Sterane®)

Solution, ophthalmic (as sodium phosphate) 0.5% (Metreton®, Optimyd®)

Tablets   1 mg, 2.5 mg, and 5 mg

Legal Status

Prescription

Prednisolone acetate/sulfacetamide sodium (Metimyd®)

See CORTICOSTEROIDS.

Prednisone (Deltasone®, Meticorten®)

Action and Use

Corticosteroid (glucocorticoid).

Dosage and Administration

Dosage is individualized to the patient and condition being treated; 5 to 75 mg daily, orally.

Cautions

See **Cortisone acetate.**

Adverse Reactions

Similar in nature to adverse reactions to cortisone acetate (see), except that there is less electrolyte disturbance.

Composition and Supply

Tablets   1 mg, 2.5 mg, 5 mg, 10 mg, 20 mg, and 50 mg

Legal Status

Prescription

Preludin®

See **Phenmetrazine hydrochloride.**

Premarin®

See **Estrogens, conjugated.**

Prepodyne® (poloxamer iodine)

See ANTI-INFECTIVES, LOCAL, miscellaneous antiseptic disinfectants.

Presamine®

See **Imipramine hydrochloride.**

Pre-Sate® (chlorphentermine hydrochloride)

See CEREBRAL STIMULANTS, anorectics.

PreSun® (para-aminobenzoic acid ointment)

See EMOLLIENT-PROTECTANTS.

Prilocaine hydrochloride (Citanest®)

See ANESTHETICS, local.

Primaquine phosphate

Action and Use
Antimalarial used to treat relapsing vivax infections.

Dosage and Administration
1 tablet daily for 14 days, orally.

Cautions
There is a danger of bone marrow depression and hemolytic anemia.

Adverse Reactions
Occasional side effects include nausea, vomiting, and abdominal pains. Toxic effects include bone marrow depression (with agranulocytopenia) and hemolytic anemia (especially in patients with glucose-6-phosphate dehydrogenase deficiency, and notably in highly pigmented persons). The drug should be discontinued if the urine becomes dark or if levels of hemoglobin, leukocytes, or erythrocytes decrease.

Composition and Supply
Tablets   26.3 mg (equivalent to 15 mg base)

Legal Status
Prescription

Primidone (Mysoline®)

Action and Use
Anticonvulsant.

Dosage and Administration
Dosage is individualized to the patient; the usual range is 250 mg to 2 g daily, orally (the total dose should not exceed 2 g per day).

Cautions
Contraindicated in patients with porphyria and in those who are hypersensitive to phenobarbital. Neonatal hemorrhage (resembling vitamin K deficiency) may occur in infants whose mothers were treated with primidone or other anticonvulsants. Recent reports suggest an association between the use of anticonvulsants by women with epilepsy and increased incidence of birth defects in children born to these women.

Adverse Reactions
Similar to adverse reactions to phenytoin sodium and phenobarbital (see).

Composition and Supply
Suspension   250 mg/5 ml
Tablets   50 mg and 250 mg

Legal Status
Prescription

Principen®
See **Ampicillin.**

Priscoline®
See **Tolazoline hydrochloride.**

Privine®
See **Naphazoline hydrochloride.**

Probana®
See INFANT FORMULAS.

Pro-Banthīne®
See **Propantheline bromide.**

Probenecid (Benemid®)

Action and Use
Uricosuric used to treat gout and to prolong plasma levels of penicillin (and its analogues and congeners).

Dosage and Administration
500 mg to 3 g daily in divided doses, orally.

Cautions
Contraindicated in children under the age of 2, in patients with blood dyscrasias or uric acid kidney stones, and in patients experiencing an acute attack of gout. Probenecid may exacerbate gout, in which case colchicine is advisable; it also may increase the plasma levels of sulfa drugs, indomethacin, and rifampin. Salicylates antagonize the activity of probenecid. Use cautiously in patients with a history of peptic ulcer.

Adverse Reactions
The more common symptoms include headache, anorexia, nausea, vomiting, hypersensitivity reactions, sore gums, flushing, dizziness, and anemia. Less common side effects include urinary frequency, dermatitis, pruritus, and fever. Hemolytic anemia may occur in patients with a genetic deficiency of glucose-6-phosphate dehydrogenase. Overdosage may produce CNS stimulation, convulsions, and death from respiratory failure.

Composition and Supply
Tablets   500 mg
Tablets   500 mg with colchicine 500 μg (ColBENEMID®)

Legal Status
Prescription

Probucol (Lorelco®)

See ANTILIPEMICS.

Procainamide hydrochloride (Pronestyl®)

Action and Use
Cardiac antiarrhythmic agent.

Dosage and Administration
Dosage is individualized to the patient: the usual range is 250 mg to 1 g every 4 to 6 hours, orally or IM; or 200 mg to 1 g (not to exceed 1 g), IV.

Cautions
This drug should be used with extreme caution; it can cause hypotension, sometimes precipitously following IV administration. There are many side effects, some of which are dangerous. The effects of cholinergic agents and muscle relaxants are potentiated.

Adverse Reactions
Occasionally, oral use may produce anorexia, nausea, vomiting, diarrhea, bitter taste, flushing, weakness, depression, giddiness, psychosis, dizziness, and hallucinations. Hypersensitivity may occur, with chills,

fever, malaise, joint and muscle pain, pruritus, angioneurotic edema, urticaria, and rash. Intravenous administration requires slow infusion and the monitoring of blood pressure and ECG. Continued use of the drug should be questioned if hypotension, progressive widening of QRS complex, or other undesirable changes occur. Rare side effects include bone marrow depression (frequent blood examinations are recommended, and the patient should be observed for sore throat and bleeding), arrhythmias, and cardiac arrest. Prolonged administration may produce a syndrome similar to systemic lupus erythematosus, with fever and arthralgia.

Composition and Supply
Capsules   250 mg, 375 mg, and 500 mg
Injection   100 mg/ml, in 10 ml vials; 500 mg/ml, in 2 ml vials

Legal Status
Prescription

Procaine hydrochloride (Novocain®)

Action and Use
Local anesthetic (injectable).

Dosage and Administration
The smallest possible dose that produces desired effect should be used. Administered by infiltration, nerve block, caudal block, or other epidural blocks.

Cautions
Use with caution in patients with cardiovascular disease or endocrine disorders. Contraindicated in patients with myasthenia gravis and in those who are receiving digitalis, cholinergic agents, or succinylcholine. Should not be used if crystals, cloudiness, or discoloration is observed. Protect the ampuls from light.

Adverse Reactions
Adverse reactions include nausea, vomiting, rapid pulse, talkativeness, syncope, respiratory difficulty, and convulsions. Overdosage or poisoning is similar to the adverse effects of tetracaine hydrochloride (see).

Composition and Supply
Injection   0.5%, 1%, and 2%, in ampuls and vials

Legal Status
Prescription

Procarbazine hydrochloride (Matulane®)

Action and Use
Antineoplastic used in the palliative management of patients with generalized Hodgkin's disease and in the treatment of those resistant to other forms of therapy.

Dosage and Administration
50 to 100 mg daily as a maintenance dose, orally.

Cautions
Procarbazine hydrochloride is highly toxic, particularly to bone marrow. Because the sedative effects may be augmented, the concomitant use of tricyclic antidepressants or adrenergic agents should be avoided. The concomitant ingestion of alcohol causes intense warmth and reddening of the face. Ripe cheese and bananas potentiate the drug.

Adverse Reactions
The most common side effects are nausea and vomiting. Less frequent side effects include anorexia, stomatitis, dry mouth, dysphagia, diarrhea, constipation, and jaundice; paresthesias, neuropathies, headache, dizziness, depression, nervousness, apprehension, insomnia, nightmares, hallucinations, falling, unsteadiness, ataxia, foot drop, decreased reflexes, and tremors; and dermatitis, pruritus, herpes, hyperpigmentation, flushing, and alopecia. Orthostatic hypotension may occasionally develop. Coma and convulsions are severe responses that may rarely occur.

Composition and Supply
Capsules   50 mg

Legal Status
Prescription

Prochlorperazine (Compazine®)

Action and Use
Major tranquilizer and antiemetic.

Dosage and Administration
Dosage is individualized to the patient and condition being treated, with a range of 5 to 150 mg daily, orally, IM, IV, or rectally.

Cautions
See **Chlorpromazine hydrochloride.**

Adverse Reactions
See **Chlorpromazine hydrochloride.**

Composition and Supply
Capsules, long-acting (as maleate)   10 mg, 15 mg, 30 mg, and 75 mg
Injection (as edisylate)   5 mg/ml, in 2 ml ampuls and 10 ml vials
Liquid concentrate, oral (as edisylate)   10 mg/ml
Suppositories   2.5 mg, 5 mg, and 25 mg
Syrup (as edisylate)   5 mg/5 ml
Tablets   5 mg, 10 mg, and 25 mg

Legal Status
Prescription

Procyclidine hydrochloride (Kemadrin®)

Action and Use
Antiparkinsonic (anticholinergic).

Dosage and Administration
2.5 to 10 mg 3 times a day (usually), orally.

Cautions
Use with caution in patients with glaucoma or tachycardia.

Adverse Reactions
Similar to adverse reactions to trihexyphenidyl hydrochloride (see).

Composition and Supply
Tablets   5 mg

Legal Status
Prescription

Profilate® (antihemophilic factor [human] VIII)

See HEMOSTATICS.

Progesterone (Corlutin®, Lipo-Lutin®, Proluton®)

Action and Use
Progestogen (see p. 60).

Dosage and Administration
5 to 50 mg daily, IM; it should never be administered IV.

Cautions
Contraindicated in patients with impaired renal function, missed or incomplete abortion, carcinoma of the breast, undiagnosed genital bleeding, or a history of thrombophlebitis, thromboembolic disorders,

cerebrovascular accident, or pulmonary embolism. Administer cautiously in patients who have had periodic attacks of asthma, migraine, or epilepsy.

Adverse Reactions

Possible side effects include thrombotic disorders (such as thrombophlebitis, cerebrovascular accident, and pulmonary embolism), abnormal liver function, and hypercalcemia. Progesterone is locally irritating; not more than 50 mg should be given in a single IM injection. When used with estrogens, it may cause nausea, vomiting, anorexia, abdominal cramps, breakthrough bleeding, headache, increase in cervical mucus, mental depression, hirsutism, change in libido, change in appetite, itching, backache, breast tenderness and engorgement, and congestive heart failure.

Composition and Supply

Injection   50 mg/ml and 100 mg/ml, in 1 ml ampuls and 10 ml vials

Legal Status

Prescription

Progynon®

See **Estradiol.**

Prolixin®

See **Fluphenazine.**

Proloid®

See **Thyroglobulin.**

Proluton®

See **Progesterone.**

Promazine hydrochloride (Sparine®)

Action and Use

Minor tranquilizer.

Dosage and Administration

25 to 200 mg every 4 to 6 hours, orally; or 50 to 150 mg, IM or IV.

Cautions

Promazine hydrochloride may cause drowsiness, orthostatic hypotension, and photosensitivity. See **Chlorpromazine** for further cautions.

Adverse Reactions
Similar to but much less severe than the adverse reactions to chlorpromazine hydrochloride (see).

Composition and Supply
Injection   25 mg/ml and 50 mg/ml, in 10 ml vials
Syrup   10 mg/5 ml
Tablets   10 mg, 25 mg, 50 mg, 100 mg, and 200 mg

Legal Status
Prescription

Promethazine hydrochloride (Phenergan®)

Action and Use
Antihistamine, antiemetic, and sedative.

Dosage and Administration
12.5 to 25 mg every 4 to 6 hours, orally; or 25 to 75 mg, IM, IV, or rectally.

Cautions
Pronounced sedation may occur. Not to be given subcutaneously or intra-arterially, since arteriospasm may result, with consequent gangrene. Use cautiously when administering intravenously. See **Chlorpromazine hydrochloride** for further cautions.

Adverse Reactions
Similar in nature to adverse reactions to chlorpromazine hydrochloride (see).

Composition and Supply
Expectorant   (see Section 1, COUGH-COLD PREPARATIONS)
Injection   25 mg/ml and 50 mg/ml, in 1 ml ampuls and 10 ml vials
Syrup   6.25 mg/5 ml and 12.5 mg/5 ml
Suppositories, rectal   12.5 mg, 25 mg, and 50 mg
Tablets   12.5 mg and 25 mg

Legal Status
Prescription

Promin® (glucosulfone sodium)

See ANTILEPROTICS.

Pronestyl®

See **Procainamide hydrochloride.**

Propantheline bromide (Pro-Banthīne®, Pro-Banthīne P.A.®)

Action and Use
Anticholinergic and antispasmodic.

Dosage and Administration
75 mg in divided doses daily, orally; 30 mg every 6 hours, IM or IV.

Cautions
Use with caution in patients with cardiac disease. Contraindicated in patients with glaucoma. See **Atropine sulfate.**

Adverse Reactions
Similar to but less pronounced than adverse reactions to atropine sulfate (see).

Composition and Supply
Injection   30 mg vials
Tablets   7.5 mg and 15 mg
Tablets, sustained-release   30 mg (*Note:* dosage is usually 2 tablets
   daily) (Pro-Banthīne P.A.®)
Tablets   7.5 mg and 15 mg with phenobarbital 15 mg (Probital®)

Legal Status
Prescription

Proparacaine hydrochloride (Alcaine®, Ophthaine®)

Action and Use
Local anesthetic for ophthalmic use.

Dosage and Administration
1 or 2 drops applied to the eye.

Cautions
Use carefully in patients with allergies, cardiac disease, hyperthyroidism, or open lesions.

Adverse Reactions
Causes relatively little burning and discomfort. Rare side effects include corneal damage, mydriasis, and contact dermatitis.

Composition and Supply
Solution, ophthalmic   0.5%

Legal Status
Prescription

Propion Gel® (propionate compound)

See ANTI-INFECTIVES, fungicides.

Propionate compound (Propion Gel®)

See ANTI-INFECTIVES, fungicides.

Propoxyphene hydrochloride (Darvon®, Dolene®)

Propoxyphene napsylate (Darvon-N®)

Action and Use
Analgesic for mild to moderate pain.

Dosage and Administration
65 mg 3 or 4 times a day, orally (Darvon®, Dolene®); 100 mg 3 or 4 times a day, orally (Darvon-N®).

Cautions
Tolerance and physical dependence may occur when large doses are used. Should be used with caution in pregnant women. The CNS-depressant effect may be additive with that of other CNS depressants, including alcohol.

Adverse Reactions
The most frequent side effects include dizziness, sedation, and vomiting, especially in ambulatory patients. Since it may impair mental or physical abilities, patients should use caution in such tasks as operating machinery or driving. Other reported adverse effects include constipation, abdominal pain, skin rash, lightheadedness, headache, weakness, euphoria, and minor visual disturbances. The effects of an overdose resemble narcotic intoxication, with respiratory depression, somnolence (progressing to coma), miosis, circulatory collapse, and possibly death.

Composition and Supply
Capsules (as hydrochloride)
    32 mg and 65 mg (Darvon®, Dolene®)
    65 mg with acetaminophen (Wygesic®)
    65 mg with aspirin (Darvon® with A.S.A.®)
    32 mg and 65 mg with aspirin compound (Darvon® Compound,
        Darvon® Compound-65, Dolene® Compound-65)
Suspension (as napsylate)   50 mg/5 ml (Darvon-N®)
Tablets (as napsylate)
    100 mg (Darvon-N®)
    50 mg with acetaminophen (Darvocet-N®)

65 mg with acetaminophen (Dolene® AP-65)
100 mg with acetaminophen (Darvocet-N® 100)
100 mg with aspirin (Darvon-N® with A.S.A.®)

Legal Status
Prescription

Propranolol hydrochloride (Inderal®)

Action and Use
Beta-adrenergic blocking agent used to treat angina pectoris, cardiac arrhythmias, and hypertension.

Dosage and Administration
The dosage is individualized to the patient's need, with a range of 30 to 240 mg daily, orally; or 500 μg to 3 mg, IV (at a rate not exceeding 1 mg/minute).

Cautions
Severe bradycardia may occur. Use with caution in patients with inadequate myocardial function or impaired liver or kidney function. The drug should not be withdrawn abruptly; in some patients this might precipitate cardiac failure. It may prevent the appearance of signs and symptoms of hypoglycemia in diabetics. Contraindicated in patients with bronchial asthma, allergic rhinitis, sinus bradycardia, cardiogenic shock, right ventricular failure (secondary to pulmonary hypertension), and congestive heart failure (unless secondary to a tachyarrhythmia), and in those receiving adrenergic-augmenting psychotropics there should be a two-week withdrawal period from such drugs before the administration of propranolol. The inotropic action of digitalis is reduced by propranolol, and both drugs are additive in depressing atrioventricular conduction.

Adverse Reactions
Common side effects include nausea, vomiting, diarrhea, and constipation. Infrequent side effects include rash, fever, pruritus, agranulocytosis, respiratory distress, purpura, weakness, fatigue, depression, hallucinations, and nightmares. Rare side effects include hypotension, bradycardia, heart block, and congestive heart failure (especially in patients with limited cardiac reserve); intensified hypoglycemia in patients with diabetes; reversible alopecia; and increased BUN levels, decreased SGOT levels, alkaline phosphatase, and paresthesias. Bronchoconstriction is possible; an asthmatic attack may result in susceptible individuals.

Composition and Supply
Injection   1 mg/ml, in 1 ml ampuls
Tablets   10 mg, 40 mg, and 80 mg

Legal Status
Prescription

Propylhexedrine (Benzedrex®)

See ADRENERGICS; NASAL DECONGESTANTS.

Propylthiouracil (PTU)

Action and Use
Thyroid depressant.

Dosage and Administration
The usual dose is 50 to 100 mg daily, orally for maintenance.

Cautions
Agranulocytosis and hepatic damage are possible. Use cautiously in pregnant women. Contraindicated in nursing mothers.

Adverse Reactions
The most common side effect is a mild purpuric papular rash. Other possible responses include agranulocytosis, pain and stiffness in the joints, myalgia, paresthesias, loss of taste, urticaria, edema of the lower extremities, headache, nausea, vomiting, depigmentation of hair, vertigo, drug fever, hepatitis, and nephritis.

Composition and Supply
Tablets   50 mg

Legal Status
Prescription

Prostaphlin®

See **Oxacillin sodium.**

Prostigmin®

See **Neostigmine.**

Protamine sulfate

Action and Use
Acts as an anticoagulant when administered alone, but in the presence of heparin forms a stable salt that results in the loss of anticoagulant activity of both drugs. Used to treat heparin overdosage.

Dosage and Administration
1 mg of protamine sulfate neutralizes approximately 86 USP units of heparin derived from lung tissue and 115 USP units of heparin derived

from intestinal mucosa. It is administered very slowly (in 1 to 3 minutes) IV as a 1% solution.

Cautions
The dosage should not exceed 50 mg of protamine sulfate activity in any 10 minute period. Facilities to treat shock should always be available.

Adverse Reactions
IV injection may cause a sudden fall in blood pressure, bradycardia, dyspnea, or transitory flushing and a feeling of warmth.

Composition and Supply
Injection   10 mg/ml, in 5 ml and 25 ml ampuls; 50 mg vials with 5 ml ampul diluent

Legal Status
Prescription

Protamine, Zinc & Iletin®

See under **Insulin.**

Protein hydrolysate injection 5% and 10% (Amigen®, Aminosol®)

See PARENTERAL ALIMENTATION.

Protopam®

See **Pralidoxime chloride.**

Protriptyline hydrochloride (Vivactil®)

Action and Use
Antidepressant.

Dosage and Administration
Dosage is individualized to the patient's requirements; the usual dose is 15 to 40 mg daily, but may range up to 60 mg, orally.

Cautions
Contraindicated in patients being treated with MAO inhibitors. See **Amitriptyline hydrochloride** for further cautions.

Adverse Reactions
See **Amitriptyline hydrochloride.**

Composition and Supply
Tablets   5 mg and 10 mg

Legal Status
Prescription

Provera®

See **Medroxyprogesterone acetate.**

Prydon® (belladonna alkaloids)

See ANTICHOLINERGICS.

Pseudoephedrine hydrochloride (Novafed®, Sudafed®)

Action and Use
Adrenergic decongestant and bronchodilator.

Dosage and Administration
Tablets and liquid: 30 to 60 mg 3 or 4 times a day.
Controlled-release capsules: 1 capsule every 12 hours.

Cautions
Use cautiously in patients with hypertension, diabetes, or thyroid disease, in patients being treated with MAO inhibitors or beta-adrenergic blocking agents, and in those with increased intraocular pressure or prostatic hypertrophy.

Adverse Reactions
Drowsiness may occur. There may be mild stimulation and palpitations in persons sensitive to adrenergic drugs. Overdosage in persons over age 60 may cause hallucinations, convulsions, central nervous system depression, and death.

Composition and Supply
Capsules, controlled-release   120 mg (Novafed®)
Liquid and syrup   30 mg/5 ml
Syrup   30 mg/5 ml with triprolidine hydrochloride 1.25 mg/5 ml
   (Actifed® syrup)
Tablets   30 mg and 60 mg
Tablets   60 mg with triprolidine hydrochloride 2.5 mg (Actifed®)

Legal Status
Prescription (capsules and 60 mg tablets)
Nonprescription (syrup and 30 mg tablets)

PSP

See **Phenolsulfonphthalein.**

444

Psyllium hydrophilic mucilloid (Effersyllium®, Konsyl®, Metamucil®)

Action and Use
Bulk cathartic and gastrointestinal demulcent.

Dosage and Administration
4 to 7 g, 1 to 3 times a day, stirred in a glass of cool water and followed by an additional glass of water.

Cautions
Use cautiously in patients on sodium restricted diets, since each dose contains 250 mg of sodium. Contraindicated in patients with fecal impaction or abdominal pain.

Adverse Reactions
Flatulence may occur, which can sometimes be relieved by increasing the fluid intake.

Composition and Supply
Powder

Legal Status
Nonprescription

PTU

See **Propylthiouracil.**

Purinethol®

See **Mercaptopurine.**

Purodigin®

See **Digitoxin.**

Pyopen®

See **Carbenicillin disodium.**

Pyrantel pamoate (Antiminth®)

See ANTHELMINTICS, pinworm.

Pyrazinamide (PZA) (Aldinamide®)

Action and Use
Antituberculotic.

Dosage and Administration
35 mg/kg orally in 3 or 4 divided doses (the maximum dose is 3 g per day).

445

Cautions
Liver damage is possible; periodic liver function tests are recommended.

Adverse Reactions
Possible side effects include jaundice, hyperuricemia, symptoms of gout, and hypersensitivity.

Composition and Supply
Tablets   500 mg

Legal Status
Prescription

Pyrethrins/piperonyl butoxide (RID™)

See ANTI-INFECTIVES, scabicide-pediculicides.

Pyribenzamine®

See **Tripelennamine hydrochloride.**

Pyridium®

See **Phenazopyridine hydrochloride.**

Pyridostigmine bromide (Mestinon®)

Action and Use
Anticholinesterase cholinergic agent used to control myasthenia gravis and to reverse the effects of curariform drugs.

Dosage and Administration
Dosage is individualized to the needs of the patient; the usual range in patients with myasthenia gravis is 60 mg to 1.5 g daily, orally, or 1/30 of the oral dose IM or IV. When used to antagonize muscle relaxants, the dosage is 10 to 20 mg, IV.

Cautions
Contraindicated in patients with intestinal or urinary obstruction. See **Physostigmine salicylate** for further cautions.

Adverse Reactions
Adverse reactions are most commonly related to overdose and are essentially cholinergic in nature (see **Physostigmine salicylate**).

Composition and Supply
Injection   5 mg/ml, in 2 ml ampuls
Tablets   60 mg
Tablets, prolonged-action   180 mg

Legal Status
Prescription

Pyridoxine hydrochloride (vitamin B₆) (Hexa-Betalin®)

Action and Use
B-complex vitamin.

Dosage and Administration
25 to 450 mg daily (depending on use), orally, IM, or IV.

Cautions
Pyridoxine hydrochloride will reverse effects of levodopa.

Adverse Reactions
Nontoxic when used in therapeutic dosage.

Composition and Supply
Injection   50 mg/ml, in 1 ml ampuls and 10 ml vials; 100 mg/ml, in
    1 ml and 5 ml ampuls and 10 ml vials
Tablets   5 mg, 10 mg, 25 mg, and 50 mg

Legal Status
Prescription (injection)
Nonprescription (tablets)

Pyrimethamine (Daraprim®)

Action and Use
Antimalarial.

Dosage and Administration
Suppression: 25 mg per week, orally.
Treatment: 25 mg daily for 2 days, orally.

Cautions
Contraindicated in pregnant women and in children under the age of
12.

Adverse Reactions
High doses may produce anorexia, nausea, vomiting, glossitis, and
rash. An overdose may produce anemia, leukopenia, and thrombo-
penia. Periodic blood examinations are recommended.

Composition and Supply
Tablets   25 mg

Pyrrobutamine compound (Co-Pyronil™)

Action and Use
Antihistamine.

Dosage and Administration
The usual dosage ranges from 1 capsule every 12 hours to 2 capsules every 4 hours, depending on symptoms.

Cautions
Drowsiness is frequent. Contraindicated in newborn or premature infants, in patients with lower respiratory disease, narrow-angle glaucoma, stenosing peptic ulcer, prostatic hypertrophy, bladder neck obstruction, or pyloroduodenal obstruction, and in those receiving MAO inhibitors. In infants and children, especially, overdosage of antihistamines may cause hallucinations, convulsions, and death. Use with caution in patients with asthma, increased intraocular pressure, or hyperthyroidism.

Adverse Reactions
The most common side effects include sedation, sleepiness, dizziness, disturbed coordination, and dryness of the mouth, nose, and throat. Other possible side effects include restlessness, insomnia, nausea, vomiting, diarrhea, constipation, hypotension, palpitations, urinary retention, hemolytic anemia, and agranulocytosis.

Composition and Supply
Capsules   pyrrobutamine phosphate 15 mg, methapyrilene hydrochloride 25 mg, and cyclopentamine hydrochloride 6.25 mg
Suspension (per 5 ml)   pyrrobutamine phosphate 7.5 mg, methapyrilene hydrochloride 12.5 mg, and cyclopentamine hydrochloride 6.25 mg

Legal Status
Prescription

Pyrvinium pamoate (Povan®)

Action and Use
Anthelmintic used to treat pinworm.

Dosage and Administration
5 mg of base per kg in one dose, repeated in 2 to 3 weeks if needed, orally.

Cautions
Contraindicated in patients with suspected intestinal obstruction or acute abdominal disease. Use cautiously in patients with renal or hepatic disease.

Adverse Reactions
The stool becomes bright red in color (the patient should be forewarned). The tablets should be swallowed immediately without chewing, to avoid staining the teeth. Occasional side effects include nausea, vomiting, and cramping. Possible side effects include diarrhea and hypersensitivity reactions (e.g., photosensitivity).

Composition and Supply
Suspension, oral   50 mg (base)/5 ml
Tablets   50 mg (base)

Legal Status
Prescription

PZA

See **Pyrazinamide.**

PZI

See under **Insulin.**

Quāālude® (methaqualone)

See SEDATIVE-HYPNOTICS, nonbarbiturates.

Quelicin®

See **Succinylcholine chloride.**

Questran®

See **Cholestyramine.**

Quibron® (theophylline/guaifenesin)

See ANTIASTHMATICS, xanthine preparations.

Quide® (piperacetazine)

See PSYCHOTROPICS, antipsychotics.

Quinacrine hydrochloride (Atabrine®)

Action and Use
Anthelmintic of choice against tapeworm.

Dosage and Administration
4 doses of 200 mg 10 minutes apart (800 mg total, orally). A saline cathartic should be given 1 hour later to insure removal of the head of the tapeworm.

Cautions
Use cautiously in patients with psoriasis or with reduced ventilation or dyspnea. Contraindicated in pregnant women, in patients receiving antimalarial therapy with primaquine, and in those with a history of psychosis.

Adverse Reactions
Possible side effects include nausea, headache, vomiting, diarrhea, and a yellow discoloration of skin and urine (which usually disappears in a few weeks after the drug is discontinued). Toxic psychosis and aplastic anemia are rare side effects with prolonged therapy.

Composition and Supply
Tablets   100 mg

Legal Status
Prescription

Quinaglute®

See under **Quinidine gluconate.**

Quinamm™

See under **Quinine sulfate.**

Quinethazone (Hydromox®)

See DIURETICS.

Quinidex®

See under **Quinidine sulfate.**

Quinidine gluconate
Quinidine sulfate

Action and Use
Antiarrhythmic.

Dosage and Administration
Regular tablets: 200 to 400 mg every 3 or 4 hours, orally.
Injection: dosage is individualized; administered IM or IV.

Cautions
Before administration, check the patient's blood pressure (and notify the physician if hypotension exists) and note the rate and rhythm of apical and radial pulses for 1 minute. Frequent quinidine plasma concentration estimates are recommended. Intravenous administration should be accompanied by cardiographic and blood pressure monitoring. Patients with hepatic or renal insufficiency or congestive heart failure should be closely observed for toxic signs. Contraindicated in patients with a history of thrombocytopenia purpura, digitalis intoxication, or atrioventricular block.

Adverse Reactions
Common side effects, especially with large doses, relate to cinchonism: nausea, vomiting, diarrhea, headache, tinnitus, vertigo, confusion, and visual disturbances. Other possible side effects include hypotension, abnormal widening of the QRS complex, evidence of second degree or complete heart block, premature ventricular contraction, ventricular fibrillation, congestive heart failure, and cardiac arrest.

Composition and Supply
Injection (as gluconate)   80 mg/ml
Injection (as sulfate)   200 mg/ml
Tablets (as sulfate)   200 mg and 300 mg (Quinora®)
Tablets, sustained-release (as gluconate)   324 mg (Quinaglute® Dura-Tabs®) (*Note:* dosage is individualized; 2 tablets every 8 to 12 hours)
Tablets, sustained-release (as sulfate)   300 mg (Quinidex® Extentabs®) (*Note:* dosage is individualized; 2 tablets every 8 to 12 hours)

Legal Status
Prescription

Quinidine polygalacturonate (Cardioquin®)

See CARDIACS, antiarrhythmics.

Quinine sulfate

Action and Use
Antimalarial and skeletal muscle relaxant used for nocturnal cramps.

Dosage and Administration
300 mg to 1 g (depending on use) every 8 hours, orally.

Cautions
Contraindicated in pregnant women and in patients with glucose-6-phosphate dehydrogenase deficiency.

Adverse Reactions

The maximum therapeutic dosage may lead to cinchonism, with head-ache, dizziness, and visual disturbances. More severe poisoning produces gastrointestinal disturbance (with nausea, vomiting, and diarrhea), renal damage (with anuria and uremia), acute hemolytic anemia, hypoprothrombinemia, purpura, agranulocytopenia, apprehension, syncope, delirium, cardiovascular disturbances, skin disruptions (with flushing, diaphoresis, rash, and angioedema), and possibly respiratory arrest.

Composition and Supply

Capsules   120 mg, 200 mg, and 300 mg

Tablets   260 mg with aminophylline 195 mg (Quinamm™) (*Note:* for nocturnal leg muscle cramps, dosage is 1 tablet upon retiring)

Legal Status

Prescription

Quinora®

See under **Quinidine sulfate.**

Quotane®

See **Dimethisoquin hydrochloride.**

Rabies vaccine

Action and Use

Vaccine (dried killed virus derived from duck embryo), used for active immunization against rabies. The World Health Organization Expert Committee on Rabies has considered various types of exposure to rabies and made the following recommendations:

I. If contact with the rabid animal has been indirect or if there has been only a lick on unabraded skin, no exposure is considered to have occurred and vaccine is not recommended.

II. If the exposure was mild, i.e., a lick on abraded skin or on mucosal surfaces, or for single bites *not* on the head, neck, face, or arm.

   A. If the animal is healthy at the time of exposure, withhold vaccine, but observe the animal for 10 days.

   B. If during the 10-day observation period the animal is proved to have rabies or becomes clinically suspicious, start vaccine immediately.

C. If the animal has signs suspicious of rabies at the time of exposure, start vaccine immediately, but stop injections if the animal is normal on the fifth day after exposure.

D. If the animal is rabid, if it escapes or is killed, or if it is unknown, give complete course of vaccine. If the biting animal is wild, also give rabies antiserum.

III. If exposure was severe (multiple bites or single bites on the head, neck, face, or arm), the indications for giving vaccine are the same as in mild exposure (see II above). In addition, in every category, the administration of rabies antiserum is recommended.

Dosage and Administration
It is recommended that the injections be given under the skin of the abdomen on alternate sides each day. Each dose should be given in a site not previously used for a vaccine or toxoid.
Postexposure immunization: 1 dose daily for 14 days, SC.
Preexposure: 4 doses of 1 ml each, SC. The first 3 doses are given 1 week apart, and the fourth is given 6 months after the third. A booster shot of 1 ml should be given every 1 to 2 years.

Cautions
Rabies vaccine should be used with caution in persons with a history of allergy, especially allergy to protein or chicken or duck eggs. Anaphylactoid reactions may occur.

Adverse Reactions
Pain and induration may occur at the injection site. Possible constitutional reactions include headache, photophobia, paresthesias, and malaise. Rare side effects include transverse myelitis, cranial or peripheral palsy, and encephalitis.

Composition and Supply
Injection   single-dose vials (dry powder) with 1 ampul of sterile water for injection

Legal Status
Prescription

Ramses® Vaginal Jelly (dodecaethyleneglycol monolaurate)

See CONTRACEPTIVES, TOPICAL.

Raudixin®

See **Rauwolfia serpentina.**

Rauwolfia serpentina (Raudixin®)

Action and Use
Antihypertensive.

Dosage and Administration
200 to 400 mg daily, orally.

Cautions
Contraindicated in patients with mental depression, colitis, or peptic ulcer.

Adverse Reactions
Common side effects include mild sedation, weakness, fatigue, nightmares, angina-like pains, arrhythmia, weight gain, increased salivation, flushing, nausea, diarrhea, nasal congestion, and epistaxis. Other reported side effects include dry mouth, insomnia, dyspnea, dysuria, pruritus, and skin eruptions. The convulsive threshold in some patients may be lowered.

Composition and Supply
Tablets   50 mg and 100 mg

Legal Status
Prescription

Rectal Medicone®-HC Suppositories
See ANTIHEMORRHOIDALS.

Redisol®
See **Cyanocobalamin injection.**

Regitine®
See **Phentolamine.**

Rela®
See **Carisoprodol.**

Renese® (polythiazide)
See DIURETICS.

Renografin®
See under **Diatrizoate meglumine.**

Reno-M-30®

See under **Diatrizoate meglumine.**

Reno-M-60®

See under **Diatrizoate meglumine.**

Renoquid® (sulfacytine)

See SULFONAMIDES.

Repoise® (butaperazine)

See PSYCHOTROPICS, antipsychotics.

Rescinnamine (Moderil®)

See ANTIHYPERTENSIVES, nondiuretic.

Reserpine (Serpasil®)

Action and Use
Antihypertensive.

Dosage and Administration
100 μg to 1 mg daily, orally; or 500 μg to 4 mg, IM.

Cautions
See **Rauwolfia serpentina.**

Adverse Reactions
See **Rauwolfia serpentina.**

Composition and Supply
Injection   2.5 mg/ml, in 2 ml ampuls
Tablets   100 μg and 250 μg

Legal Status
Prescription

Reserpine/chlorothiazide (Diupres®)

See ANTIHYPERTENSIVES, combinations.

Reserpine/hydrochlorothiazide (Hydropres®)

See ANTIHYPERTENSIVES, combinations.

Resorcinol

Action and Use
Antiseptic and keratolytic used to treat various diseases of the skin.

Dosage and Administration
Apply to the skin 2 or 3 times a day.

Cautions
Resorcinol should not come into contact with the eyes, and it should not be applied to large areas of the skin.

Adverse Reactions
Ingestion or percutaneous absorption may cause tinnitus, tachycardia, tachypnea, diaphoresis, methemoglobinemia, vascular collapse, coma, convulsions, and death. Application to gray, blonde, or white hair may darken the hair; this problem can often be prevented by using resorcinol monoacetate.

Composition and Supply
Lotion   5%
Solution   10%

Legal Status
Prescription

Respaire®

See **Acetylcysteine.**

Respihaler®

See under **Dexamethasone.**

Retin-A®

See **Tretinoin.**

Rezipas®

See **Aminosalicylic acid.**

R-Gene™ 10

See **Arginine hydrochloride.**

Rheomacrodex® (dextran 40)

See ELECTROLYTE SOLUTIONS AND WATER-BALANCE AGENTS, plasma extenders.

RhoGAM®

See **Globulin, Rh₀ (D) immune human.**

Rhulicream® (menthol preparation)

See ANTIPRURITICS, topical preparations.

Riboflavin (vitamin B₂, vitamin G)

Action and Use
B-complex vitamin.

Dosage and Administration
2 to 10 mg per day, orally.

Cautions
Protect from light.

Adverse Reactions
None.

Composition and Supply
Injection   5 mg/ml and 10 mg/ml, in 1 ml ampuls and 10 ml vials
Tablets   1 mg, 5 mg, 10 mg, 25 mg, and 50 mg

Legal Status
Prescription (injection)
Nonprescription (tablets)

RID™ (pyrethrins/piperonyl butoxide)

See ANTI-INFECTIVES, scabicide-pediculicides.

Rifadin®

See **Rifampin.**

Rifamate™ (rifampin/isoniazid)

See ANTITUBERCULOTICS.

Rifampin (Rifadin®, Rimactane®)

Action and Use
Antitubercular antibiotic; the drug of choice in the treatment of asymptomatic carriers of *Neisseria meningitidis.*

Dosage and Administration
600 mg daily in a single dose, taken orally 1 hour before or 2 hours after a meal.

Cautions

There may be teratogenic effects. Rifampin increases the requirement for coumarin-type anticoagulants; it may change the therapeutic effect of oral contraceptives, methadone, digitalis preparations, oral hypoglycemics, and corticosteroids, especially when given concomitantly with other antitubercular agents. The patient should be warned that the urine, feces, saliva, sputum, sweat, and tears may be colored red-orange or brownish red.

Adverse Reactions

The most common side effects include liver dysfunction (with jaundice), anorexia, nausea, vomiting, diarrhea, and cramps. Occasional side effects include drowsiness, fatigue, headache, dizziness, visual disturbances, ataxia, confusion, lack of concentration, numbness, pain in the extremities, muscular weakness, and hypersensitivity (fever, pruritus, urticaria, eosinophilia, and sore mouth and tongue). Rare side effects include hemolysis, hemoglobinuria, hematuria, and renal failure.

Composition and Supply

Capsules   300 mg

Legal Status

Prescription

Rifampin/isoniazid (Rifamate™, Rimactazid®)

See ANTITUBERCULOTICS.

Rimactane®

See **Rifampin.**

Rimactazid® (rifampin/isoniazid)

See ANTITUBERCULOTICS.

Ringer's injection

See ELECTROLYTE SOLUTIONS AND WATER-BALANCE AGENTS, replacement solutions.

Ringer's injection, lactated

See ELECTROLYTE SOLUTIONS AND WATER-BALANCE AGENTS, replacement solutions.

Ringer's solution

See IRRIGATING SOLUTIONS.

Riopan®

See **Magaldrate.**

Ritalin®

See **Methylphenidate hydrochloride.**

Robalate® (dihydroxyaluminum aminoacetate)

See ANTACIDS.

Robaxin®

See **Methocarbamol.**

Robaxisal®

See under **Methocarbamol.**

Robinul®

See **Glycopyrrolate.**

Robitussin®

See **Guaifenesin.**

Rocky Mountain spotted fever vaccine

Action and Use
Used for active immunization against Rocky Mountain spotted fever.

Dosage and Administration
3 injections, 1 ml each, at 7 to 10 day intervals, SC.

Cautions
People with allergies to egg, chicken, or chicken feathers may react unfavorably.

Adverse Reactions
Pain and induration at injection site may occur.

Composition and Supply
Injection   3 ml, 15 ml, and 20 ml vials

Legal Status
Prescription

Rondomycin® (methacycline hydrochloride)

See ANTIBIOTICS, tetracyclines.

Roniacol®

See **Nicotinyl alcohol.**

Rose water ointment

See EMOLLIENT-PROTECTANTS.

Rubella and mumps virus vaccine, live (Bivax®)

See BIOLOGICALS, vaccines.

Rubella virus vaccine, live (Cendevax®, Meruvax®)

Action and Use
Used for active immunization against rubella (German measles).

Dosage and Administration
0.5 ml (500 μl) (1,000 TCID$_{50}$), SC.

Cautions
Contraindicated in patients with febrile illness, leukemia, generalized malignancy, lowered resistance (resulting from disease, drugs, or irradiation), or hypersensitivity to rabbits (Cendevax®), chickens or ducks (Meruvax®), or neomycin; in patients being treated with steroids (except in replacement therapy); and in pregnant women. In women of childbearing age, the possibility of pregnancy occurring in the 3 months following vaccination must be eliminated by appropriate means. Vaccination should be deferred for at least 3 months following blood or plasma transfusions or after the administration of more than 0.02 ml (20 μl) of human immune serum globulin per pound of body weight. Schedule tuberculin tests before vaccination to avoid a possible false-negative response.

Adverse Reactions
Possible side effects include rash, fever, lymphadenopathy (especially in postpubertal females), and mild local reactions (such as erythema, induration, and tenderness). Thrombocytopenic purpura sometimes occurs. Arthritis, arthralgia, and peripheral neuritis with pain are other possible reactions.

Composition and Supply
Injection   10 ml and 50 ml multiple-dose vials, and single-dose syringes (*Note:* store at 2° to 8° C and avoid exposure to light before and after reconstitution)

Legal Status
Prescription

Rubramin PC®

See **Cyanocobalamin injection.**

Salicylic acid

Action and Use
Keratolytic aid in hyperkeratotic skin disorders.

Dosage and Administration
Applied topically.

Cautions
Salicylic acid is highly caustic and should be kept away from eyes and other sensitive areas.

Adverse Reactions
Overuse may cause inflammation and skin ulcerations.

Composition and Supply
Various preparations ranging from 1% to 20% (depending on specific use)

Legal Status
Prescription

Sanorex® (mazindol)

See CEREBRAL STIMULANTS, anorectics.

Sansert®

See **Methysergide maleate.**

Santyl®

See **Collagenase.**

Scopolamine hydrobromide (hyoscine)

Action and Use
Anticholinergic used as a preanesthetic medication.

Dosage and Administration
300 to 600 μg, IM or IV.

Cautions
See **Atropine sulfate.**

Adverse Reactions
See **Atropine sulfate.**

Composition and Supply
Injection 400 μg and 600 μg/ml, in 1 ml ampuls

Legal Status
Prescription

Sebizon®

See **Sulfacetamide sodium.**

Secobarbital sodium (Seconal®)

Action and Use
Short-acting barbiturate.

Dosage and Administration
100 to 300 mg (depending on use), orally, rectally, **IM**, or **IV**.

Cautions
Respiratory depression and dependence may occur. Secobarbital sodium is incompatible with bacteriostatic agents and Ringer's lactate solution. See **Amobarbital** for further cautions.

Adverse Reactions
See **Amobarbital.**

Composition and Supply
Capsules 30 mg, 50 mg, and 100 mg
Elixir 22 mg/5 ml
Injection 50 mg/ml, in 2 ml syringes and 20 ml vials
Suppositories 30 mg, 60 mg, 120 mg, and 200 mg

Legal Status
Schedule II

Secobarbital sodium/amobarbital sodium (Tuinal®)

See SEDATIVE-HYPNOTICS, barbiturates.

Seconal®

See **Secobarbital sodium.**

Secretin (Secretin–Boots)

See DIAGNOSTICS, pancreatic function.

Selenium sulfide (Exsel®, Selsun®)

Action and Use
Used to treat seborrheic dermatitis, including dandruff.

Dosage and Administration
Applied topically as shampoo.

Cautions
Keep out of the eyes. Toxic if taken internally. Do not use in the presence of inflammation or exudation.

Adverse Reactions
Irritation is an occasional side effect. Discoloration and increased hair loss may occur.

Composition and Supply
Lotion   2.5% (Selsun®)
Lotion   1% (Selsun Blue®)

Legal Status
Prescription (Selsun®)
Nonprescription (Selsun Blue®)

Selsun®

See **Selenium sulfide.**

Semicid® (nonoxynol 9)

See CONTRACEPTIVES, TOPICAL.

Senna concentrate (Senokot®)

Action and Use
Senna concentrate contains anthraquinone glycosides (sennoside A and B); in the colon these change to laxative aglycones, which stimulate peristalsis via Auerbach's plexus. Indicated in the management of functional constipation.

Dosage and Administration
Granules: 5 ml (to a maximum of 10 ml), twice a day.
Syrup: 10 to 15 ml (maximum, 15 ml), twice a day.
Tablets: 2 tablets (maximum, 4 tablets), twice a day.
Capsules: 1 or 2 capsules (maximum, 3 capsules), twice a day.
Suppositories: 1 suppository moistened with water and inserted high in the rectum.

Cautions
Contraindicated in patients with nausea, vomiting, or abdominal pain.

Adverse Reactions
None.

Composition and Supply
Capsules   senna concentrate with dioctyl sodium sulfosuccinate (Senokap® DSS)
Granules
Syrup
Tablets
Tablets   senna concentrate with diocytl sodium sulfosuccinate (Senokot® S)

Legal Status
Nonprescription

Senokot®

See **Senna concentrate.**

Septra®

See **Trimethoprim/sulfamethoxazole.**

Septra® DS

See under **Trimethoprim/sulfamethoxazole.**

Ser-Ap-Es®

See under **Hydralazine hydrochloride.**

Serax®

See **Oxazepam.**

Serentil® (mesoridazine)

See PSYCHOTROPICS, antipsychotics.

Seromycin® (cycloserine)

See ANTIBIOTICS, miscellaneous; ANTITUBERCULOTICS.

Serpasil®

See **Reserpine.**

Silicote® (dimethicone)

See EMOLLIENT-PROTECTANTS.

Silvadene®

See **Silver sulfadiazene.**

Silver nitrate

Action and Use
Antiseptic, astringent, and cauterizing agent.

Dosage and Administration
Astringent: 0.1 to 1% solution.
Burns: soaked dressings (0.5% solution).
Cautery: pencils or cones (dipped in water)
Eyes of newborns: 2 drops of ophthalmic solution in each eye.

Cautions
The use of strengths greater than 1% in eye is hazardous. Irrigation of eyes is not recommended after instillation of ophthalmic solution. Protect crystals and solution from light.

Adverse Reactions
When wet dressings are applied to burns, the dressings must not be allowed to dry or irritation will occur. Extensive use of silver nitrate on burns may cause electrolyte imbalance. It produces temporary brown-black tissue stains when applied to the skin.

Composition and Supply
Solution, astringent   0.1% to 1%
Solution, for burns   0.5%
Solution, ophthalmic   1%, in wax ampuls
Sticks (toughened silver nitrate)

Legal Status
Prescription

Silver sulfadiazine (Silvadene®)

Action and Use
Sulfonamide used in the prevention and treatment of infections associated with second- and third-degree burns.

Dosage and Administration
1 or 2 times daily, topically.

Cautions
Contraindicated in pregnant women at term and in premature infants or newborns younger than 1 month of age. Extensive use may cause the absorption of sulfadiazine and cause the characteristic adverse reactions of sulfonamides.

Adverse Reactions
Systemic sulfonamide reactions may occur if this medication is used improperly (see **Sulfisoxazole**).

Composition and Supply
Cream   1%

Legal Status
Prescription

Simethicone (Mylicon®)

Action and Use
Defoaming agent used to treat flatulence, gastric bloating, and postoperative gas pains.

Dosage and Administration
150 to 400 mg daily in divided doses after meals and at bedtime, orally.

Cautions
The tablets should be well chewed.

Adverse Reactions
None.

Composition and Supply
Drops   40 mg/0.6 ml
Tablets   40 mg and 80 mg

Legal Status
Nonprescription

Simethicone/pancreatin (Phazyme®)

See ANTIFLATULENTS.

Similac®

See INFANT FORMULAS.

Similac® PM

See INFANT FORMULAS.

Sinemet®

See under **Levodopa.**

Sinequan®

See **Doxepin hydrochloride.**

Sinografin® (iodipamide meglumine/diatrizoate meglumine)

See **DIAGNOSTICS**, roentgenography.

Sintrom® (acenocoumarol)

See **ANTICOAGULANTS.**

Sinutab® Tablets

See COUGH-COLD PREPARATIONS, common cold preparations.

Sitosterols (Cytellin®)

Action and Use
Antilipemic agent used in adjunctive treatment of hypercholesterolemia and hyperbetalipoproteinemia.

Dosage and Administration
9 to 36 g daily in divided doses, taken before meals, orally.

Cautions
Sitosterols may interfere with the absorption of other substances and
drugs in addition to cholesterol.

Adverse Reactions
There is a mild laxative effect.

Composition and Supply
Suspension, oral   1 g/5 ml

Legal Status
Prescription

Skelaxin® (metaxalone)

See SKELETAL MUSCLE RELAXANTS.

SK-Penicillin VK™

See **Penicillin V potassium.**

Slow-K®

See **Potassium chloride oral.**

SMA®

See INFANT FORMULAS.

Smallpox vaccine

Action and Use
Used for active immunization against smallpox.

Dosage and Administration
The vaccine is administered on the upper arm over the insertion of the deltoid muscle by multiple pressure, puncture, or scratch techniques. In nonimmune individuals, a papule appears in 3 to 5 days, followed by a vesicle and a pustule (the crust falls off by about the twenty-first day).

Cautions
Routine immunization is not recommended. Contraindicated in patients with serious acute illness, eczema or other forms of chronic dermatitis, bacterial respiratory or skin infections, leukemia, lymphoma or other reticuloendothelial malignancies, or dysgammaglobulinemia; in persons receiving immunosuppressive drugs; and in pregnant women. Do not bathe the reaction site or crust.

Adverse Reactions
Lymphadenopathy, fever, and malaise are frequent side effects. Possible complications include accidental infection, generalized vaccinia, eczema, and vaccinia necrosum. Postvaccinal encephalitis and congenital vaccinia are rare side effects.

Composition and Supply
Injection   vials (25 doses), or capillary tubes (1, 5, and 10 doses) (*Note:* protect from heat and light and store according to the manufacturer's directions)

Legal Status
Prescription

Sodium bicarbonate (baking soda)

Action and Use
Systemic antacid and urinary alkalizer.

Dosage and Administration
When used in acidosis: as indicated, IV.
When used as a urinary alkalizer: 4 g initially, followed by 1 to 2 g every 4 hours, orally.

Cautions
Rapid injection is dangerous and can be fatal. Excessive oral use can lead to alkalosis. Contraindicated in patients with hypertension or edema. Do not use as an antidote for acid poisoning, because it may cause perforation of the stomach.

Adverse Reactions
Side effects include gastric distention, flatulence, belching, and acid rebound. Metabolic alkalosis may occur, especially in patients who have impaired kidney function. Hypernatremia (and edema) is possible in patients with heart disease.

Composition and Supply
Injection   7.5%, in 50 ml ampuls
Tablets   300 mg, 500 mg, and 600 mg

Legal Status
Prescription (injection)
Nonprescription (tablets)

Sodium bicarbonate/citric acid/aspirin (Alka-Seltzer® Effervescent Pain Reliever and Antacid)

See ANALGESICS, nonnarcotic; ANTACIDS.

Sodium borate compound

See MOUTHWASHES.

Sodium chloride (0.45% and 0.9% for irrigation)

See IRRIGATING SOLUTIONS.

Sodium citrate

Action and Use
Expectorant, alkalizing agent, and anticoagulant used in blood collection.

Dosage and Administration
Alkalizing agent: 1 to 2 g every 2 to 4 hours, orally.
Expectorant: doses of 100 mg, orally.

Cautions
Excessive use can cause alkalosis. Intravenous use may cause hypocalcemia.

Adverse Reactions
None with proper use.

Composition and Supply
Capsules   500 mg
Liquid (various expectorant formulations)   100 mg/5 ml
Solution, anticoagulant citrate dextrose

Legal Status
Nonprescription (except for parenteral forms)

Sodium citrate/potassium citrate (Polycitra®)

See ELECTROLYTE SOLUTIONS AND WATER-BALANCE AGENTS, alkalizing agents.

Sodium dehydrocholate (Decholin® Sodium)

See under **Dehydrocholic acid.**

Sodium dextrothyroxine (Choloxin®)

Action and Use
Antilipemic used to reduce serum cholesterol and triglycerides. Also indicated in the treatment of hypothyroidism in cardiac patients who cannot tolerate other thyroid preparations.

Dosage and Administration
Hypercholesterolemia: 1 to 2 mg per day initially, gradually increased to 4 to 8 mg per day for maintenance, orally.
Hypothyroidism: 1 mg per day initially, gradually increased to 4 mg for maintenance, orally.

Cautions
Contraindicated in euthyroid patients who have advanced liver or kidney disease, heart disease, or hypertension, or who are pregnant. Sodium dextrothyroxine may potentiate the effects of anticoagulants, increase blood sugar levels in diabetics, depress uptake of iodine 131, and raise serum protein bound iodine levels.

Adverse Reactions
The most common effects include insomnia, palpitations, nervousness, tremors, weight loss, diuresis, and menstrual irregularities. Other possible adverse reactions include nausea, vomiting, diarrhea, headache, dizziness, tinnitus, malaise, perspiration, muscle pain, arrhythmias, and myocardial infarction.

Composition and Supply
Tablets   2 mg and 4 mg

Legal Status
Prescription

Sodium fluoride (Fluoritab®, Luride®, Pediaflor®)

Action and Use
Prophylactic agent used to reduce the incidence of dental caries.

Dosage and Administration
In areas where the water is supplied with 0.2 parts or less fluoride per million: 500 μg daily from birth to 3 years of age and 1 mg daily for those older than 3 years of age.
In areas where the water is supplied with 0.2 to 0.6 parts fluoride per million: 250 μg daily from birth to 3 years of age and 1 mg daily for those older than 3 years of age.

Cautions
Do not use supplementary sodium fluoride in areas where the water contains 0.7 parts per million of fluoride.

Adverse Reactions
Excess fluoride may cause dental fluorosis.

Composition and Supply
Liquid   fluoride (as sodium fluoride) 1 mg/ml
Tablets   fluoride (as sodium fluoride) 1 mg

Legal Status
Prescription

Sodium hypochlorite solution, diluted (Dakin's solution)

Action and Use
Antiseptic and disinfectant.

Dosage and Administration
Applied topically as wet dressings or irrigation.

Cautions
Sodium hypochlorite solution delays clotting. It is unstable and must be freshly prepared.

Adverse Reactions
Irritation may occur.

Composition and Supply
Solution   0.5%

Legal Status
Nonprescription

Sodium iodide I 131 (Oriodide®, Theriodide®)

See ANTITHYROIDS; ANTINEOPLASTICS, radioisotopes.

Sodium lactate

See ELECTROLYTE SOLUTIONS AND WATER-BALANCE AGENTS, alkalizing agents.

Sodium lauryl sulfoacetate (Lowila® Cake)

Action and Use
Anionic wetting agent (soap substitute) used in various dermatitic and eczematous conditions.

Dosage and Administration
Applied topically, like soap.

Cautions
Problems are rare.

Adverse Reactions
Relatively nonirritating.

Composition and Supply
Cake   sodium lauryl sulfoacetate with dextrin, boric acid, urea, sorbitol, mineral oil, peg 14 M, lactic acid, cellulose gum, dioctyl sodium sulfosuccinate, and fragrance

Legal Status
Nonprescription

Sodium nitroprusside (Nipride®)

Action and Use
Antihypertensive used in hypertensive crises.

Dosage and Administration
0.5 to 8 μg per kg per minute, by IV infusion.

Cautions
Contraindicated in patients with compensatory hypertension. Monitor the patient, checking the flow rate and blood pressure continuously to avoid overdose (which will cause rapid hypotension). The maximum dose should not exceed 800 μg per minute. Only dextrose injection 5% should be used to prepare solutions, and solutions should be protected from light by wrapping in aluminum foil. Solutions more than 4 hours old should be discarded.

Adverse Reactions
Acute toxicity may occur, especially with rapid injection; this may cause nausea, vomiting, diaphoresis, restlessness, headache, apprehension, dizziness, palpitations, and substernal discomfort. Hypothyroidism is a rare side effect.

Composition and Supply
Injection   50 mg vials

Legal Status
Prescription

Sodium perborate

See MOUTHWASHES.

Sodium phosphate and biphosphate enema (Fleet® Brand Enema)

See CATHARTICS.

Sodium phosphate and biphosphate oral solution (Fleet® Brand Phospho-Soda®)

See CATHARTICS.

Sodium phosphate P 32 (Phosphotope®)

See ANTINEOPLASTICS, radioisotopes.

Sodium polystyrene sulfonate (Kayexalate®)

Action and Use
Potassium-removing agent (ion exchange resin) used to treat hyperkalemia.

Dosage and Administration
15 g in 150 to 200 ml of water 1 to 4 times a day, orally; 30 g suspended in 200 ml of 1% methycellulose, 10% dextrose, or 25% sorbitol solution, rectally.

Cautions
Serious potassium deficiency is possible; it is therefore imperative that serum potassium levels be determined at least daily. Use with caution in patients who cannot tolerate even a small increase in sodium loads.

Adverse Reactions
Possible side effects include gastric irritation, anorexia, nausea and vomiting, and diarrhea. In the elderly, large doses may cause fecal impaction.

473

Composition and Supply
Powder

Legal Status
Prescription

Sodium Sulamyd®

See **Sulfacetamide sodium.**

Sodium tetradecyl sulfate (Sotradecol®)

Action and Use
Sclerosing agent.

Dosage and Administration
0.5 ml (500 μl) to 2 ml, IV; 10 ml maximum single dose.

Cautions
Should not be used if the solution has a precipitate. Contraindicated in pregnant women, in bedridden persons, and in patients with acute superficial thrombophlebitis, varicosities caused by pelvic or abdominal tumors, underlying arterial disease, diabetes mellitus, thyrotoxicosis, tuberculosis, asthma, sepsis, neoplasms, blood dyscrasias, or acute respiratory or skin diseases. Use with caution in women taking antiovulatory drugs.

Adverse Reactions
There may be pain at the injection site; sloughing of tissue may result if extravasation occurs. A small, permanent discoloration may occur at injection site. Allergic reactions and anaphylaxis are possible.

Composition and Supply
Injection   1% and 3%, in 2 ml ampuls

Legal Status
Prescription

Sodium thiosulfate

Action and Use
Antifungal agent; antidote for cyanide poisoning used in conjunction with sodium nitrite (see p. 556).

Dosage and Administration
Antifungal agent: The lotion is applied as directed.
Cyanide antidote: see p. 556.

Cautions
Injection may suppress the blood clotting mechanism.

Adverse Reactions
Hypersensitivity may occur.

Composition and Supply
Injection   25%
Lotion   5% to 25%

Legal Status
Prescription

Sodium thiosulfate/salicylic acid/2-propanol (Tinver®)

See ANTI-INFECTIVES, fungicides.

Sodium warfarin (Coumadin®, Panwarfin®)

Action and Use
Sodium warfarin is an anticoagulant indicated for the prophylaxis and treatment of venous thrombosis and its extension, the treatment of atrial fibrillation with embolization, the prophylaxis and treatment of pulmonary embolism, and as an adjunct in the treatment of coronary occlusion. The drug is possibly effective as an adjunct in the treatment of cerebral ischemic attacks.

Dosage and Administration
The administration and dosage of sodium warfarin must be individualized for each patient, and periodic determination of prothrombin time or other suitable coagulation test is essential. Satisfactory levels are 1½ to 2½ times the normal prothrombin time.
Induction: Usually 40 to 60 mg for one dose only given orally, IV, or IM.
Maintenance: Usually, 2 to 10 mg daily, orally.

Cautions
Sodium warfarin is a potent and potentially dangerous drug. Contraindications include pregnancy, hemorrhagic tendencies, blood dyscrasias, recent or contemplated surgery, bleeding tendencies, threatened abortion, spinal puncture, polyarthritis, vitamin C deficiency, major lumbar regional block anesthesia, and malignant hypertension. The following may be associated with increased risks: lactation, vitamin K deficiency, moderate to severe hepatic or renal insufficiency, infectious diseases, surgery or trauma resulting in large exposed raw surfaces, indwelling catheters, moderate to severe hypertension, severe diabetes, polycythemia vera, allergic and anaphylactic disorders. Drugs that increase the effect of sodium warfarin include: salicylates, chloral hydrate, clofibrate, disulfiram, phenylbutazone, methylpheni-

date, propylthiouracil, *d*-thyroxine, androgenic anabolic steroids, and antibiotics that affect intestinal flora. Drugs that decrease the effect of sodium warfarin include: barbiturates, ethchlorvynol, glutethimide, and griseofulvin. Sodium warfarin potentiates phenytoin and tolbutamide. The occurrence of bleeding calls for the administration of fresh whole blood and/or phytonadione (p. 417).

Adverse Reactions
Possible minor or major hemorrhage from any tissue or organ. Much less frequent side effects include abdominal cramping, nausea, diarrhea, urticaria, alopecia, dermatitis, and fever.

Composition and Supply
Injection   50 mg vial accompanied by 2 ml ampul sterile water
Tablets   2 mg, 2.5 mg, 5 mg, 7.5 mg, 10 mg, and 25 mg

Legal Status
Prescription

Solarcaine® (menthol preparation)

See ANTIPRURITICS, topical preparations.

Solbar® (oxybenzone/dioxybenzone)

See EMOLLIENT-PROTECTANTS.

Solganal®

See **Aurothioglucose.**

Solu-B-Forte® (S-B-F®)

See VITAMINS, MULTIPLE, parenteral.

Solu-Cortef®

See **Hydrocortisone.**

Solu-Medrol®

See under **Methylprednisolone.**

Soma®

See **Carisoprodol.**

Somnos®

See **Chloral hydrate.**

Somophyllin®

See under **Aminophylline.**

Sonilyn® (sulfachloropyridazine)

See SULFONAMIDES.

Sopor® (methaqualone)

See SEDATIVE-HYPNOTICS, nonbarbiturates.

Sopronol® (sodium proprionate/sodium and zinc caprolates)

See ANTI-INFECTIVES, LOCAL, fungicides.

Sorate®

See **Isosorbide dinitrate.**

Sorbitol 3.3%

See IRRIGATING SOLUTIONS.

Sorbitrate®

See **Isosorbide dinitrate.**

Sotradecol®

See **Sodium tetradecyl sulfate.**

Soxomide®

See **Sulfisoxazole.**

Sparine®

See **Promazine hydrochloride.**

Spectinomycin hydrochloride (Trobicin®)

Action and Use
An antibiotic, spectinomycin hydrochloride is an alternative to penicillin in the treatment of acute gonorrhea when penicillin-resistant organisms are involved or when the patient is allergic to penicillin.

Dosage and Administration
2 to 4 g, IM.

Cautions
Not effective in the treatment of syphilis. Clinical effectiveness should be monitored to detect evidence of developing resistance by *Neisseria gonorrhoeae.*

Adverse Reactions
Occasional side effects include urticaria, fever, chills, dizziness, insomnia, decreased levels of hemoglobin and hematocrit, and increased levels of alkaline phosphatase and SGPT. Injection is painful; the injection should be made deeply, and the sites rotated.

Composition and Supply
Injection   2 g and 4 g vials with accompanying diluent

Legal Status
Prescription

Spironolactone (Aldactone®)

Action and Use
Potassium-sparing diuretic used in treating essential hypertension and edema.

Dosage and Administration
Hypertension: 25 mg 2 to 4 times a day (initially), orally.
Edema: 25 mg 4 times a day (initially), orally.

Cautions
Patients receiving potassium supplements may develop hyperkalemia. Use cautiously in patients with impaired renal function or hepatic disease. The action of other antihypertensive agents is potentiated.

Adverse Reactions
Possible side effects include cramping, diarrhea, drowsiness, headache, lethargy, ataxia, mental confusion, urticaria, skin eruptions, gynecomastia, impotence, and mild androgenic manifestations. Reactions reported in association with thiazides include thrombocytopenia, agranulocytosis, paresthesias, acute pancreatitis, jaundice, dizziness, vertigo, photosensitivity, orthostatic hypertension, muscle spasm, and restlessness.

Composition and Supply
Tablets   25 mg
Tablets   25 mg with hydrochlorothiazide 25 mg (Aldactazide®)
(*Note:* dosage is 1 to 8 tablets daily, depending on use, in divided doses)

Legal Status
Prescription

Sporostacin®

See **Chlordantoin.**

SSKI (saturated solution of potassium chloride)

See **Potassium iodide solution.**

Stanozolol (Winstrol®)

See ANDROGENS.

Staphcillin®

See **Methicillin sodium.**

Starch

Action and Use
Dusting powder and protectant.

Dosage and Administration
Dry: apply as a dusting powder.
Soaking bath: 1 cup of powder is mixed with 4 cups of water, and then added to a tubful of lukewarm water; use for 30 minutes.

Cautions
Powder should not be inhaled, and should not be used on raw surfaces.

Adverse Reactions
Starch turns to a dark color when in contact with iodine or iodine-releasing compounds, such as povidone-iodine.

Composition and Supply
Powder

Legal Status
Nonprescription

Stelazine®

See **Trifluoperazine hydrochloride.**

Sterane®

See under **Prednisolone.**

Sterile water

See IRRIGATING SOLUTIONS.

Stibophen (Fuadin®)

See ANTHELMINTICS, schistosomiasis.

Stilbestrol

See **Diethylstilbestrol.**

Stilphostrol®

See **Diethylstilbestrol diphosphate.**

Stoxil®

See **Idoxuridine.**

Streptokinase/streptodornase (Varidase®)

Action and Use
Proteolytic enzyme combination used in the liquefaction of clotted blood or fibrinous or purulent accumulations resulting from trauma or infection.

Dosage and Administration
Applied topically or by local injection.

Cautions
Should not be used in patients with active hemorrhage or acute cellulitis.

Adverse Reactions
Pyrogenic reactions are possible. Allergic reactions may rarely occur.

Composition and Supply
Powder streptokinase 100,000 units per vial and streptodornase 25,000 units per vial
Jelly streptokinase 100,000 units per 15 ml and streptodornase 25,000 units per 15 ml

Legal Status
Prescription

Streptomycin sulfate

Action and Use
Antibiotic used in patients with tuberculosis, tularemia, plague, and bacterial endocarditis.

Dosage and Administration
2 to 4 g daily in divided doses, IM.

Cautions
In the treatment of tuberculosis, this medication should be used only in combination with other antituberculotics. Damage to the eighth

cranial nerve may occur, resulting in deafness and severe vertigo. Use with caution in pregnant women.

Adverse Reactions
Possible side effects include paresthesias of lips and extremities, allergic reactions, renal damage, and superinfection. Pain may occur at the injection site.

Composition and Supply
Injection   1 g vials

Legal Status
Prescription

Stresscaps®

See VITAMINS, MULTIPLE, oral.

Sublimaze®

See **Fentanyl citrate.**

Suby's solution G

See IRRIGATING SOLUTIONS.

Succinylcholine chloride (Anectine®, Quelicin®, Sucostrin®)

Action and Use
Skeletal muscle relaxant.

Dosage and Administration
Short procedures: 10 to 30 mg, IV, over 10 to 30 seconds.
Prolonged procedures: dilute and give by IV infusion according to the manufacturer's direction.

Cautions
Respiratory paralysis is possible. Use with caution in patients concomitantly being treated with cyclophosphamide, phenelzine, phenothiazines, or thiotepa. Contraindicated in patients using echothiophate, isofluorophate, or demecarium. Neostigmine and edrophonium should not be used to counteract the effects of succinylcholine.

Adverse Reactions
See **Pancuronium bromide.**

Composition and Supply
Injection   500 mg and 1 g, in vials of dry powder
Injection   20 mg/ml, in 10 ml vials

Legal Status
Prescription

Sucostrin®

See **Succinylcholine chloride.**

Sudafed®

See **Pseudoephedrine hydrochloride.**

Suladyne® (sulfamethizole/sulfadiazine/phenazopyridine hydrochloride)

See SULFONAMIDES.

Sulfacetamide sodium (Sebizon®, Sodium Sulamyd®)

Action and Use
Sulfonamide anti-infective.

Dosage and Administration
Ointment: applied to lower lid at bedtime.
Drops: 1 or 2 drops every 2 to 4 hours.

Cautions
Use cautiously in patients with known sensitivity to sulfonamide. The solution is incompatible with silver preparations. Discolored solution should be discarded.

Adverse Reactions
Sensitivity may develop.

Composition and Supply
Ointment, ophthalmic   10%
Solution, ophthalmic   10%, 15%, and 30%

Legal Status
Prescription

Sulfachloropyridazine (Sonilyn®)

See SULFONAMIDES.

Sulfacytine (Renoquid®)

See SULFONAMIDES.

Sulfadiazine

See ANTIPROTOZOALS, antitrypanosomals; SULFONAMIDES.

Sulfameter (Sulla®)

See SULFONAMIDES.

Sulfamethizole (Thiosulfil®)

Action and Use
Sulfonamide used to treat urinary tract infections.

Dosage and Administration
2 to 4 g daily, orally.

Cautions
See **Sulfisoxazole.**

Adverse Reactions
See **Sulfisoxazole.**

Composition and Supply
Suspension   250 mg/5 ml
Tablets   250 mg and 500 mg

Legal Status
Prescription

Sulfamethizole/sulfadiazine/phenazopyridine hydrochloride (Suladyne®)

See SULFONAMIDES.

Sulfamethoxazole (Gantanol®)

Action and Use
Sulfonamide.

Dosage and Administration
2 g initially, followed by 1 g twice a day, orally.

Cautions
See **Sulfisoxazole.**

Adverse Reactions
See **Sulfisoxazole.**

Composition and Supply
Suspension   500 mg/5 ml
Tablets   500 mg
Tablets   500 mg with phenazopyridine hydrochloride 100 mg (Azo
  Gantanol®)

Legal Status
Prescription

Sulfamethoxypyridazine (Midicel®)

See SULFONAMIDES.

Sulfamylon®

See **Mafenide acetate cream.**

Sulfasalazine (Azulfidine®)

Action and Use
Sulfonamide used to treat ulcerative colitis.

Dosage and Administration
3 to 4 g per day, initially, followed by 500 mg 4 times a day for maintenance, orally.

Cautions
See **Sulfisoxazole.**

Adverse Reactions
See **Sulfisoxazole.**

Composition and Supply
Tablets 500 mg

Legal Status
Prescription

Sulfathalidine®

See **Phthalylsulfathiazole.**

Sulfinpyrazone (Anturane®)

Action and Use
Potent uricosuric agent used in maintenance therapy in chronic gout.

Dosage and Administration
Initial dosage: 200 to 400 mg in 2 divided doses, with meals or milk.
Maintenance dosage: 400 mg daily in 2 divided doses, as above; the dosage may be increased to 800 mg daily if necessary.

Cautions
Contraindicated in patients with active peptic ulcer. Sulfinpyrazone should not be administered concurrently with salicylates, since they antagonize its action. It may potentiate action of coumarin anticoagulants, sulfonamides, hypoglycemic sulfonylurea agents, and insulin.

The patient should be aware that there may be acute exacerbations early in the course of therapy; these usually subside with time.

Adverse Reactions
The main adverse reactions involve gastric symptoms; these are relieved by food, milk, or antacids. Adequate fluid intake and alkalization of urine are needed to avoid urolithiasis and renal colic (intake and output should be recorded). Hematopoiesis may be depressed (periodic blood counts are recommended). The effects of an overdose include nausea, vomiting, diarrhea, abdominal pain, ataxia, labored respirations, convulsions, and coma. Possible late symptoms include anemia, jaundice, and ulceration.

Composition and Supply
Tablets   100 mg
Capsules   200 mg

Legal Status
Prescription

Sulfisoxazole (Gantrisin®, Soxomide®)

Action and Use
Sulfonamide.

Dosage and Administration
Oral: 2 to 4 g initially, followed by 2 to 4 g daily in divided doses.
Parenteral: 100 mg/kg/24 hours in divided doses, SC, IM, or IV (as 5% solution for SC and IV, and 40% solution for IM); the initial dose is one-half of the 24-hour dose.
Ophthalmic: 2 or 3 drops of solution in the eye 3 or more times daily; or a small amount of ointment in lower conjunctival sac 1 to 3 times daily and at bedtime.
Vaginal: 2 to 5 ml of 10% cream for up to 2 weeks.

Cautions
Hypersensitivity and hematologic and renal toxicity are possible. Adequate fluid intake should be maintained. Contraindicated in patients with hypersensitivity to sulfonamides, infants under 2 months of age (except in the treatment of congenital toxoplasmosis), pregnant women at term, and nursing mothers.

Adverse Reactions
Possible side effects include nausea, vomiting, diarrhea, jaundice, and hepatitis (periodic liver function tests are recommended). Other reported side effects include dizziness, restlessness, irritability, confusion, ataxia, vertigo, headache, depression, and skin involvement (such as vascular lesions or dermatitis). Drug fever, especially during the second week of therapy, is an occasional side effect, with head-

ache, chills, malaise, joint pains, bronchospasm, conjunctivitis, and lupus erythematosus phenomenon. Pancytopenia may occur (periodic blood tests are recommended). Topical preparations may produce irritation, pruritus, urticaria, and vulvitis.

Composition and Supply
Cream, vaginal   10%
Injection (as diolamine)   40%, in 5 ml and 10 ml ampuls
Ointment and solution, ophthalmic (as diolamine)   4%
Suspension   500 mg/5 ml
Tablets   500 mg
Tablets   500 mg with phenazopyridine hydrochloride 50 g (Azo Gantrisin®) (*Note:* dosage is 4 to 6 tablets initially followed by 2 tablets 4 times a day for up to 3 days; the patient should be warned that phenazopyridine turns the urine orange-red)

Legal Status
Prescription

Sulfobromophthalein sodium (Bromsulphalein®, BSP®)

Action and Use
Diagnostic agent used in the assessment of liver function; in a normal test, 5% or less of the injected material remains in the blood at end of 45 minutes.

Dosage and Administration
5 mg/kg, IV (slowly) up to a maximum of 500 mg.

Cautions
Should be administered only by a person capable of dealing with an acute anaphylactoid reaction. Use with extreme caution in patients with a history of allergy and in those who have had these tests repeatedly. Store ampuls in a warm place to prevent crystallization.

Adverse Reactions
Hypersensitivity is possible. Extravasation may occur, which may induce local irritation and allergic reactions. Ice should be applied and the patient's arm elevated if extravasation occurs.

Composition and Supply
Injection   50 mg/ml, in 3 ml and 7.5 ml ampuls

Legal Status
Prescription

Sulfoxone sodium (Diasone®)

See ANTILEPROTICS.

Sulfur, colloidal (present in Bensulfoid®, Collosul®)

See KERATOLYTICS.

Sulfurated lime solution (Vleminckx's solution)

See KERATOLYTICS.

Sulla® (sulfameter)

See SULFONAMIDES.

Sumycin®

See **Tetracycline hydrochloride.**

Suramin (Antrypol®, Germanin®, Naphuride®)

See ANTIPROTOZOALS, antitrypanosomals.

Surfacaine®

See **Cyclomethycaine sulfate.**

Surfadil® (titanium dioxide preparation)

See EMOLLIENT-PROTECTANTS.

Surfak®

See **Dioctyl calcium sulfosuccinate.**

Surgicel™ Absorbable Hemostat

See **Cellulose, oxidized regenerated.**

Surital®

See **Thiamylal sodium.**

Sustacal®

See FOOD FORMULATIONS.

Sustagen®

See FOOD FORMULATIONS.

Sutilains (Travase®)

Action and Use
Proteolytic enzyme used for biochemical debridement.

Dosage and Administration
Ointment applied 3 or 4 times a day.

Cautions
Keep away from the eyes. Contraindicated in wounds communicating with major cavities, in areas exposing nervous tissue, in neoplastic ulcers, and in pregnant women. Inactivated by several detergents and antiseptics, including benzalkonium chloride, hexachlorophene, iodine, and nitrofurazone. Moist tissue is essential to the effectiveness of the drug.

Adverse Reactions
Occasional side effects include mild transient pain, paresthesias, bleeding, and dermatitis.

Composition and Supply
Ointment   82,000 units/g (*Note:* store at 2° to 8°C)

Legal Status
Prescription

Symmetrel®

See **Amantadine hydrochloride.**

Synalar®

See **Fluocinolone acetonide.**

Synemol®

See **Fluocinolone acetonide.**

Synkayvite®

See **Menadiol sodium diphosphate.**

Synthroid®

See **Levothyroxine sodium.**

Syntocinon®

See **Oxytocin.**

Syntocinon® Nasal Spray

See under **Oxytocin.**

Tacaryl® (methdilazine hydrochloride)

See ANTIPRURITICS, systemic preparations.

Tace®

See **Chlorotrianisene.**

Tagament®

See **Cimetidine.**

Talbutal (Lotusate®)

See SEDATIVE-HYPNOTICS, barbiturates.

Talc (talcum)

See EMOLLIENT-PROTECTANTS.

Talwin®

See **Pentazocine.**

Talwin® Compound

See under **Pentazocine.**

Tamoxifen citrate (Nolvadex®)

See ANTINEOPLASTICS, antimetabolites.

Tandearil®

See **Oxyphenbutazone.**

TAO® (troleandomycin)

See ANTIBIOTICS, miscellaneous.

Tapazole®

See **Methimazole.**

Tartar emetic

See **Antimony potassium tartrate.**

Tedral® (theophylline/ephedrine/phenobarbital)

See ANTIASTHMATICS, xanthine preparations.

Tegopen®

See **Cloxacillin sodium.**

Tegretol®

See **Carbamazepine.**

Teldrin®

See **Chlorpheniramine maleate.**

Telepaque®

See **Iopanoic acid.**

Temaril®

See **Trimeprazine tartrate.**

Tempra®

See **Acetaminophen.**

Tensilon®

See **Edrophonium chloride.**

Tenuate®

See **Diethylpropion hydrochloride.**

Tepanil®

See **Diethylpropion hydrochloride.**

Terbutaline sulfate (Brethine®, Bricanyl®)

Action and Use
Beta-adrenergic bronchodilator.

Dosage and Administration
Oral: 2.5 to 5 mg 3 times a day at 6 hour intervals.
Parenteral: 250 µg, IM. A second dose (250 µg) is given 15 to 30 minutes later if needed.

Cautions
The total parenteral dose of 500 µg should not be exceeded within a 4 hour period. Use with caution in patients with diabetes mellitus,

hypertension, hyperthyroidism, or heart problems. Contraindicated in persons with known hypersensitivity to sympathomimetic amines.

Adverse Reactions
Possible side effects include nervousness, weakness, drowsiness, dizziness, tremors, and tachycardia. Other reported side effects include headache, nausea, vomiting, and anxiety.

Composition and Supply
Injection   1 mg/ml, in 2 ml ampuls
Tablets   2.5 mg and 5 mg

Legal Status
Prescription

Terfonyl® (trisulfapyrimidines)

See SULFONAMIDES.

Terpin hydrate/codeine

Action and Use
Expectorant and antitussive.

Dosage and Administration
5 to 10 ml every 3 to 4 hours, orally.

Cautions
This medication has a high alcoholic content; do not administer it in large doses. Codeine is habit-forming.

Adverse Reactions
There is a bitter taste. See **Codeine** for further adverse reactions.

Composition and Supply
Elixir   terpin hydrate 85 mg/5 ml and codeine 10 mg/5 ml

Legal Status
Schedule V

Terramycin®

See **Oxytetracycline.**

Teslac®

See **Testolactone.**

Tessalon®

See **Benzonatate.**

Tes-Tape®

See DIAGNOSTICS, urine (glucose).

Testolactone (Teslac®)

Action and Use
Antineoplastic used as an adjunct in the palliative treatment of advanced or disseminated breast cancer in postmenopausal women.

Dosage and Administration
250 mg 4 times a day, orally; 100 mg 3 times a week IM.

Cautions
Plasma calcium levels should be routinely determined. Contraindicated in pregnant women and in men with breast cancer.

Adverse Reactions
Possible side effects include maculopapular erythema, hypertension, paresthesias, acute pain of the extremities, glossitis, anorexia, nausea, and vomiting. Pain may occur at the injection site, with local inflammation or irritation.

Composition and Supply
Injection   100 mg/ml, in 5 ml vials
Tablets   50 mg and 250 mg

Legal Status
Prescription

Testosterone cypionate (Depo®-Testosterone)

See ANDROGENS.

Testosterone enanthate (Delatestryl®)

Action and Use
Long-acting androgen.

Dosage and Administration
Male hypogonadism: 200 to 400 mg every 4 weeks, IM.
Oligospermia: 100 to 200 mg every 4 to 6 weeks, IM.

Cautions
See **Fluoxymesterone.**

Adverse Reactions
See **Fluoxymesterone.**

Composition and Supply
Injection   200 mg/ml, in 1 ml disposable syringes and 5 ml vials

Legal Status
Prescription

Testosterone enanthate/estradiol valerate (Deladumone®)

See ANDROGENS; ESTROGENS.

Testosterone propionate

Action and Use
Androgen.

Dosage and Administration
10 to 50 mg 2 to 6 times a week, IM; or 5 to 40 mg daily (depending on use), sublingually or buccally.

Cautions
See **Fluoxymesterone.**

Adverse Reactions
See **Fluoxymesterone.**

Composition and Supply
Injection   25 mg/ml, 50 mg/ml, and 100 mg/ml
Tablets, buccal   10 mg (Oreton® Propionate)

Legal Status
Prescription

Testred®

See **Methyltestosterone.**

Tetanus antitoxin

See BIOLOGICALS.

Tetanus immune human globulin (Ar-Tet®, Homo-Tet®, Hyper-Tet®, IMMU-Tetanus®)

Action and Use
Provides tetanus antibody (antitoxin); indicated for the prophylaxis and treatment of tetanus.

Dosage and Administration
Prophylaxis: 250 to 500 units, IM.
Treatment: 500 units initially IM, followed by daily doses of 500 to 1,000 units, for a total dosage of 3,000 to 6,000 units.

Cautions
Should not be given IV. Use with caution in patients with a history of allergic reaction following the administration of human gamma globulin.

Adverse Reactions
Possible side effects include urticaria, angioedema, and local pain and tenderness at the injection site. Anaphylactic reactions have been reported.

Composition and Supply
Injection   250 unit vials and disposable syringes

Legal Status
Prescription

Tetanus toxoid, adsorbed

Action and Use
Used for active immunization against tetanus.

Dosage and Administration
Primary immunization: two 0.5 ml doses at an interval of not less than 1 month, administered deep SC or IM, at sites away from previous immunization.
Booster dose: 0.5 ml, deep SC or IM.

Cautions
Avoid administration in patients with acute infectious illnesses.

Adverse Reactions
A stinging sensation may occur immediately after the injection. A mild to moderate local reaction, induration, and tenderness for about 24 hours may also occur. Fever and malaise may occur. Sometimes a small subcutaneous nodule forms at injection site, but this gradually disappears in a few weeks.

Composition and Supply
Syringes, disposable   0.5 ml (500 μl)
Vials, multidose   5 ml

Legal Status
Prescription

Tetracaine hydrochloride (Pontocaine®)

Action and Use
Local anesthetic.

Dosage and Administration
Topical, in the eye: ophthalmic solution or ointment is instilled.
Topical, in the nose, throat, or mouth: solution is instilled.
Injection: dosage and routes vary with procedure.

Cautions
Use cautiously in patients with diseases of the cerebrospinal system, suppuration at the site of puncture, shock, profound anemia, cachexia, sepsis with positive blood culture, hypertension, hypotension, visceral perforation, bowel strangulation, acute peritonitis, gastrointestinal hemorrhage, cardiac decompensation, massive pleural effusion, or increased intra-abdominal pressure, and in highly nervous and sensitive persons. Protect the ampuls from light and store under refrigeration. Not to be used if crystals, cloudiness, or discoloration occurs.

Adverse Reactions
More potent and more toxic than procaine hydrochloride (see); toxic effects are rare because low concentrations are used. Eye drops may produce a brief burning sensation and can cause epithelial damage with prolonged use. Possible systemic repercussions include hypotension, nausea, vomiting, restlessness, pallor, diaphoresis, weak pulse, respiratory depression, and convulsions.

Composition and Supply
Injection   0.15%, 0.2%, 0.3%, and 1%
Ointment, ophthalmic   0.5%
Solution   2%
Solution, ophthalmic   0.5%

Legal Status
Prescription

Tetrachloroethylene

Action and Use
Anthelmintic used in the treatment of hookworm, especially *Necator americanus.*

Dosage and Administration
0.12 ml/kg (maximum 5 ml) as a single oral dose in the morning after an overnight fast; may be repeated in 1 week..

Cautions

Fats, oils, and alcohol enhance absorption and should be avoided throughout therapy. Use with caution in small or severely ill children, in debilitated persons, in pregnant women, and in patients with anemia, liver disease, or alcoholism. Store the drug in a cool place to prevent the formation of toxic substances.

Adverse Reactions

Side effects include a burning sensation in the stomach, abdominal cramps, nausea, vomiting, dizziness, and drowsiness. The patient should rest 2 to 4 hours after the administration of the drug. Effects on the central nervous system may be manifested by headache, vertigo, inebriation, and, rarely, loss of consciousness.

Composition and Supply

Capsules   200 μl, 500 μl, 1 ml, and 2.5 ml

Legal Status

Prescription

Tetracycline/amphotericin B (Mysteclin-F®)

See ANTIBIOTICS, tetracyclines.

Tetracycline hydrochloride (Achromycin®, Achromycin® V, Cyclopar®, Panmycin®, Sumycin®, Tetracyn®)

Tetracycline phosphate complex (Tetrex®)

Action and Use

Broad-spectrum antibiotic.

Dosage and Administration

Oral: 250 to 500 mg every 6 hours.
Parenteral: 250 mg once every 24 hours, IM (deep); or 250 to 500 mg every 12 hours, IV (not to exceed 500 mg every 6 hours).
Topical: ointment or ophthalmic suspension is applied.

Cautions

Photosensitivity occurs frequently. Antacids and iron preparations interfere with absorption and should not be given concomitantly with tetracycline. (Food also interferes with absorption of the drug.) It depresses the prothrombin levels; patients being treated with anticoagulants may require downward adjustment of dosage. The use of tetracycline during tooth development (during the last half of pregnancy and in infants and children up to 8 years of age) may cause permanent discoloration of teeth. Contraindicated in patients with renal insufficiency. There is a high risk of sensitization with topical administration, except in the case of eye preparations. Outdated, unused, or degraded tetracycline should be discarded to avoid renal toxicity. The drug should be stored in airtight containers in a cool place.

Adverse Reactions

The most frequent side effects include abdominal discomfort, nausea, and vomiting (divided doses may relieve the symptoms). Superinfection, as a result of the overgrowth of nonsusceptible organisms, may take the form of candidiasis (with inflammation of the mouth and throat, anal itch, and vaginitis) and staphylococcal enterocolitis (which produces diarrhea late in therapy). Rarely, allergic reactions may occur, including rash, fever, eosinophilia, and photosensitivity (the patient should be advised to stay out of sunlight while being treated). Increased intracranial pressure and bulging fontanels may occur in young infants. Anaphylaxis is possible. Liver damage has occurred in patients with impaired kidney function and in pregnant women receiving high daily doses. Other possible side effects include negative nitrogen balance, weight loss, urinary loss of sodium, and a rise in BUN. Long-term treatment may produce anemia, purpura, and alteration of leukocytes. Intramuscular injections given deeply to avoid poor absorption and pain at the injection site. Thrombophlebitis may occur at the site of intravenous injections.

Composition and Supply

Tetracycline hydrochloride
Capsules   100 mg, 250 mg, and 500 mg
Capsules   250 mg with nystatin 250,000 units (Achrostatin® V)
Drops, pediatric   100 mg/20 drops (1 ml)
Injection, IM   100 mg and 250 mg vials
Injection, IV   250 mg and 500 mg vials
Ointment   3%
Ointment, ophthalmic   1%
Suspension, oral   250 mg/5 ml
Tablets   250 mg and 500 mg

Tetracycline phosphate complex
Capsules   250 mg
Capsules, long-acting   500 mg (Tetrex® BidCAPS®)
Syrup   125 mg/5 ml

Legal Status
Prescription

Tetracycline phosphate complex/sulfamethizole/ phenazopyridine hydrochloride (Azotrex®)

See URINARY ANTISEPTICS.

Tetracyn®

See **Tetracycline hydrochloride.**

Tetrahydrozoline hydrochloride (Tyzine®, Visine®)

Action and Use
Adrenergic vasoconstrictor used in the eye and nose.

Dosage and Administration
Eye: 1 or 2 drops of ophthalmic solution 2 or 3 times a day.
Nose, in adults: 2 to 4 drops of 0.1% solution as needed (but never more often than every 3 hours).
Nose, in children 2 to 6 years old: 2 or 3 drops of 0.05% solution in each nostril (never more often than every 3 hours).

Cautions
Contraindicated in children under 2 years of age, in patients with glaucoma or other serious eye disease, and in patients undergoing therapy with MAO inhibitors. If relief does not occur within 48 hours, or if irritation or redness persists or increases, the drug should be discontinued. Use cautiously in patients with hypotension, shock, cardiovascular disorders, metabolic or endocrine disorders (e.g., hyperthyroidism and diabetes). Long-term therapy with glucocorticoids used concurrently with sympathomimetics results in increased ocular pressure. In children, an overdose may produce profound sedation.

Adverse Reactions
Local irritation may be observed on occasion. Nose drops may produce burning, stinging, sneezing, dryness, headache, drowsiness, weakness, tremors, lightheadedness, insomnia, and palpitations. Rare systemic toxic effects include nervousness, tachycardia, and insomnia.

Composition and Supply
Drops, nasal, pediatric   0.05%
Solution, nasal   0.1%
Solution, ophthalmic   0.05%

Legal Status
Prescription (Tyzine®)
Nonprescription (Visine®)

Tetrex®

See **Tetracycline phosphate complex.**

Tetrex® BidCAPS®

See under **Tetracycline phosphate complex.**

Tham (tromethamine)

See ELECTROLYTE SOLUTIONS AND WATER-BALANCE AGENTS, alkalizing agents.

Theolair™ (theophylline)

See ANTIASTHMATICS, xanthine preparations.

Theophylline (Aerolate®, Elixophyllin®, Theolair™)

See ANTIASTHMATICS, xanthine preparations.

Theophylline ethylenediamine

See **Aminophylline.**

Theophylline/ephedrine/hydroxyzine (Marax®)

See ANTIASTHMATICS, xanthine preparations.

Theophylline/ephedrine/phenobarbital (Tedral®)

See ANTIASTHMATICS, xanthine preparations.

Theophylline/guaifenesin (Quibron®)

See ANTIASTHMATICS, xanthine preparations.

Theragran®-M Tablets

See VITAMINS, MULTIPLE, oral.

Theriodide® (sodium iodide I 131)

See ANTITHYROIDS.

Thiabendazole (Mintezol®)

Action and Use
Broad-spectrum anthelmintic.

Dosage and Administration
50 mg/kg per day, in 2 doses, orally, for 3 days.

Cautions
Use with caution in patients with liver dysfunction. Activities requiring mental alertness should be prohibited during therapy.

Adverse Reactions
Common but mild and transient symptoms occur 3 to 4 hours after ingestion and last 2 to 8 hours. The side effects include dizziness, anorexia, nausea, vomiting, abdominal cramping, diarrhea, headache, drowsiness, lethargy, giddiness, and pruritus; these effects are decreased if the drug is given after meals. There are infrequent allergic reactions. Rare side effects include tinnitus, collapse, abnormal sensations in the eyes, numbness, hyperglycemia, xanthopsia, enuresis, bradycardia, lowered systolic blood pressure, and a transitory rise in cephalin flocculation and SGOT.

Composition and Supply
Suspension   500 mg/5 ml
Tablets, chewable   500 mg

Legal Status
Prescription

Thiamine hydrochloride (vitamin B₁)

Action and Use
Used in the treatment of thiamine deficiency.

Dosage and Administration
10 to 30 mg 3 times a day, orally; or 50 mg 3 times a day, IM.

Cautions
Intravenous use can lead to serious sensitivity reactions.

Adverse Reactions
A slight transitory vasodilatation and hypotension may occur after rapid IV administration. Hypersensitivity may occur. An overdose may produce symptoms of toxicity, including weakness, dyspnea, and respiratory failure.

Composition and Supply
Injection   50 mg/ml, in 5 ml, 10 ml, and 30 ml vials; 100 mg/ml, in 1 ml, 5 ml, 10 ml, and 30 ml vials
Injection   100 mg prefilled syringe (Tubex®)
Tablets   5 mg, 10 mg, 15 mg, 25 mg, and 50 mg

Legal Status
Prescription (injection)
Nonprescription (tablets)

Thiamylal sodium (Surital®)

Action and Use
Ultrashort-acting barbiturate used for hypnosis and anesthesia.

Dosage and Administration
An initial injection of 3 to 6 ml of 2.5% solution, IV, is generally sufficient to produce short periods of surgical anesthesia. The rate of injection is about 1 ml every 5 seconds.

Cautions
See **Thiopental sodium.**

Adverse Reactions
See **Thiopental sodium.**

Composition and Supply
Injection   1 g, 5 g, and 10 g vials (*Note:* the contents should be reconstituted with sterile water, isotonic sodium chloride, or 5% dextrose)

Legal Status
Schedule III

Thiethylperazine (Torecan®)

See ANTIEMETICS.

Thimerosal (Merthiolate®)

See ANTI-INFECTIVES, LOCAL, miscellaneous antiseptic-disinfectants.

Thioguanine (Thioguanine, Tabloid® Brand)

Action and Use
Antineoplastic used to treat acute leukemia.

Dosage and Administration
Dosage is carefully adjusted to the patient; the dose ranges from 2 to 3 mg/kg (maximum dose is 20 mg), orally.

Cautions
There is a danger of bone marrow depression; blood counts should be determined weekly.

Adverse Reactions
Stomatitis may occur with use of this drug.

Composition and Supply
Tablets 40 mg

Legal Status
Prescription

Thiomerin®

See **Mercaptomerin sodium.**

Thiopental sodium (Pentothal®)

Action and Use
Ultrashort-acting barbiturate used for hypnosis and anesthesia.

Dosage and Administration
2 to 3 ml of 2.5% solution at 20 to 40 second intervals, depending on
the reaction of the patient.

Cautions
Contraindicated in patients with status asthmaticus or porphyria. Use
with caution in patients with cardiovascular disease, hypotension,
excessive premedication, Addison's disease, liver or kidney dysfunction, myxedema, increased blood urea, severe anemia, increased intracranial pressure, or myasthenia gravis. Keep resuscitation and endo-
tracheal intubation equipment and oxygen available. A patent airway
should be maintained at all times. Extravasation should be avoided.
The solution deteriorates very rapidly.

Adverse Reactions
Side effects include respiratory depression, myocardial depression,
arrhythmias, prolonged somnolence, sneezing, coughing, bronchospasm, laryngospasm, and shivering.

Composition and Supply
Injection 500 mg and 1 g vials and 2.5 g, 5 g, and 10 g containers
(*Note:* the contents should be reconstituted with sterile water, iso-
tonic sodium chloride, or 5% dextrose)

Legal Status
Schedule III

Thioridazine hydrochloride (Mellaril®)

Action and Use
Major tranquilizer for use in psychotic disorders and depressive neuroses.

Dosage and Administration
Dosage is individualized to the patient; the dosage range is 30 to 800 mg daily in divided doses, orally.

Cautions
Cross-sensitivity with other phenothiazine drugs may develop. See **Chlorpromazine hydrochloride** for further cautions.

Adverse Reactions
The most common side effects include ataxia, sedation, hypotension, dry mouth, blurred vision, nausea, vomiting, edema, and impotence. Cardiographic alterations and pigmentary retinopathy may occur, especially with large doses. See **Chlorpromazine hydrochloride** for further adverse reactions.

Composition and Supply
Concentrate   30 mg/ml and 100 mg/ml
Tablets   10 mg, 15 mg, 25 mg, 50 mg, 100 mg, 150 mg, and 200 mg

Legal Status
Prescription

Thiosulfil®

See **Sulfamethizole.**

Thiotepa

Action and Use
Antineoplastic.

Dosage and Administration
Topical: 60 mg in 30 to 60 ml distilled water instilled into the bladder by catheter.
Local injection: 45 to 60 mg initially.
IV: half the dose for local injection.

Cautions
There is a danger of gastrointestinal perforation. Thiotepa may cause cumulative toxic effects in blood-forming tissues. Irreversible aplastic anemia has been known to develop. Contraindicated in patients with hepatic or renal impairment.

Adverse Reactions
Occasional side effects include headache, fever, allergic reactions, and mild anemia. Other possible side effects include local pain, tightness of throat, dizziness, anorexia, and weeping from a subcutaneous lesion (as a result of the breakdown of tumor tissue). Thiotepa may interfere with spermatogenesis and ovarian function. Lesions in a heavily ir-

radiated area may show a slow or lessened response, accompanied by an enhanced toxic reaction caused by the radiomimetic effect of thiotepa. Hyperuricemia (with uric acid nephropathy) and anaphylactic reaction may occur.

Composition and Supply
15 mg vials

Legal Status
Prescription

Thiothixene hydrochloride (Navane®)

Action and Use
Major tranquilizer.

Dosage and Administration
6 to 60 mg daily in divided doses, orally; or 16 to 20 mg daily in divided doses, IM.

Cautions
Drowsiness and possibly syncope may occur. The action of CNS depressants, anticholinergics, and hypotensive agents may be potentiated.

Adverse Reactions
Side effects include blurred vision, hypotension, tachycardia, and dizziness.

Composition and Supply
Capsules   1 mg, 2 mg, 5 mg, 10 mg, and 20 mg
Injection   2 mg/ml
Liquid, oral   5 mg/ml

Legal Status
Prescription

Thiphenamil hydrochloride (Trocinate®)

See ANTIDIARRHEALS; ANTISPASMODICS.

Thorazine®

See **Chlorpromazine hydrochloride.**

Thrombin

Action and Use
Local hemostatic agent used to treat capillary bleeding.

Dosage and Administration
Administered topically as a powder or a solution (1,000 to 2,000 units/ml).

Cautions
Thrombin solutions should never be injected.

Adverse Reactions
Allergic reaction may occur following the use of thrombin in the treatment of epistaxis.

Composition and Supply
Vials   1,000 units, 5,000 units, and 10,000 units

Legal Status
Prescription

Thymol iodide

See ANTI-INFECTIVES, LOCAL, miscellaneous antiseptic-disinfectants.

Thyroglobulin (Proloid®)

Action and Use
Thyroid hormone preparation, containing levothyroxine and liothyronine.

Dosage and Administration
15 to 60 mg initially, and gradually increased to maintenance dose as required, orally. The usual maintenance dose is 32 to 190 mg daily.

Cautions
See **Thyroid.**

Adverse Reactions
See **Thyroid.**

Composition and Supply
Tablets   15 mg, 30 mg, 60 mg, 100 mg, 200 mg, and 300 mg

Legal Status
Prescription

Thyroid

Action and Use
Thyroid extract.

Dosage and Administration

15 to 60 mg daily, initially, and gradually increased to maintenance dose as required, orally. The usual maintenance dose is 32 to 190 mg daily.

Cautions

Hyperthyroidism may result from overdosage. Use with caution in patients taking insulin or oral hypoglycemic agents, and in those with a history of angina pectoris, recent myocardial infarction, congestive heart failure, or hypertension. Contraindicated in patients with uncorrected adrenal insufficiency or hypopituitarism unless the adrenal deficiency is first corrected by the administration of adequate doses of cortisone or hydrocortisone. Patients taking coumarin anticoagulants may require a one-third reduction in dosage with any thyroid preparation.

Adverse Reactions

The patient should be instructed about the dosage schedule and the signs of hyperthyroidism (the instructions should be in written form if the patient has severe hypothyroidism). One of the first symptoms of an overdose is an increase in the pulse rate; the pulse should always be taken before the administration of thyroid, and the physician should be consulted if the pulse is 100 or more beats per minute. The other signs of an overdose include tachycardia, cardiac arrhythmias, elevated pulse pressure, angina type chest pains, dyspnea, congestive heart failure, excessive sweating, intolerance to heat, fever, flushing, nervousness, irritability, insomnia, headache, increased gastrointestinal motility, abdominal cramps, diarrhea, nausea, increased appetite, loss of weight, and menstrual irregularities.

Composition and Supply

Tablets   15 mg, 30 mg, 60 mg, 120 mg, 200 mg, and 300 mg

Legal Status

Prescription

Thyrolar® (liotrix)

See THYROID PREPARATIONS.

Thyrotropin (Thytropar®)

See DIAGNOSTICS, thyroid function test.

Thytropar® (thyrotropin)

See DIAGNOSTICS, thyroid function test.

Ticar®

See **Ticarcillin disodium.**

Ticarcillin disodium (Ticar®)

Action and Use
Ticarcillin disodium is a semisynthetic injectable penicillin primarily indicated in gram-negative infections, including *Pseudomonas aeruginosa, Escherichia coli,* and *Proteus* species (both indole-positive and indole-negative).

Dosage and Administration
Bacterial septicemia, respiratory tract infections, and skin and soft tissue infections: 3 g by IV infusion every 3, 4, or 6 hours, depending on body weight and the severity of the infection.
Urinary tract infections (complicated): usual dosage, 3 g 4 times a day by IV infusion.
Urinary tract infections (uncomplicated): 1 g IM or direct IV every 6 hours.

Cautions
Contraindicated in patients with a history of allergic reaction to any of the penicillins. Also see **Penicillin G potassium.**

Adverse Reactions
See **Penicillin G potassium.**

Composition and Supply
Bottles, piggyback   3 g and 6 g (*Note:* 3 g and 6 g bottles should be reconstituted with a minimum of 30 ml and 60 ml, respectively, of Sterile Water for Injection)
Vials   1 g, 3 g, and 6 g (*Note:* for IM use each gram of ticarcillin disodium should be reconstituted with 2 ml of Sterile Water for Injection or 1% lidocaine hydrochloride (without epinephrine); for IV use reconstitute each gram with at least 4 ml of Sterile Water for Injection)

Legal Status
Prescription

Tigan®

See **Trimethobenzamide hydrochloride.**

Tinactin®

See **Tolnaftate.**

Tindal® (acetophenazine maleate)

See PSYCHOTROPICS, antipsychotics.

Tinver® (sodium thiosulfate/salicylic acid/2-propanol)

See ANTI-INFECTIVES, fungicides.

Titanium dioxide preparations (A-Fil®, Surfadil®)

See EMOLLIENT-PROTECTANTS.

Titralac® (calcium carbonate/glycine)

See ANTACIDS.

Tobramycin sulfate (Nebcin®)

Action and Use
Aminoglycoside antibiotic indicated in serious infections caused by *Pseudomonas aeruginosa, Proteus* species, *Escherichia coli, Klebsiella-Enterobacter-Serratia* group, *Citrobacter* species, *Providencia* species, staphylococci, and streptococci.

Dosage and Administration
Serious infections: 3 mg/kg per day in 3 equal doses every 8 hours, IM or IV.
Life-threatening infections: up to 5 mg/kg per day in 3 or 4 equal doses, IM or IV; this dosage should be reduced as soon as possible.

Cautions
Since this drug has the potential for ototoxicity and nephrotoxicity, both renal and eighth-nerve function should be closely monitored in patients with known or suspected renal or otic impairment. Concurrent use of other ototoxic or nephrotoxic drugs should be avoided. Use with caution in premature and newborn infants. Cross-sensitivity among the aminoglycosides has been demonstrated.

Adverse Reactions
Reported adverse reactions include nephrotoxicity, neurotoxicity, blood dyscrasias, fever, rash, itching, urticaria, nausea, vomiting, headache, lethargy, and increased SGOT and SGPT levels.

Composition and Supply
Injection   40 mg/ml, in 2 ml ampuls and 1.5 ml and 2 ml disposable single-dose syringes
Injection, pediatric   10 mg/ml, in 2 ml ampuls

Legal Status
Prescription

Tofranil®

See **Imipramine hydrochloride.**

Tokols® (vitamin E)

See VITAMINS, fat-soluble.

Tolazamide (Tolinase®)

Action and Use
Oral hypoglycemic agent.

Dosage and Administration
100 mg to 1 g daily in 1 or 2 doses, orally.

Cautions
See **Chlorpropamide.**

Adverse Reactions
See **Chlorpropamide.**

Composition and Supply
Tablets   100 mg and 250 mg

Legal Status
Prescription

Tolazoline hydrochloride (Priscoline®)

Action and Use
Antiadrenergic vasodilator used in the treatment of peripheral vascular diseases.

Dosage and Administration
100 to 300 mg daily in divided doses, orally; or 40 to 200 mg in divided doses, SC, IM, or IV.

Cautions
Contraindicated following a cerebrovascular accident and in patients with known or suspected coronary artery disease. Peptic ulcer may be aggravated. A sharp drop in blood pressure and collapse may occur.

Adverse Reactions
Side effects include flushing, palpitations, weakness, cardiac arrhythmias, anginal pain, hypertension, nausea, vomiting, epigastric discomfort, and diarrhea.

Composition and Supply
Injection   25 mg/ml, in 10 ml vials
Tablets   25 mg
Tablets, long-acting   80 mg (Lontabs®) (*Note:* the usual dosage is 1
tablet every 12 hours)

Legal Status
Prescription

Tolbutamide (Orinase®)

Action and Use
Oral hypoglycemic agent.

Dosage and Administration
500 mg to 2 g daily in divided doses after meals, orally.

Cautions
See **Chlorpropamide.**

Adverse Reactions
See **Chlorpropamide.**

Composition and Supply
Tablets   500 mg

Legal Status
Prescription

Tolbutamide sodium (Orinase® Diagnostic)

See DIAGNOSTICS, diabetes mellitus.

Tolectin®

See **Tolmetin sodium.**

Tolinase®

See **Tolazamide.**

Tolmetin sodium (Tolectin®)

Action and Use
Nonsteroidal anti-inflammatory agent useful in the treatment of rheumatoid arthritis.

Dosage and Administration
600 mg to 1.8 g daily in divided doses, orally (doses larger than 2 g daily are not recommended).

Cautions
See **Fenoprofen calcium.**

Adverse Reactions
See **Fenoprofen calcium.**

Composition and Supply
Tablets   200 mg

Legal Status
Prescription

Tolnaftate (Tinactin®)

Action and Use
Antifungal.

Dosage and Administration
Applied twice daily, topically.

Cautions
Ineffective against *Candida albicans.*

Adverse Reactions
Transient pruritus may occur.

Composition and Supply
Cream   1%
Powder   1%
Solution   1%

Legal Status
Nonprescription

Topic® (benzyl alcohol/menthol/camphor)

See ANTIPRURITICS, topical preparations.

Topicort® (desoximetasone)

See CORTICOSTEROIDS.

Torecan® (thiethylperazine)

See ANTIEMETICS.

Tral® (hexocyclium methylsulfate)

See ANTICHOLINERGICS.

Tranxene®

See **Clorazepate dipotassium.**

Tranylcypromine (Parnate®)

See PSYCHOTROPICS, MAO inhibitors.

Trasentine® (adiphenine hydrochloride)

See ANTICHOLINERGICS.

Travase®

See **Sutilains.**

Travasol® (amino acid injection)

See PARENTERAL ALIMENTATION.

Travert® (fructose 5% and 10%)

See PARENTERAL ALIMENTATION.

Trecator® SC (ethionamide)

See ANTITUBERCULOTICS.

Tremin®

See **Trihexyphenidyl hydrochloride.**

Trest® (methixene hydrochloride)

See ANTICHOLINERGICS.

Tretinoin (Retin-A®)

Action and Use
Used in the dermatologic treatment of acne vulgaris, primarily grades I, II, and III.

Dosage and Administration
Applied topically, once a day before retiring.

Cautions
Avoid contact with the eyes, mouth, angles of nose, and mucous membranes. Use cautiously when a concomitant topical medication is being administered, because of possible interactions. Severe inflammatory reactions are possible.

Adverse Reactions

The skin of certain sensitive individuals may become red, edematous, blistered, or crusted. Heightened sensitivity to sunlight may occur.

Composition and Supply

Cream   0.05% and 0.1%
Gel   0.025%
Liquid   0.05%
Saturated swabs   0.05%

Legal Status

Prescription

Triamcinolone (Aristocort®, Kenacort®)

Triamcinolone acetonide (Aristocort® A, Kenalog®)

Triamcinolone hexacetonide (Aristospan®)

Action and Use

Glucocorticoid.

Dosage and Administration

Initial oral dosage: 4 to 48 mg daily (individualized to the patient).
Initial parenteral (IM) dosage: one-third to one-half of the oral dose.
Intra-articular and intralesional dosage: 5 to 40 mg.
Topical application: creams, lotions, ointments, and oral paste.

Cautions

Similar to cautions for cortisone acetate (see).

Adverse Reactions

Similar to adverse reactions to cortisone acetate, except that there is little or no mineralocorticoid action when triamcinolone is given in therapeutic doses.

Composition and Supply

Cream and ointment (as acetonide)   0.025%, 0.1%, 0.5%
Injection, intra-articular (as hexacetonide)   20 mg/ml, in 5 ml vials
Injection, intralesional (as diacetate)   25 mg/ml, in 5 ml vials
Injection, intralesional (as hexacetonide)   5 mg/ml, in 12.5 ml vials
Injection, parenteral (as diacetate)   40 mg/ml, in 5 ml vials
Lotion (as acetonide)   0.025% and 0.1%
Paste (as acetonide)   0.1% (Kenalog® in Orabase®)
Syrup   2 mg/ml
Tablets   1 mg, 2 mg, 8 mg, and 16 mg

Legal Status

Prescription

Triaminic® Expectorant

See COUGH-COLD PREPARATIONS, cough preparations.

Triaminicin® (phenylpropanolamine hydrochloride/chlorpheniramine maleate)

See NASAL DECONGESTANTS.

Triaminicol® Cough Syrup

See COUGH-COLD PREPARATIONS, cough preparations.

Triamterene (Dyrenium®)

Action and Use
Diuretic used alone or with other diuretics for added effect or for potassium-conserving potential.

Dosage and Administration
100 mg twice daily, orally, after meals, is the usual starting dose. When triamterene is combined with other diuretics, the total daily dosage of each agent should usually be lowered initially.

Cautions
Potassium supplements should not be given to patients receiving triamterene alone. Contraindicated in patients with severe kidney disease or hyperkalemia.

Adverse Reactions
Possible side effects include nausea, vomiting, diarrhea, weakness, headache, dry mouth, anaphylaxis, photosensitivity, and rash. Triamterene may elevate serum uric acid levels, especially in persons predisposed to gouty arthritis.

Composition and Supply
Capsules   50 mg and 100 mg
Capsules   50 mg and hydrochlorthiazide 25 mg (Dyazide®)

Legal Status
Prescription

Triavil®

See **Perphenazine/amitriptyline hydrochloride.**

Trichlormethiazide (Naqua®)

See DIURETICS.

Trichloroacetic acid

See KERATOLYTICS.

Trichloroethylene (Trilene®)

See ANESTHETICS, general.

Triclofos (Triclos®)

See SEDATIVE-HYPNOTICS, nonbarbiturates.

Triclos® (triclofos)

See SEDATIVE-HYPNOTICS, nonbarbiturates.

Tricofuron® (furazolidone/nifuroxime)

See ANTIPROTOZOALS.

Tridesilon® (desonide)

See CORTICOSTEROIDS.

Tridione®

See **Trimethadione.**

Triethanolamine polypeptide oleate condensate (Cerumenex®)

See CERUMINOLYTICS.

Trifluoperazine hydrochloride (Stelazine®)

Action and Use
Major tranquilizer.

Dosage and Administration
In patients with mild anxiety: 1 to 4 mg daily, orally.
In psychotic patients: 15 to 30 mg daily, orally or IM.

Cautions
See **Chlorpromazine hydrochloride.**

Adverse Reactions
The most common side effects include sedation, ataxia, constipation, dermatitis, hypotension, antiemesis, blurred vision, tachycardia, nasal congestion, extrapyramidal effects, and photosensitivity. See **Chlorpromazine hydrochloride** for further adverse reactions.

Composition and Supply

Injection   2 mg/ml, in 10 ml vials (*Note:* the exposure of parenteral preparations to light may cause discoloration; discard the liquid if it is markedly discolored)

Liquid, oral   10 mg/ml

Tablets   1 mg, 2 mg, 5 mg, and 10 mg

Legal Status
Prescription

Triflupromazine (Vesprin®)

See ANTIEMETICS; PSYCHOTROPICS, antipsychotics.

Trihexyphenidyl hydrochloride (Artane®, Tremin®)

Action and Use
Anticholinergic muscle relaxant used in the treatment of parkinsonism and in the prevention or control of extrapyramidal disorders caused by CNS drugs.

Dosage and Administration
The starting dose is 1 mg daily, increased to 6 to 10 mg daily in divided doses, orally.

Cautions
Use with caution in patients with glaucoma or obstructive disease of the gastrointestinal or genitourinary tract and in elderly males with possible prostatic hypertrophy. Intraocular pressure should be carefully monitored.

Adverse Reactions
Dry mouth, blurred vision, constipation, urinary retention, tachycardia, headache, dizziness, nausea, vomiting, nervousness, and dilated pupils are possible side effects. Patients with arteriosclerosis may experience confusion, agitation, nausea, and vomiting. Older patients may experience confusion, agitation, and disorientation. Overdosage: drowsiness, delirium, ataxia, hallucinations, somnolence, and coma.

Composition and Supply
Capsules, sustained-release   5 mg (Artane® Sequels®) (*Note:* these are usually given as a single dose after breakfast)

Elixir   2 mg/ml

Tablets   2 mg and 5 mg

Legal Status
Prescription

Tri-Immunol®

See **Diphtheria toxoid/tetanus toxoid/pertussis vaccine, adsorbed.**

Trilafon®

See **Perphenazine.**

Trilene® (trichloroethylene)

See ANESTHETICS, general.

Trimeprazine tartrate (Temaril®)

Action and Use
Phenothiazine (with antihistaminic properties) used as an antipruritic agent.

Dosage and Administration
The usual dosage is 2.5 mg 4 times a day, orally; 5 mg sustained-release capsule twice a day.

Cautions
Drowsiness may occur. See **Chlorpromazine hydrochloride** for further cautions.

Adverse Reactions
See **Chlorpromazine hydrochloride.**

Composition and Supply
Capsules, sustained-release   5 mg (Temaril® Spansule®)
Syrup   2.5 mg/5 ml
Tablets   2.5 mg

Legal Status
Prescription

Trimethadione (Tridione®)

Action and Use
Anticonvulsant used in the treatment of petit mal seizures refractory to other drugs.

Dosage and Administration
300 to 600 mg 3 or 4 times a day, orally.

Cautions
Contraindicated in patients with hepatic or renal disease or optic nerve disorders. There is a risk of blood dyscrasias. Use with caution in pregnant women, because of the danger of birth defects.

Adverse Reactions

Serious untoward effects are possible, including gastric irritation, nausea, anorexia, weight loss, skin eruptions, headache, vertigo, drowsiness, paresthesias, fatigue, personality changes, light sensitivity, and defects in vision.

Composition and Supply

Capsules   300 mg
Solution, oral   200 mg/5 ml
Tablets, chewable   150 mg

Legal Status

Prescription

Trimethaphan camsylate (Arfonad®)

See ANTIHYPERTENSIVES, nondiuretic.

Trimethobenzamide hydrochloride (Tigan®)

Action and Use

Antiemetic.

Dosage and Administration

250 mg 3 or 4 times a day, orally; or 200 mg 3 or 4 times a day, IM or rectally.

Cautions

The parenteral form is contraindicated in children; the suppository is contraindicated in premature and newborn infants. The suppository is also contraindicated in persons sensitive to benzocaine, which is an adjunctive ingredient.

Adverse Reactions

Occasional side effects include dizziness, diarrhea, blood dyscrasias, blurred vision, coma, convulsions, depression, disorientation, and skin reactions. Rare but possible reactions include drowsiness, hypotension, and parkinsonian symptoms. Irritation may occur after rectal administration. Pain may occur at the injection site.

Composition and Supply

Capsules   100 mg and 250 mg
Injection   100 mg/ml, in 2 ml ampuls and syringes
Suppositories   100 mg and 200 mg

Legal Status

Prescription

Trimethoprim/sulfamethoxazole (Bactrim™, Septra®)

Action and Use
Urinary antibacterial with the synergistic action of trimethoprim and sulfamethoxazole.

Dosage and Administration
2 tablets (plain) or 1 tablet (double strength) every 12 hours for 10 to 14 days.

Cautions
Contraindicated in patients with hypersensitivity to trimethoprim or sulfonamides, in pregnant women, and in nursing mothers. Deaths from hypersensitivity reactions have been associated with sulfonamides. Use with caution in patients with impaired renal or hepatic function, possible folate deficiency, severe allergy, bronchial asthma, or glucose-6-phosphate dehydrogenase deficiency. Not recommended for children under 12.

Adverse Reactions
Possible side effects include blood dyscrasias and allergic gastrointestinal or CNS reactions (see **Sulfisoxazole**).

Composition and Supply
Suspension   trimethoprim 40 mg/5 ml and sulfamethoxazole 200 mg/5 ml
Tablets   trimethoprim 80 mg and sulfamethoxazole 400 mg
Tablets, double strength   trimethoprim 160 mg and sulfamethoxazole 800 mg (Bactrim® DS, Septra® DS)

Legal Status
Prescription

Triniad Plus 30™

See under **Isoniazid.**

Trinsicon® (intrinsic factor/cyanocobalamin/ferrous fumarate/ascorbic acid)

See HEMATINICS.

Triogen®

See **Diphtheria toxoid/tetanus toxoid/pertussis vaccine, adsorbed**.

Tripelennamine hydrochloride (Pyribenzamine®)

Action and Use
Antihistamine.

Dosage and Administration
25 to 50 mg every 4 to 6 hours, orally, topically.

Cautions
Drowsiness is likely. See **Brompheniramine maleate.**

Adverse Reactions
See **Brompheniramine maleate.**

Composition and Supply
Elixir (as the citrate)   37.5 mg/5 ml
Ointment and cream   2%
Tablets   25 mg and 50 mg
Tablets, long-acting   50 mg and 100 mg (Pyribenzamine®
   Lontabs®)

Legal Status
Prescription

Triprolidine hydrochloride (Actidil®)

Action and Use
Antihistamine.

Dosage and Administration
2.5 mg 2 or 3 times a day, orally.

Cautions
Drowsiness, dizziness, and gastrointestinal disturbances may occur.
See **Brompheniramine maleate.**

Adverse Reactions
See **Brompheniramine maleate.**

Composition and Supply
Syrup   1.25 mg/5 ml
Tablets   2.5 mg

Legal Status
Prescription

Tri-Solgen®

See **Diphtheria toxoid/tetanus toxoid/pertussis vaccine, adsorbed.**

Trisulfapyrimidines (Terfonyl®)

See SULFONAMIDES.

Triten® (dimethindine maleate)

See ANTIHISTAMINES.

Triva® Combination (oxyquinoline sulfate)

See ANTIPROTOZOALS, antitrichomonials.

Trobicin®

See **Spectinomycin hydrochloride.**

Trocinate® (thiphenamil hydrochloride)

See ANTIDIARRHEALS; ANTISPASMODICS.

Troleandomycin (TAO®)

See ANTIBIOTICS, miscellaneous.

Tromethamine (Tham)

See ELECTROLYTE SOLUTIONS AND WATER-BALANCE AGENTS, alkalizing agents.

Tromexan® (ethyl biscoumacetate)

See ANTICOAGULANTS.

Tronothane®

See **Pramoxine hydrochloride.**

Tropicamide (Mydriacyl®)

Action and Use
Mydriatic.

Dosage and Administration
In mydriasis: 1 or 2 drops of 0.5% solution; may be repeated every 30 minutes.
In cycloplegia: 1 or 2 drops of 1% solution, given in 2 instillations, 5 to 25 minutes apart.

Cautions
Contraindicated in patients with glaucoma.

Adverse Reactions
There may occasionally be swelling of the eyelids and conjunctivitis. See **Atropine sulfate** for further adverse reactions.

Composition and Supply
Solution, ophthalmic   0.5% and 1%

Legal Status
Prescription

Trypsin-chymotrypsin (Chymoral®)

See ANTI-INFLAMMATORY ENZYMES.

Tuberculin, old

Tuberculin, purified protein derivative (PPD) (Aplisol®, Tubersol®)

Action and Use
Sterile liquid containing the growth products of *Mycobacterium tuberculosis* used in the diagnosis of tuberculosis. Injection under or into the skin has no effect in nontuberculous persons but causes inflammation at injection site in persons allergic to tuberculin and/or having an inactive or active infection.

Dosage and Administration
Old tuberculin: Multiple-puncture technique (e.g., tine test); 4 mm or more of induration constitutes a positive test.
PPD: 5 Tuberculin Units (0.1 ml) administered intradermally; 10 mm or more of induration constitutes a positive test.

Cautions
Reactivity to the test may be depressed or suppressed for as long as 4 to 6 weeks in individuals who have recently been immunized with certain viral vaccines (e.g., measles or influenza), who have had viral infections (rubeola, influenza, mumps, and probably others), or who are receiving corticosteroids or immunosuppressive agents.

Adverse Reactions
Ulceration or necrosis may occur at the injection site in very sensitive persons.

Composition and Supply
Old tuberculin
Multiple-puncture devices
PPD
10 test and 50 test vials   5 Tuberculin Units/test
10 test vials   1 Tuberculin Unit/test and 250 Tuberculin Units/test

Legal Status
Prescription

Tuberculosis vaccine

See **BCG vaccine.**

Tubersol®

See **Tuberculin,** purified protein derivative (PPD).

Tubocurarine chloride

Action and Use
Skeletal muscle relaxant.

Dosage and Administration
100 to 300 μg/kg as an adjunct to general anesthesia.

Cautions
Tubocurarine chloride is a potent and toxic drug that may cause possible asphyxia. It is potentiated by ether, cyclopropane, methoxyflurane, and other anesthetics, necessitating a reduction in dosage. Contraindicated in patients with hepatic or renal impairment or respiratory disorders.

Adverse Reactions
Prolonged apnea, bronchospasm, and hypotension may occur. The antidote is neostigmine or edrophonium chloride.

Composition and Supply
Injection   3 mg/ml and 15 mg/ml

Legal Status
Prescription

Tuinal® (secobarbital sodium/amobarbital sodium)

See SEDATIVE-HYPNOTICS, barbiturates.

Tussend® Expectorant

See COUGH-COLD PREPARATIONS, cough preparations.

Tuss-Ornade® Spansule® Capsules

See COUGH-COLD PREPARATIONS, common cold preparations.

Tylenol®

See **Acetaminophen.**

Tylosterone®

See **Diethylstilbestrol/methyltestosterone.**

Tylox™ (oxycodone/acetaminophen)

See ANALGESICS, narcotic.

Tyloxapol (Alevaire®)

See MUCOLYTICS.

Tympagesic® (antipyrine/benzocaine/phenylephrine)

See ANESTHETICS, local.

Typhoid vaccine

Action and Use
Used to achieve active immunization against typhoid fever and to produce artificial fever.

Dosage and Administration
Primary immunization: 1.5 ml in 3 doses of 0.5 ml (500 µl) each, 1 to 4 weeks apart, SC.
Booster dosage: 0.5 ml (500 µl) every 1 or 2 years.

Cautions
Contraindicated in patients with acute illness. The use of typhoid vaccine for fever therapy is contraindicated in elderly, cachectic, arteriosclerotic, or anemic patients and in those with cardiac disease.

Adverse Reactions
Side effects include inflammation, fever, malaise, headache, and edema and pain at the injection site.

Composition and Supply
Vaccine   1.5 ml, 5 ml, and 20 ml vial

Legal Status
Prescription

Typhus vaccine

Action and Use
Used for active immunization against epidemic typhus.

Dosage and Administration
Primary immunization: 2 injections, 1 ml each, at 7 to 10 day intervals.
Booster doses: 1 ml every 6 months.

Cautions
Should not be given during acute illness. Contraindicated in those with known sensitivity to eggs.

Adverse Reactions
Local and systemic reactions may occur, including anaphylaxis (in those sensitive to eggs) and postvaccinal neurological disorders.

Composition and Supply
Injection   1 ml ampuls, 20 ml vials

Legal Status
Prescription

Tyropanoate sodium (Bilopaque®)

See DIAGNOSTICS, roentgenography.

Tyzine®

See **Tetrahydrozoline hydrochloride.**

Ultra Tears®

See **Hydroxypropyl methylcellulose.**

Undecylenic acid/zinc undecylenate (Desenex®)

Action and Use
Antifungal agent used to treat athlete's foot and ringworm of the body (exclusive of nails and hairy areas).

Dosage and Administration
Applied topically, twice a day.

Cautions
Not to be used near the eyes.

Adverse Reactions
None when used as directed.

Composition and Supply
Ointment   zinc undecylenate 20% and undecylenic acid 5%
Powder   zinc undecylenate 20% and undecylenic acid 5%

Legal Status
Nonprescription

525

Uniad Plus 5™

See under **Isoniazid.**

Unipen®

See **Nafcillin sodium.**

Unitensin® (cryptenamine tannate)

See ANTIHYPERTENSIVES, nondiuretic.

Unna's boot (zinc gelatin)

See under **Zinc oxide.**

Uracid®

See **Methionine.**

Uranap®

See **Methionine.**

Urea, sterile (Ureaphil®)

Action and Use
Osmotic diuretic used to reduce intracranial pressure (in the control of cerebral edema) and intraocular pressure (in the control of acute glaucoma).

Dosage and Administration
1.0 to 1.5 g (3.3 to 5 ml)—as 30% solution—per kg of body weight by slow IV infusion; the rate should not exceed 4 ml (60 drops) per minute.

Cautions
Contraindicated in patients with kidney disease, severe dehydration, or active intracranial bleeding. Urea may cause electrolyte depletion. Unused drug should be discarded.

Adverse Reactions
Common side effects include vomiting, headache, hypotension, confusion, and tachycardia. Avoid infusion into the leg veins of elderly patients to prevent the possibility of thrombophlebitis and blood clot formation. Extravasation may cause local irritation, leading occasionally to tissue necrosis.

Composition and Supply
Injection   40 g per Abbott Non-Vac® single-dose container (*Note:* the desired diluent is added directly to the contents of the container)

Legal Status
Prescription

Urea preparations (Aquacare®, Carmol®)

See EMOLLIENT-PROTECTANTS; KERATOLYTICS.

Ureaphil®

See **Urea, sterile.**

Urecholine®

See **Bethanechol chloride.**

Urex®

See **Methenamine hippurate.**

Urispas®

See **Flavoxate hydrochloride.**

Urobiotic® (oxytetracycline hydrochloride/sulfamethizole/phenazopyridine hydrochloride)

See URINARY ANTISEPTICS.

Urokinase (Abbokinase®)

See Anticoagulants.

Urolene Blue®

See **Methylene blue.**

Utibid®

See **Oxolinic acid.**

Vagisec® (polyoxyethylene nonyl phenol/sodium edetate/sodium dioctyl sulfosuccinate)

See ANTIPROTOZOALS, antitrichomonials.

Valadol®

See **Acetaminophen.**

Valisone®

See **Betamethazone.**

Valium®

See **Diazepam.**

Valmid® (ethinamate)

See SEDATIVE-HYPNOTICS, nonbarbiturates.

Valproic acid (Depakene®)

See ANTICONVULSANTS.

Vanceril®

See **Beclomethasone dipropionate.**

Vancocin®

See **Vancomycin hydrochloride.**

Vancomycin hydrochloride (Vancocin®)

Action and Use
Antibiotic especially effective against staphylococci; should be used only when other antibiotics are ineffective or the patient is allergic to them.

Dosage and Administration
In staphylococcal enterocolitis: 500 mg every 6 hours, orally.
In other infections: 500 mg every 6 hours, IV.

Cautions
Vancomycin hydrochloride is ototoxic and nephrotoxic.

Adverse Reactions
Reported side effects include nausea, chills, fever, urticaria, macular rashes, eosinophilia, and anaphylactoid reactions.

Composition and Supply
Injection   500 mg (dry powder), in 10 ml ampuls
Solution, oral   10 g in screw-top container

Legal Status
Prescription

Vanobid®

See **Candicidin.**

Vanoxide® (benzoyl peroxide preparation)

See KERATOLYTICS.

Varidase®

See **Streptokinase/streptodornase.**

Vaseline®

See under **Petrolatum.**

Vasodilan®

See **Isoxsuprine hydrochloride.**

Vasopressin (Pitressin®)

Action and Use
Antidiuretic hormone used for replacement therapy in diabetes insipidus.

Dosage and Administration
Vasopressin: 1 ml SC or IM.
Vasopressin tannate: 0.3 ml (300 µl) to 1 ml, as needed, IM.

Cautions
Contraindicated in patients with epilepsy, angina pectoris, coronary thrombosis, toxemia of pregnancy, cardiovascular disease with hypertension, goiter with cardiac complications, or arteriosclerosis. Prolonged rotation of suspension (tannate in oil) is essential for full therapeutic effect.

Adverse Reactions
Possible side effects include sweating, vertigo, tremors, circumoral pallor, headache, passage of flatus, nausea, vomiting, intestinal and uterine cramps, water retention, and occasionally water intoxication. Spasm of coronary arteries may occur; vasopressin should be used cautiously in patients with inadequate coronary circulation. Other reported responses include urticaria, anaphylactic shock, bronchial constriction, and cardiac arrest.

Composition and Supply
Injection (vasopressin)   0.5 ml (500 µl) ampuls (10 units) and 1 ml ampuls (20 units)
Injection (vasopressin tannate)   5 units/ml, in 1 ml ampuls

Legal Status
Prescription

Vasospan®

See **Papaverine hydrochloride.**

Vasoxyl® (methoxamine hydrochloride)

See ADRENERGICS.

V-Cillin® (penicillin V)

See ANTIBIOTICS, penicillins.

V-Cillin® K

See **Penicillin V potassium.**

Vectrin®

See **Minocycline hydrochloride.**

Veetids®

See **Penicillin V potassium.**

Velban®

See **Vinblastine sulfate.**

Velosef® (cephradine)

See ANTIBIOTICS, cephalosporins.

Veracillin®

See **Dicloxacillin sodium.**

Vercyte® (pipobroman)

See ANTINEOPLASTICS, alkylating agents.

Vermox®

See **Mebendazole.**

Verstran® (prazepam)

See PSYCHOTROPICS, tranquilizers, minor.

Vesprin® (triflupromazine)

See ANTIEMETICS; PSYCHOTROPICS, antipsychotics.

Vibramycin®

See **Doxycycline.**

Vidarabine (Vira-A®)

Action and Use
Antiviral purine nucleoside effective in acute keratoconjunctivitis and recurrent epithelial keratitis due to herpes simplex virus types 1 and 2. Also effective in superficial keratitis that has not responded to iodoxuridine or when iodoxuridine hypersensitivity or toxic reactions occur.

Dosage and Administration
One-half inch of ointment is applied to the lower conjunctival sac 5 times daily at 3-hour intervals.

Cautions
Should be used only in herpes simplex keratoconjunctivitis. The patient should be warned of a possible visual haze.

Adverse Reactions
Possible side effects include irritation, burning, lacrimation, pain, photophobia, and sensitivity. Secondary glaucoma, uveitis, corneal vascularization, and stromal edema are reported problems that appear to be disease-related.

Composition and Supply
Ointment   3%

Legal Status
Prescription

Vi-Daylin® ADC Drops

See VITAMINS, MULTIPLE, oral.

Vi-Dom-A®

See **Vitamin A.**

Vigran® Capsules

See VITAMINS, MULTIPLE, oral.

Vinblastine sulfate (Velban®)

Action and Use
Antineoplastic; its use is limited to Hodgkin's disease and choriocarcinoma resistant to other therapy.

Dosage and Administration
100 μg (initial dose) to 500 μg (maximum dose) given no more frequently than every 7 days, IV.

Cautions
Contraindicated in leukopenic patients and in those who have an infection.

Adverse Reactions
Nausea, vomiting, leukopenia, and alopecia may occur.

Composition and Supply
Injection   10 mg vials

Legal Status
Prescription

Vincristine sulfate (Oncovin®)

Action and Use
Antineoplastic used to treat acute leukemia, Hodgkin's disease, lymphosarcoma, neuroblastoma, and Wilms' tumor.

Dosage and Administration
1.4 mg/m² per week, IV.

Cautions
Neurotoxicity, which may be permanent, includes areflexia, peripheral neuritis, weakness, ataxia, paresthesias, footdrop, ptosis, double vision, polyuria, and dysuria. Some marrow depression may occur (observe the patient for signs of infection and bleeding).

Adverse Reactions
Prominent side effects include leukopenia, alopecia, nausea, vomiting, oral ulcers, diarrhea, constipation, and abdominal cramps. Extravasation may cause irritation.

Composition and Supply
Injection   1 mg and 5 mg vials

Legal Status
Prescription

Vinethene® (vinyl ether)

See ANESTHETICS, general.

Vinyl ether (Vinethene®)

See ANESTHETICS, general.

Viocin®

See **Viomycin sulfate.**

Vioform®

See **Iodochlorhydroxyquin.**

Viokase® (pancreatin)

See DIGESTANTS.

Viomycin sulfate (Viocin®)

Action and Use
Antituberculotic indicated only when the primary drugs (isoniazid, streptomycin, and aminosalicylic acid) have failed.

Dosage and Administration
2 g in divided doses every 12 hours, IM.

Cautions
Use with extreme caution; use lower dosages in patients with impaired renal function. Viomycin sulfate is potentially ototoxic and should not be used in combination with other ototoxic drugs. It is not recommended for children except in life-threatening situations.

Adverse Reactions
Possible side effects include impaired renal function, tinnitus and vertigo, and hypersensitivity reactions (namely, rash, drug fever, and laryngeal edema).

Composition and Supply
Injection   1 g and 5 g vials

Legal Status
Prescription

Vi-Penta® F Multivitamin Drops

See VITAMINS, MULTIPLE, oral.

Vira-A®

See **Vidarabine.**

Visine®

See **Tetrahydrozoline hydrochloride.**

Vistaril®

See **Hydroxyzine.**

Vitamin A (Aquasol A®, Vi-Dom-A®)

Action and Use
Used for replacement in vitamin A deficiencies (evidenced by nyctalopia, keratinization of epithelial cells, retarded growth, xerophthalmia, keratomalacia, weakness, and/or increased susceptibility of mucous membranes to infection).

Dosage and Administration
25,000 units per day, orally.

Cautions
Overdosage may produce hypervitaminosis A.

Adverse Reactions
Early symptoms of overdosage include irritability, anorexia, pruritus, myalgia, loss of body hair, nystagmus, gingivitis, hepatosplenomegaly, lymph node enlargement, and jaundice. With prolonged or extreme overdosage there are bone lesions due to accelerated resorption and new bone formation; the bones continue to grow in length but not in thickness, which causes increased susceptibility to fracture. Other possible reactions include cutaneous lesions, temporary thickening of the skin, exophthalmos, and hypoprothrombinemia.

Composition and Supply
Capsules   5,000 units, 25,000 units, 50,000 units, and 100,000 units
Injection   50,000 units/ml and 100,000 units/ml
Solution   50,000 units/ml

Legal Status
Nonprescription (except for injection)

Vitamin B₁

See **Thiamine hydrochloride.**

Vitamin B₂

See **Riboflavin.**

Vitamin B₆

See **Pyridoxine hydrochloride.**

Vitamin B₁₂

See **Cyanocobalamin injection.**

Vitamin C

See **Ascorbic acid.**

Vitamin D

See **Ergocalciferol.**

Vitamin D₂

See **Ergocalciferol.**

Vitamin E (Aquasol® E, Tokols®)

See VITAMINS, fat-soluble.

Vitamin G

See **Riboflavin.**

Vitamin K

See **Menadiol sodium diphosphate.**

Vitamin K₁

See **Phytonadione.**

Vivactil®

See **Protriptyline hydrochloride.**

Vivonex®

See FOOD FORMULATIONS.

Vleminckx's solution (sulfurated lime solution)

See KERATOLYTICS.

VōSol® Otic Solution (acetic acid)

See ANTI-INFECTIVES, LOCAL, miscellaneous, antiseptic-disinfectants.

Vontrol® (diphenidol)

See ANTIEMETICS.

Voranil® (clortermine hydrochloride)

See CEREBRAL STIMULANTS, anorectics.

Warfarin sodium

See **Sodium warfarin.**

Whitfield's ointment

See **Benzoic acid/salicylic acid.**

Winstrol® (stanozolol)

See ANDROGENS.

Wintergreen oil

See **Methyl salicylate.**

Witch hazel

See ASTRINGENTS.

Wycillin®

See **Penicillin G procaine.**

Wydase®

See **Hyaluronidase.**

Wygesic®

See under **Propoxyphene hydrochloride.**

Xylocaine®

See **Lidocaine hydrochloride.**

Xylometazoline hydrochloride (Otrivin®)

Action and Use
Adrenergic nasal decongestant.

Dosage and Administration
2 or 3 drops or 2 sprays 3 or 4 times a day.

Cautions

Contraindicated in patients with narrow-angle glaucoma and in those who are receiving MAO inhibitors or tricyclic antidepressants. Use with caution in patients with hypertension, heart disease, angina pectoris, hyperthyroidism, or advanced arteriosclerosis.

Adverse Reactions

Stinging, burning, dryness of nasal mucosa, and sneezing may occur. Prolonged or excessive use may produce rebound congestion. Possible systemic effects, especially in infants, include arrhythmias, hypertension, headache, lightheadedness, nervousness, insomnia, blurred vision, and drowsiness.

Composition and Supply

Solution   0.05% and 0.1%

Legal Status

Nonprescription

Yellow fever vaccine

See BIOLOGICALS, vaccines.

Yomesan® (niclosamide)

See ANTHELMINTICS, tapeworm.

Zactane®

See **Ethoheptazine.**

Zanchol®

See **Florantyrone.**

Zarontin®

See **Ethosuximide.**

Zaroxolyn® (metolazone)

See DIURETICS.

Zephiran®

See **Benzalkonium chloride.**

Zinc gelatin (Unna's boot)

See under **Zinc oxide.**

Zinc oxide

Action and Use
Astringent and protectant.

Dosage and Administration
Applied topically.

Cautions
For external use only.

Adverse Reactions
There are none of consequence.

Composition and Supply
Ointment   20%
Paste   25%
Paste   25% with salicylic acid (Lassar's paste)
Zinc gelatin   10% with gelatin 15% and glycerin 40% (Unna's boot)

Legal Status
Nonprescription

Zinc sulfate

Action and Use
Astringent and local anti-infective.

Dosage and Administration
1 or 2 drops of ophthalmic solution applied in the eye 2 or 3 times a day.

Cautions
Concentrations greater than 0.2% may irritate the eyes.

Adverse Reactions
Irritation may occur even at usual therapeutic concentrations.

Composition and Supply
Drops and eyewash   0.2%
Ointment, opthalmic   10%

Legal Status
Nonprescription

Zyloprim®

See **Allopurinol.**

Section 3
Appendixes

1. Notes on Drug Administration

Oral Route

1. The oral route is generally the safest, easiest, and most economical way of giving a drug; however, certain drugs cannot be given orally because of poor absorption or digestive destruction.
2. Tablets and capsules are swallowed easily by most persons if placed on the back of the tongue and washed down with fluid.
3. Most drugs are absorbed in 30 to 90 minutes; drugs in solution are absorbed more readily than in solid form, and a relatively empty gastrointestinal tract enhances absorption. Controlled-release preparations may be used for prolonged action.
4. Drugs irritating to gastric mucosa are best given with food or antacids; drugs destroyed by gastric juice may be given as enteric-coated capsules or tablets.
5. Certain compounds may be given as chewable tablets or similar formulations.

Sublingual and Buccal Routes

1. The sublingual and buccal routes are indicated for certain drugs that may be destroyed by digestive juices, altered by the liver, or urgently needed for self-administration.
2. The tablets must dissolve readily and should be held in place until absorption is effected.
3. The tablets must not be swallowed, and fluid should not be taken until the drug has been absorbed.

Rectal Route

1. The rectal route is indicated for local and, on occasion, systemic effect; systemic absorption is generally erratic.
2. Suppositories are superior to retention enemas; the latter are usually given at a volume of 25 to 75 ml.

Intradermal (Intracutaneous) Route

1. The intradermal route is commonly used for diagnosis, anesthesia, and determination of sensitivity to antigens and antiserums.
2. The area to be treated is cleansed with alcohol, and a fine needle (25 or 26 gauge) is inserted as superficially as possible. No more than 0.1 ml of fluid should be injected, to minimize discomfort.

Subcutaneous Route

1. Subcutaneous (hypodermic) injections are generally limited to small quantities (0.2 to 2 ml) of soluble and nonirritating medication. Preferred sites are the lateral aspects of the upper arms and

the anterior portions of the midthighs. Peak action usually occurs in about 30 minutes.

2. The injection site is cleansed with alcohol, and the needle (22 gauge or smaller) is inserted at an angle of 45 to 60 degrees through all layers of skin. Gentle aspiration should be attempted to avoid injection into a vein.

Intramuscular Route

1. The intramuscular route is commonly used when prompt action is desirable or when the drug is irritating to subcutaneous tissues. Preparations given IM include solutions or suspensions in water or oil; suspensions result in prolonged action.

2. The skin is cleansed with alcohol or other suitable antiseptic, and the needle (length 1 to 3 inches, 19 to 22 gauge) is inserted at a right angle into the muscle. Preferred sites are the deltoid of the upper arm and the upper outer angle of the upper lateral quadrant of the buttocks and the lateral side of the thigh (using the vastus lateralis). Gentle aspiration should be attempted to avoid injection into a vein.

3. Iron preparations, such as iron dextran (Imferon®), may discolor the skin and should never be injected into the arm or other exposed areas. To avoid injection or leakage into the subcutaneous tissue, a Z-track technique (displacement of the skin laterally prior to injection) should be used.

Intravenous Route

Injection
1. An intravenous injection (bolus) is used when rapid action is desired or when there is some reason why the drug cannot be given by other parenteral routes. The preparations (solutions) must be completely clear.

2. The injection site should be cleansed with an antiseptic and the limb placed in a comfortable position. The most commonly used veins are the basilic and median cephalic at the bend of the elbow.

3. The tourniquet is drawn tightly around the middle of the arm to distend the vein, and all air is expelled from the syringe. The needle is inserted quickly through the skin (bevel upward)—parallel and lateral to the vein—and then introduced into the vein at an oblique angle. Once blood enters the syringe the tourniquet is removed and the injection is made very slowly.

Infusion
1. Intravenous infusions are employed to bolster blood volume, restore fluids and electrolytes, and supply nutrition. Preferred sites include the veins of the forearm, external jugular vein, femoral

vein, and scalp veins in infants; the superior vena cava is used in hyperalimentation.

2. The amount of fluid ranges from 500 ml to 3 liters, and the rate of flow usually averages about 3 ml per minute. Extravasation, due to faulty venipuncture or displacement of the needle or cannula, is a common complication.

3. Infusion reactions are caused by elements contained in the fluid, specific incompatibility of recipient, and method of administration. The following steps will minimize or prevent reactions: avoid too rapid administration, replace air in the tubing with solution before injecting, avoid constant use of the same vein, reduce fluid volume, and ensure that the needle remains constantly in the vein.

Nose Drops

Nose drops are usually employed to effect vasoconstriction. Preparations that contain oil may cause lipid pneumonia. The drops should be instilled by having the patient lie down with the head tilted far back and turned slightly to the affected side.

Ophthalmic Preparations

Eye drops and ointments are used for mydriasis, miosis, anesthesia, and chemotherapy. Discolored or cloudy solutions should not be used, and due care must be exercised to keep the dropper or ointment tube from contact with the eye. As the patient looks upward, the medication is introduced into the lower conjunctival sac; the drops should not fall more than 1 inch, and the ointment should be spread in small amounts from the inner to the outer canthus. Apply finger compression to nasolacrimal ducts for 1 to 2 minutes to minimize drainage and subsequent absorption via nasal mucosa.

Ear Drops

Ear drops are employed for chemotherapy and analgesia. Instillations are made with the pinna gently pulled downward in adults and backward in infants. They are best given warmed to body temperature, and drops should fall on the side of the canal. The presense of eardrum damage calls for great care to prevent infection.

2. Federal Controlled Substances Act of 1970*

With the enactment of the Controlled Substances Act of 1970, the Drug Enforcement Administration (formerly the Bureau of Narcotics and Dangerous Drugs) came into being. This agency, a division of the Justice Department, is responsible for execution of the provisions of said act. The law is a lengthy document that deals with registration requirements, procurement, storage and security, distribution, administration, records and record keeping, and penalties for noncompliance. In its present state, the law encompasses all narcotic and nonnarcotic drugs that have a potential for abuse and places these drugs in five categories or *schedules* according to the extent of this potential. Some states have enacted their own laws and created additional schedules; when such regulations are more stringent than the federal, the local regulations *take precedence.* Massachusetts, for example, enacted a Controlled Substance Act based on the federal law but created a sixth schedule to encompass all other prescription drugs.

The federal schedules are as follows:

Schedule I
Drugs of highest abuse potential with no legal medical use (outlawed). Examples are heroin, lysergic acid diethylamide (LSD), marijuana, and Δ-9 tetrahydrocannabinol (THC).

Schedule II
Drugs of high abuse potential that may lead to severe psychological or physical dependence but with less abuse potential than those of Schedule I. Examples of drugs in Schedule II are opiates, amphetamines, short-acting barbiturates, cocaine, meperidine hydrochloride, methylphenidate hydrochloride, and oxycodone.

Schedule III
Drugs with an abuse potential less than that of drugs in Schedules I and II. Schedule III drugs may lead to moderate or low physical dependence or to high psychological dependence. Examples are codeine combinations (except cough preparations), butabarbital sodium, methyprylon, nalorphine hydrochloride, paregoric, certain amphetamine combinations, and Hycodan®.

Schedule IV
Drugs with a lower potential for abuse than those in Schedule III. Abuse may lead to limited physical or psychological dependence. Examples are phenobarbital, chloral hydrate, diethylpropion hydro-

*Comprehensive Drug Abuse Prevention and Control Act of 1970.

chloride, paraldehyde, flurazepam hydrochloride, chlordiazepoxide, diazepam, and meprobamate.

Schedule V
Drugs with an abuse potential less than that of those drugs in Schedule IV, including preparations containing limited quantities of narcotic drugs in combination with one or more nonnarcotic ingredients, the latter in sufficient amounts to confer valuable medicinal properties over and above the narcotic alone. Examples are cough syrups containing codeine and certain antidiarrheal agents, such as Lomotil® and Parepectolen®. Some Schedule V preparations are OTC (e.g., Parepectolen® and Lomotil®), but no more than 240 ml or 48 solid dosage units of any substance containing opium, and no more than 120 ml or 24 solid dosage units of any controlled substance, may be dispensed at retail to the same purchaser in any given 48 hour period without a prescription. Purchasers must be 18 years of age or older and must identify themselves.

Prescriptions for controlled drugs (Schedules II to V) must contain the full name and address of the patient, the Drug Enforcement Agency number of the prescribing doctor, the signature of prescribing doctor, and the date. Prescriptions for Schedule II drugs are not refillable; Schedules III and IV drugs may be refilled up to five times within six months of initial issuance; Schedule V drugs may be refilled as authorized by the prescribing physician. In the hospital setting it is of critical importance that accurate records be maintained (especially for Schedules II and III) and that all information relative to a controlled drug be noted in the proper place.

3. Poisoning

GENERAL PRINCIPLES

Acute poisoning and overdosage are emergency situations in which sound first aid and medical treatment are often one and the same. At the very least, their purposes are complementary, and it behooves the nurse to have a working knowledge of the general principles. Knowing exactly what to do can save the patient's life. In overview, the management of acute poisoning and overdosage involves (1) removal of the poison, (2) "antidoting," (3) promotion of elimination, and (4) supportive measures. However, not all these steps may be called for, and the order in no way suggests priority. In the symptomatic patient, support of vital functions is the first concern, while in the asymptomatic patient, removal of the poison may very well be all the treatment that is needed.

Swallowed Poisons

In the asymptomatic situation the amount of poison (or drug) ingested is less than noticeably toxic or else sufficient time has not elapsed for full absorption. Symptoms may be delayed as long as 6 hours after ingestion of toxic amounts of a substance; the average time is between ½ and 2 hours. Alcohol speeds depressant intoxication (from narcotics, hypnotics, sedatives, and tranquilizers), and simultaneous ingestion of alcohol and depressants often affects the vital signs in a matter of about 15 minutes.

Clues to the drug or poison involved may come from the history or from nearby objects—for example, capsules on the floor or odor of paint remover on the breath. Information on household and industrial chemicals can be obtained at poison control centers throughout the country. Also, ingredients and first aid measures are often printed on the container.

Evacuation of the Stomach
As first aid, induce vomiting immediately *except* when: (1) the patient is in coma or unconscious, (2) the patient is in convulsion, (3) the patient has swallowed kerosene, gasoline, lighter fluid, or other petroleum products, or (4) the patient has swallowed a corrosive substance.

The most effective technique is first to give water (2 cups to children under 5 years and up to 1 quart for other patients) and then to induce vomiting by giving an emetic. The emetic of choice is ipecac syrup (15 to 20 ml for children and 30 to 45 ml for adults) given in warm water and repeated in 15 minutes if necessary. If ipecac is not available, induce vomiting by inserting finger into patient's throat. When retching and vomiting begin, place the patient face down with the head lower than the hips to prevent aspiration, which often results in pneumonia.

Gastric lavage may be used *except* in corrosive poisoning (in which case, esophageal or gastric perforation might occur) and in strychnine poisoning (since convulsions may be induced by attempts to pass the stomach tube). With the patient in a head-low position, tap water or normal saline is gradually introduced into the stomach with a large caliber tube and then siphoned off. The total fluid volume to be used should be about 3 liters beyond the volume needed to obtain a clear return.

Antidotes

General purpose antidotes include activated charcoal, milk (or egg white), and potassium permanganate (1 : 10,000). Activated charcoal (given after emesis or gastric lavage at a dose of 100 g suspended in 6 oz of water) adsorbs a vast number of drugs and poisons, most of which are not to any practical extent "desorbed" in the intestine. Thus, it may be "left in place," whereas other oral antidotes should be removed via emesis or lavage (except when contraindicated). Milk and egg white both form insoluble precipitates with heavy metal salts, neutralize acids and alkalies, and counteract corrosive poisons. Potassium permanganate oxidizes atropine, morphine, strychnine, and other alkaloids.

Specific antidotes should be used if possible. These include agents that deactivate drugs or poisons chemically or else counteract their effects physiologically. For example, sodium chloride forms insoluble silver chloride in silver nitrate poisoning, and atropine (an anticholinergic) stems the effects of pilocarpine (a cholinergic). Major antidotes used in the hospital include levallorphan, dimercaprol (BAL), penicillamine, calcium disodium edetate, deferoxamine mesylate, pralidoxime chloride, pentobarbital, amyl nitrite, sodium nitrite, and sodium thiosulfate.

Elimination

The elimination of some drugs and poisons can be enhanced either by normal excretory pathways or by dialysis. Hydration is important, and sufficient fluids should be given to promote the output of urine (but not, of course, at the expense of overloading the circulation). Also, alkalization of the urine helps in the excretion of certain agents, notably salicylates and long-acting barbiturates. Dialysis (peritoneal dialysis or hemodialysis) may be lifesaving in cases involving dialyzable poisons. Stool elimination (in the absence of diarrhea) may be promoted by the use of saline cathartics (e.g., magnesium sulfate).

Supportive Measures

The support of vital functions—always of first concern in the symptomatic patient—does not basically differ from the management of other acute medical problems. In the event of CNS depression and shock, intravenous fluids (e.g., lactated Ringer's injection), artificial respiration, and oxygen may be needed. CNS stimulation may call for a tranquilizer (e.g., diazepam) or intravenous barbiturate (e.g., pentobarbital sodium). Cerebral edema (commonly seen in depressant and carbon monoxide poisoning) is treated with hypertonic diuretics (namely, mannitol or urea), and renal failure (in nephrotoxic poisoning) yields to dialysis.

Inhaled Poisons

Carry the patient (do not let patient walk!) to fresh air immediately, loosen all tight clothing, keep the patient warm and lying down, and apply artificial respiration if breathing has stopped or is irregular. Do not give alcohol in any form.

Skin Contamination

Drench with water (from a shower, hose, or faucet) immediately, and apply stream of water to skin as contaminated garments are removed. Thoroughly wash the skin with soap and water. Organic solvents should be used judiciously, since they may increase absorption of the poison.

Eye Contamination

Hold the eyelids open and wash with a gentle stream of water immediately. Continue washing until the physician arrives. Do not use antidotes.

Chemical Burns

Wash with running water immediately (except in the case of phosphorus burns) and cover with a loosely applied clean cloth. Keep the patient warm and lying down until the physician arrives. Phosphorus burns should be immersed immediately in water (to avoid contact with air) and particles of phosphorus removed gently with water. Burn is then treated with 1 percent copper sulfate solution to neutralize any residual particles.

COMMON POISONS*

Acetone†

Signs and Symptoms
Inhalation produces bronchial irritation and pulmonary congestion; ingested acetone produces gastrointestinal symptoms; both inhalation and ingestion produce hypotension, slow pulse, respiratory depression, and fall in body temperature. Extreme intoxication results in ketosis and possibly death. Deliberate inhalation (glue-sniffing) produces euphoria and drunkenness.

Treatment
Emesis or gastric lavage; treat for metabolic acidosis; support respiration; give oxygen and fluids.

Acids (e.g., hydrochloric, nitric, and sulfuric acids)

Signs and Symptoms
Nausea and vomiting ("coffee ground" vomitus); burning pain in mouth, throat, and abdomen; erosion of mucous membranes (first turning white, then colored); dysphagia; diarrhea; shock; circulatory collapse; strictures. Death may result from asphyxia.

Treatment
Avoid gastric lavage, emesis, and sodium bicarbonate or other alkaline carbonates (the liberated carbon dioxide may cause gastric distention or rupture); give water or milk to dilute poison; keep the patient warm and quiet and give morphine sulfate (8 to 15 mg SC) for pain; use corticosteroids to reduce fibrosis and possible strictures. Perforation calls for antibiotics and emergency surgery.

Alcohol (ethyl alcohol [ethanol], whiskey, brandy, and other liquors)

Signs and Symptoms
Excitement followed by depression, delirium, inebriation, coma. Death may result from respiratory failure.

Treatment
Gastric lavage or emetics (avoid apomorphine hydrochloride); cathartics; artificial respiration; IV glucose. Change the patient's position frequently to prevent pneumonia. Dialysis should be used in potentially lethal cases.

*Acute poisoning unless indicated otherwise.
†Widely used as an organic solvent.

Alcohol, Denatured

Alcohol (see) rendered poisonous by addition of methyl alcohol (see).

Alcohol, Isopropyl

Signs and Symptoms
Dizziness; hypotension; flushed face; headache; depression; nausea and vomiting; acidosis; coma. Death may result from respiratory failure.

Treatment
The same as for alcohol, plus sodium bicarbonate to combat acidosis —4 mEq/kg every 4 hours as needed.

Alcohol, Methyl (methanol, wood alcohol)

Signs and Symptoms
Violent gastrointestinal upset; depression; headache; dilated pupils; inebriation; delirium; blindness; acidosis; coma. Death may result from respiratory or circulatory failure.

Treatment
Gastric lavage with 5% sodium bicarbonate. Combat acidosis with IV sodium bicarbonate (as used in poisoning with isopropyl alcohol), and give IV ethyl alcohol (which inhibits the formation of formic acid, its highly toxic metabolite)—750 μg/kg initially, then 500 μg/kg every 4 hours. Other measures are the same as those for ethyl alcohol.

Alkalis*

Signs and Symptoms
Nausea and vomiting; burning pain from mouth to stomach; dysphagia; mucous membranes soapy and white, then becoming brown, edematous, and ulcerated; pulse fast and weak; respiration rapid; collapse; eventual esophageal strictures.

Treatment
Avoid gastric lavage and emesis; give water or milk to dilute poison. Other measures are the same as those for corrosive acids.

Amphetamines (e.g., amphetamine sulfate, dextroamphetamine sulfate)

Signs and Symptoms
CNS stimulation; hyperflexia; dilated pupils; sweating; convulsions; hypertension; arrhythmias; sometimes coma.

*Ammonia water, potassium hydroxide (potash), sodium hydroxide (caustic soda, lye), sodium carbonate (washing soda), detergent powders.

Treatment
Gastric lavage; sedation with a barbiturate and/or tranquilizer; hypothermia; combat cerebral edema; dialysis.

Antihistamines (e.g., diphenhydramine hydrochloride)

Signs and Symptoms
CNS depression followed by excitement; dizziness; blurred vision; delirium; tremors and convulsions.

Treatment
Gastric lavage or emetics; artificial respiration and oxygen. Support blood pressure, control seizures, and use cold packs for hyperpyrexia.

Arsenic Compounds

Signs and Symptoms
Constriction of throat and intense gastric pain, followed by projectile vomiting of a "rice-water" fluid; diarrhea with bloody, rice-water stools; coma, convulsions, and collapse.

Treatment
Gastric lavage with 1% sodium thiosulfate or warm water; milk or other demulcents; dimercaprol 3 to 5 mg/kg IM every 4 hours on days 1 and 2, every 6 hours on day 3, then every 12 hours for 10 days or more; morphine sulfate 15 mg SC for pain; IV fluids for dehydration.

Barbiturates (e.g., phenobarbital)

Signs and Symptoms
Mental depression (often preceded by excitement and hallucinations); stupor; coma; respiratory depression; oliguria; hypotension; shock. Death may result from respiratory failure or pneumonia.

Treatment
Gastric lavage if the patient is seen within 4 hours after ingestion; respiratory and circulatory support; IV fluids to promote diuresis (in the case of phenobarbital, the urine should be alkalized); frequent turning and positive-pressure inhalation to prevent pneumonia; frequent tracheal suction; dialysis in potentially lethal situations. *Note:* analeptics are of no value and may be harmful.

Barium Compounds (soluble*)

Signs and Symptoms
Violent abdominal pain; nausea and vomiting; diarrhea; tremors; convulsions; hypertension; arrhythmias. Death may occur as a result of cardiac arrest.

Treatment
Prompt gastric lavage; magnesium sulfate or sodium sulfate to produce insoluble, nontoxic barium sulfate; morphine sulfate 15 mg SC for pain and sedatives to control convulsions; quinidine to prevent ventricular fibrillation.

Belladonna, Atropine, and Related Anticholinergics

Signs and Symptoms
Burning and dryness of the mouth; intense thirst; visual disturbances; widely dilated pupils (not responsive to light); weakness; giddiness; staggering gait; mental confusion; excitement; fever; delirium.

Treatment
Gastric lavage or emetics; activated charcoal; pentobarbital sodium (or other short-acting barbiturate) to control excitement or delirium; assisted respiration and oxygen; catheterization for urinary retention; sponging; darkened room.

Boric Acid

Signs and Symptoms
Erythema and exfoliation of the skin; nausea and vomiting; debilitation; dehydration; subnormal temperature; cyanosis; convulsions.

Treatment
Gastric lavage; barbiturates to control convulsions; IV fluids; dialysis in potentially lethal cases.

Bromides

Signs and Symptoms
Acute poisoning: profound CNS depression; collapse.
Bromism (chronic poisoning): acne-like dermatitis; foul breath; gastrointestinal disturbances; mental depression; speech disturbances; ataxia; malnutrition.

*Barium sulfate is nontoxic because of its extreme insolubility.

553

Treatment
Acute poisoning: stomach lavage and emesis; supportive measures.
Bromism: sodium chloride, 4 to 8 g per day, orally; forced fluids; diuretics; dialysis in severe cases.

Camphor and Camphorated Oil

Signs and Symptoms
Nausea and vomiting; headache; excitement; clammy skin; weak, rapid pulse; epileptiform convulsions; circulatory collapse.

Treatment.
Gastric lavage or emesis; saline cathartics; short-acting barbiturate (pentobarbital sodium 300 mg IV), chloral hydrate (2 g in olive oil rectally), or ether inhalation for convulsions; general supportive measures.

Carbon Monoxide

Signs and Symptoms
Headache; vertigo; vomiting; bounding pulse; dilated pupils; dusky skin; cherry red lips and nails; convulsions; muscle twitchings; respiratory depression; coma.

Treatment
Remove to fresh air; artificial respiration and 100% oxygen; avoid chilling; osmotic diuretics for cerebral edema; phlebotomy followed by blood transfusions in severe cases; complete rest for at least 24 hours.

Carbon Tetrachloride

Signs and Symptoms
Inhaled: irregular, shallow respiration; dilated pupils; cold, clammy skin; slow, weak pulse; deep narcosis; hypotension. Death may occur due to cardiac or respiratory failure.
Swallowed: headache; abdominal pain; hiccough; vomiting; diarrhea; inebriation; convulsions; narcosis; circulatory collapse; delayed jaundice; liver and kidney damage.

Treatment
Swallowed poison: gastric lavage or emesis; saline cathartics; fluids and osmotic diuretics; low-fat, high-carbohydrate, high-protein diet and large doses of methionine (3 to 5 g per day IV) to protect liver; avoid alcohol.
Inhaled poison: the same as for swallowed poisoning plus artificial respiration and oxygen.

Chloral Hydrate

Signs and Symptoms

Nausea and vomiting; deep sleep; stupor; coma; hypotension; slow, weak pulse; slow respiration; cyanosis. Death is usually due to respiratory depression.

Treatment

The same as for barbiturates.

Chlorinated Organic Insecticides*

Signs and Symptoms

Salivation; nausea and vomiting; abdominal pain; restlessness; hyper-irritability; incoordination; muscle spasms and tremors; convulsions, followed by depression, collapse, cyanosis, and dyspnea. Death may occur due to respiratory failure.

Treatment

Gastric lavage or emesis; saline cathartics; IV pentobarbital sodium plus calcium gluconate to combat stimulation and convulsions. *Note:* avoid use of epinephrine, milk, and oily cathartics and demulcents.

Cholinergics (e.g., neostigmine bromide, bethanechol chloride)

Signs and Symptoms

Vomiting; violent purging; abdominal pain; mydriasis followed by miosis; sweating; salivation; lacrimation; slow heart; respiration first accelerated, then slow and weak; hypotension; pulmonary edema; dyspnea; muscular twitchings. Death may occur from respiratory or cardiac failure.

Treatment

Emesis or gastric lavage with potassium permanganate 1 : 10,000 (this deactivates poisons through oxidation); atropine sulfate 600 μg to 1 mg SC or, in severe cases, IV, repeated every 30 minutes if necessary; supportive measures as indicated.

Cocaine and Related Local Anesthetics†

Signs and Symptoms

Stimulation, then depression; hallucinations; sweating; fever; numbness; vertigo; dyspnea; convulsions; cyanosis; coma and delirium; respiratory failure.

*Gamma benzene hexachloride (Gamene®, Kwell®) (see p. 260 for medicinal uses), as well as the insecticides aldrin, Bulan®, chlordane, DDT, dieldrin, Dilan®, endrin, heptachlor, methoxychlor, Prolan®, and toxaphene.
†Those anesthetics that act as CNS stimulants systemically.

Treatment
Tourniquet above site of injection; if the cocaine was taken orally, gastric lavage with potassium permanganate 1 : 10,000; artificial respiration and oxygen; tranquilizer or short-acting barbiturate (IV) for excitement or delirium.

Copper and Zinc Salts

Signs and Symptoms
Salivation; metallic taste; nausea and vomiting; severe abdominal pain; diarrhea with bloody stools; shallow, rapid respiration; headache; cold, clammy skin; delirium; convulsion; coma; collapse.

Treatment
Gastric lavage with 0.1% potassium ferrocyanide (to produce insoluble ferrocyanide salt) or milk, egg white, or milk of magnesia; demulcents; morphine sulfate 15 mg SC for pain; artificial respiration; calcium disodium edetate for severe cases (15 to 25 mg/kg IV every 12 hours for 5 days, then additional courses, if needed, with 2 day rest periods).

Coumarin Anticoagulants (e.g., sodium warfarin)

Signs and Symptoms
Gastrointestinal irritation; bleeding, hemorrhage.

Treatment
Mild bleeding: phytonadione (vitamin K_1) 5 to 10 mg orally.
Moderate bleeding: phytonadione 10 to 20 mg IM and, if necessary, a second dose 24 to 48 hours later.
Severe bleeding: antihemophilic (human) factor IX complex (Konȳne®), 1 bottle dissolved in 20 ml saline given IV over 15 to 30 minutes.
Massive bleeding: whole blood.

Cyanides*

Signs and Symptoms
Immediate gastrointestinal, mental, and respiratory symptoms; eyes protruding and dilated; blood-tinted foam on lips; coma and respiratory arrest.

Treatment
Immediate inhalation of amyl nitrite† for 15 to 30 seconds every 2 or 3 minutes, followed in order by (1) 3% sodium nitrite† IV at a dose

---

*Including bitter almond oil, wild cherry syrup, and seeds of apple, peach, plum, cherry, and chokecherry.
†Nitrites produce methemoglobin, which competes with the respiratory enzyme ferricytochrome oxidase for cyanide ion.

of 10 ml (given over a period of 2 to 5 minutes) and (2), through the same needle, 50 ml of 25% sodium thiosulfate (thiosulfate converts cyanide to nontoxic thiocyanate); repeat in 1 hour with half doses and again in another hour if needed.

Digitalis and Its Glycosides

Signs and Symptoms
Nausea and vomiting; abdominal pain; drowsiness; dizziness; visual disturbances; mental confusion; hallucination; delirium; tremors; possible convulsions; cardiac arrhythmias, ranging from sinus brady-cardia to ventricular tachycardia, the latter possibly terminating in ventricular fibrillation, cardiac standstill, and death.

Treatment
Prompt gastric lavage or emesis; potassium, atropine, procainamide, or quinidine to control cardiac rate and rhythm disorders; sedatives and IV fluids for restlessness and dehydration; calcium disodium edetate may reverse digitalis effects (it acts by chelating calcium, a potentiator of digitalis).

Fluorides*

Signs and Symptoms
Salivation; hematemesis; abdominal cramps; weakness; cardiac failure; shallow respiration; and eventual respiratory failure; possible epileptiform convulsions.

Treatment
Emesis or gastric lavage and leave aluminum hydroxide gel in stomach; 10 ml IV 10% calcium gluconate; IV glucose and saline; treat shock.

Formaldehyde (formalin)

Signs and Symptoms
Swallowed poison: irritation and pain in the mouth, throat, and stomach; nausea and vomiting; diarrhea; dyspnea; vertigo; fast, weak pulse; oliguria or anuria; convulsions; collapse; coma.
Inhaled poison: intense irritation of eyes and nose; headache; suffocation; edema of glottis; pneumonia.

Treatment
Swallowed poison: 250 ml 0.2% ammonia water (which converts formaldehyde to nontoxic methenamine) followed by gastric lavage; milk or egg white as demulcents; sodium bicarbonate or sodium lactate IV to combat acidosis (resulting from formation of formic acid).

*See p. 471 for medicinal uses of sodium fluoride.

Inhaled poison: oxygen and fresh air; inhalation of ammonia water or aromatic ammonia spirit; flush eyes with saline.

Glutethimide (Doriden®)

Signs and Symptoms
Similar to those for barbiturates (see); frequent fluctuations of consciousness may be misleading.

Treatment
Supportive and similar to that for barbiturate poisoning (see); poorly dialyzed.

Gold Compounds

Signs and Symptoms
Pruritus; dermatitis; stomatitis; gastrointestinal discomfort; albuminuria; hematuria; agranulocytosis; thrombocytopenia; aplastic anemia.

Treatment
Penicillamine, 500 mg twice a day; prednisone, 15 to 20 mg a day orally in divided doses.

Hydrocarbon Products*

Signs and Symptoms
Inhaled poisons: giddiness; mydriasis; dyspnea; cyanosis; coma; respiratory failure.
Swallowed poisons: burning in mouth and stomach; nausea and vomiting; cold skin; tremors; weak pulse; fall in temperature; dyspnea; convulsions; unconsciousness; aspiration pneumonia.

Treatment
Gastric lavage (if swallowed); artificial respiration and oxygen. *Do not* use emetics (they may cause aspiration pneumonia) or adrenergic vasopressors (ventricular fibrillation might result).

Hypochlorites (bleaches, Dakin's solution)

Signs and Symptoms
Inflammation, corrosion, and burning of mucosa; vomiting; edema of throat, glottis, and larynx with respiratory obstruction; circulatory collapse; possible coma.

*Kerosene, gasoline, benzene, lighter fluid, petroleum ether, naphtha, etc.

Treatment
Emesis or gastric lavage with 1% sodium thiosulfate*; milk; demulcents; morphine for pain; IV fluids for shock; tracheostomy if necessary.

Iodine (e.g., iodine tincture)

Signs and Symptoms
Brownish discoloration of lips and oral mucosa; intense thirst; vomiting; bloody stools; pallor; dyspnea; painful micturition; convulsions; collapse.

Treatment
Gastric lavage with soluble starch or 1 to 5 percent sodium thiosulfate*; frequent gruels of starch, flour, or rice; egg white; morphine sulfate 15 mg SC for pain; IV fluids for acid-base balance.

Iron Salts (e.g., ferrous sulfate)

Signs and Symptoms
Corrosion of gastrointestinal mucosa; vomiting; diarrhea; melena; weak pulse, tachycardia; hypotension; shock.

Treatment
Milk, then emesis and gastric lavage, leaving 10 g deferoxamine in stomach; in severe cases, deferoxamine (which chelates iron) 20 mg/kg IM every 4 hours or, in presence of shock, 40 mg/kg IV over a 4 hour period, then 20 mg/kg IV drip every 12 hours; exchange transfusion.

Lead and Its Compounds

Signs and Symptoms
Gastrointestinal and mental disturbances; restlessness; headache; anemia; basophilic stippling of red cells; possible black "lead line" on gums.

Treatment
Gastric lavage, leaving 30 g of magnesium sulfate in stomach; milk, egg white, or other demulcent; calcium gluconate 1 g IV for spasms; de-leading with calcium disodium edetate 15 to 25 mg/kg every 12 hours for 5 days by slow IV, then additional courses, with 2 day rest periods, as indicated.

*Starch and thiosulfate neutralize and convert these poisons to nontoxic compounds.

Mercury Compounds

Signs and Symptoms
Excessive salivation; foul breath; sore gums; metallic taste; gastrointestinal upset with bloody diarrhea; circulatory and respiratory depression; severe nephrosis (first with increased then diminished quantity of urine containing albumin and blood casts); anuria; convulsions; coma; collapse.

Treatment
Milk, egg whites, or activated charcoal followed by copious gastric lavage; dimercaprol 3 to 5 mg/kg IM every 4 hours on the first and second days, every 6 hours on the third day, and every 12 hours for a week or more; artificial kidney for renal failure.

Naphthalene (mothballs, crystals)

Signs and Symptoms
Abdominal cramps; nausea and vomiting; CNS depression; motor instability; brown or black urine; hemolytic anemia; convulsions; coma; possible damage to liver and kidneys.

Treatment
Gastric lavage or emesis; demulcents; blood transfusions and urine alkalization for hemolysis; diet high in carbohydrate and vitamins to promote regeneration of liver tissue.

Narcotics (e.g., morphine)

Signs and Symptoms
CNS depression varying from drowsiness to deep coma is most common, but excitement and convulsions sometimes occur (e.g., with codeine and meperidine); pupils constrict to pinpoint size usually, but may dilate due to asphyxia; skin initially cold and pale, then cyanotic; circulatory collapse; respiratory failure.

Treatment
Gastric lavage with 1 : 10,000 potassium permanganate; activated charcoal; saline cathartic; external heat; oxygen; IV fluids; frequent turning; nalorphine 100 μg/kg or levallorphan 20 μg/kg IV if respiration is depressed.

Nicotine and Tobacco

Signs and Symptoms
Mild poisoning: dizziness; violent nausea and vomiting; headache; perspiration; general weakness; cardiac irregularities.

"Full" *poisoning:* the same as for mild poisoning, plus intense hot or burning sensation in upper gastrointestinal tract; excitement; dyspnea; cardiac slowing and acceleration; cold, clammy skin; profuse salivation; visual disturbances; diarrhea; convulsions. Death may occur very quickly due to cardiac standstill or respiratory failure.

Treatment

Prompt gastric lavage with potassium permanganate 1 : 10,000, followed by large dose of activated charcoal; artificial respiration and oxygen; short-acting barbiturates for convulsions.

Nitrites and Nitrates (e.g., amyl nitrite, nitroglycerin)

Signs and Symptoms

Gastrointestinal upset; cyanosis (methemoglobinemia) beginning around lips, spreading to fingers and toes, the face, and eventually the entire body; possible respiratory failure. Coma and death may occur in severe intoxication.

Treatment

Gastric lavage or emesis; artificial respiration and oxygen; Trendelenburg position if the patient is hypotensive; methylene blue (as 1% solution) 1 to 2 mg/kg IV.

Organophosphate Insecticides*

Signs and Symptoms

Insidious onset following exposure via ingestion or inhalation or through the skin. The first effects are giddiness, constriction in chest, and pinpoint pupils; then in 2 to 8 hours (approximately in this order) nausea, abdominal cramps, vomiting, diarrhea, muscular twitchings, pulmonary edema, coma, convulsions, and possibly death may occur.

Treatment

Atropine sulfate 2 to 4 mg IM or IV repeated every 10 minutes until signs of atropine poisoning appear; some degree of atropinization should be maintained for at least 48 hours; pralidoxime chloride (started at the same time as atropine) 25 to 50 mg/kg IV and repeated after 12 hours; artificial respiration and oxygen as needed.

*Including Chlorthion®, demeton, Diazinon®, Dipterex®, HETP, malathion, nerve gas agents, OMPA, parathion, TEPP (the action of all such agents is due to cholinesterase inhibition).

Oxalic Acid and Oxalates

Signs and Symptoms
Gastrointestinal upset; dysphagia; erosion of mouth, throat, and stomach; hematemesis; twitching of facial muscles; extreme thirst; mydriasis; collapse.

Treatment
Magnesium sulfate, milk of magnesia, magnesium oxide, lime water, or ordinary chalk (in a small amount of water) to produce insoluble oxalate; gastric lavage only if oral or esophageal erosion is slight or absent; 10 to 20 ml 10% calcium gluconate IV to combat hypocalcemia; milk or other demulcents; IV fluids and other supportive measures as indicated.

Paraldehyde

Signs and Symptoms
Marked odor on breath; excitement; rapid pulse; pinpoint pupils; slow respiration; unconsciousness; collapse; respiratory failure.

Treatment
Gastric lavage or emesis; artificial respiration and oxygen.

Paradichlorobenzene

Signs and Symptoms
Abdominal pain; nausea and vomiting; diarrhea.

Treatment
Gastric lavage or emesis; fluids and other supportive measures.

Phenacetin*

Signs and Symptoms
Methemoglobinemia with cyanosis and severe anemia; CNS depression; respiratory difficulty; vascular collapse.

Treatment
Gastric lavage or emetics; oxygen and artificial respiration; blood transfusions; methylene blue (1% solution) 1 to 2 mg/kg IV.

*Common ingredient in a number of analgesic mixtures, for example, APC, Empirin® Compound.

Phenols (e.g., carbolic acid, cresol, and related compounds)

Signs and Symptoms
Burning pain from mouth to stomach; vomiting; bloody diarrhea; headache and dizziness; cold, clammy skin; oliguria; hematuria and fall in body temperature and blood pressure; collapse and coma. Death may result from respiratory failure or possibly pulmonary edema or aspiration pneumonia.

Treatment
On skin: neutralize with 50% alcohol or castor oil, followed by thorough rinsing.
Swallowed: activated charcoal or, preferably, olive oil at once, followed by extensive lavage with water, or preferably, olive oil (avoid use of other oils); leave some olive oil in the stomach and give egg white for demulcent effect; artificial respiration and oxygen; morphine sulfate 15 mg SC for pain.

Phosphorus (white or yellow)

Signs and Symptoms
Burning in mouth, esophagus, and stomach; nausea and hematemesis; diarrhea; hemorrhagic manifestations; destruction of liver and kidney tissues.

Treatment
Prompt gastric lavage with 0.2% copper sulfate (which forms insoluble copper phosphide) followed by 50 g of sodium phosphate for catharsis; mineral oil to coat the stomach; morphine sulfate 15 mg SC for pain; IV fluids to maintain circulation and fluid balance; high-carbohydrate, high-protein diet plus IV amino acids; *avoid* milk, oils, and fats in diet for at least a week, since fats and oils enhance the absorption of phosphorus.

Salicylates (e.g., aspirin, methyl salicylate)

Signs and Symptoms
Rapid, deep, pauseless breathing; vomiting; tinnitus; visual disturbances; profuse sweating; fever; confusion; skin eruptions; delirium; circulatory collapse; coma; convulsions; oliguria or anuria; hemorrhage.

Treatment
Emesis or gastric lavage; saline cathartics; oral or IV fluids, depending on severity; plasma or blood for shock; sodium bicarbonate for acidosis (if it occurs); tepid water (not alcohol) sponging for fever; vitamin K_1 for bleeding (due to hypoprothrombinemia); hemodialysis in the event of renal failure.

Silver Salts (namely, silver nitrate or lunar caustic)

Signs and Symptoms
Stains on lips; burning pain in the mouth and stomach; vomiting; purging; cramps; weak, thready pulse; respiratory depression; circulatory collapse; convulsions; paralysis; coma.

Treatment
Sodium chloride (which forms insoluble silver chloride) in water, followed by emesis or gastric lavage; milk or other demulcent; short-acting barbiturate (e.g., pentobarbital sodium 200 mg IV) to control convulsions and analgesics for pain.

Strychnine

Signs and Symptoms
Stiffness in the muscles of face and neck; twitchings of face and limbs; violent convulsions varying from a few minutes to an hour. Death may result from asphyxia.

Treatment
Control convulsions with diazepam IV (2 to 6 mg/M^2 of body surface area), pentobarbital sodium IV (300 to 700 mg), paraldehyde IM (1 to 4 ml), or inhalation anesthetic; gastric lavage (once convulsions are under control) with 1 : 10,000 potassium permanganate followed by a large dose of activated charcoal; artificial respiration and oxygen; absolute darkness and absolute quiet.

Thallium Compounds (namely, ant poison, rat poison, roach poison)

Signs and Symptoms
Severe abdominal pain accompanied by vomiting and bloody diarrhea; ulcerative stomatitis and possible gingival line similar to that caused by lead; paresthesias; ptosis; strabismus; mydriasis; facial palsies; skin lesions (eruptions, ecchymoses, petechiae); liver and kidney damage; delirium; convulsions; respiratory failure.

Treatment
Emetics or gastric lavage with 1% sodium or potassium iodide followed by repeated doses of activated charcoal; potassium chloride 5 to 25 g per day, orally; sodium iodide (300 mg to 1 g IV). Treat shock and convulsions (barbiturates or diazepam); chelation with diphenylthoicarbazone 10 mg/kg, orally.

Tranquilizers

Signs and Symptoms
The most common effects are CNS depression (ranging from sedation to coma), respiratory depression, and hypotension; initial sedation

with phenothiazine derivatives, sometimes followed by restlessness and, occasionally, convulsions; respiratory depression marked in event of concomitant ingestion of alcohol, barbiturates, or narcotics.

Treatment

Essentially the same as for barbiturate poisoning. Vasopressors are used, but norepinephrine is contraindicated in cases involving phenothiazines.

4. Drug Interactions

Drugs Enhancing Sedative-Hypnotic Action

    alcohol
    anesthesia (general and regional)
    antihistamines
    chloramphenicol
    griseofulvin
    muscle relaxants
    narcotics
    rauwolfia alkaloids
    tranquilizers

Drugs Enhancing Coumarin-Anticoagulant Action

    acetaminophen
    aminosalicylic acid
    androgens
    anesthetics
    antibiotics
    antilipemics
    anti-inflammatory agents
    antineoplastics
    aspirin
    cathartics
    chloral hydrate
    chloramphenicol
    clofibrate
    diazepam
    estrogens
    ethacrynic acid
    glucagon
    guanethidine
    heparin
    indomethacin
    levothyroxine
    MAO inhibitors
    methyldopa
    methylphenidate
    mineral oil
    narcotics
    oxyphenbutazone
    phenylbutazone
    phenytoin
    probenecid
    quinidine

reserpine
sulfonamides
tetracyclines
thiouracil
thioureas
thyroid preparations

Drugs Diminishing Coumarin-Anticoagulant Action

acidifying agents
ACTH
adrenocorticosteroids
aminocaproic acid
antacids in large doses
anticonvulsants
antihistamines
barbiturates
chlordiazepoxide
chlorpromazine
cholestyramine
digitalis
diphenhydramine
estrogens
ethchlorvynol
furosemide
glutethimide
griseofulvin
haloperidol
meprobamate
phytonadione (vitamin K_1)

Drugs Counteracting Heparin Action

antihistamines
digitalis
hydroxyzine
nicotine
penicillin
phenothiazine

Drugs Enhancing Sulfonylurea-Hypoglycemic Action

anabolic agents
anticoagulants
aspirin
chloramphenicol
clofibrate
cyclophosphamide
ethacrynic acid

insulin
MAO inhibitors
oxyphenbutazone
phenothiazines
phenylbutazone
probenecid
propranolol
salicylates
sulfonamides

Drugs Diminishing Sulfonylurea-Hypoglycemic Action

alcohol
chlorpromazine
corticosteroids
epinephrine
estrogens
ethchlorvynol
furosemide
oral contraceptives
thiazides
thyroid preparations

Drugs Enhancing Insulin Action

alcohol
anabolic steroids
anticoagulants
antineoplastics
cyclophosphamide
guanethidine
isoniazid
MAO inhibitors
oxyphenbutazone
phenylbutazone
propranolol
salicylates
sulfonamides
sulfonylureas

Drugs Diminishing Insulin Action

corticosteroids
dextrothyroxine
epinephrine
phenytoin
thiazide diuretics
thyroid preparations

Drugs Enhancing Curariform Action

aminoglycosides
chlorthalidone
diazepam
polymyxin B
procaine
thiazides

Drug Combinations Causing Hypertension and Hypertensive Crises

furazolidone with adrenergics
furazolidone with methyldopa
furazolidone with tyramine
guanethidine with adrenergics
guanethidine with tricyclic antidepressants
levarterenol with reserpine
MAO inhibitors with adrenergics
MAO inhibitors with levodopa
MAO inhibitors with methyldopa
MAO inhibitors with tyramine
methyldopa with adrenergics

Drugs Enhancing Antihypertensive Action

anesthetics
diazepam
ethacrynic acid
furosemide
haloperidol
isoniazid
MAO inhibitors
procainamide
propranolol
reserpine
spironolactone
thiazides
vasodilators

Drugs Enhancing Atropine Action

antihistamines
antiparkinsonics
isoniazid
MAO inhibitors
meperidine
phenothiazines
tricyclic antidepressants

Drugs Enhancing Phenytoin Action

aspirin (large doses)
barbiturates
benzodiazepine derivatives
chloramphenicol
dicumarol
estrogens
methylphenidate
phenylbutazone
prochlorperazine
sulfisoxazole

Drugs Diminishing Probenecid Action

aspirin-salicylates
ethacrynic acid

Drugs Enhancing Methotrexate Toxicity

antineoplastics
barbiturates
chloramphenicol
PABA
phenytoin
salicylates
sulfonamides
tetracyclines
tranquilizers
triamterene

Miscellaneous Interactions*

adrenergics with tricyclic antidepressants: enhanced effect
alcohol with griseofulvin: enhanced effect
alcohol with metronidazole: "disulfiram effect" (see p. 217)
aminoglycosides with ethacrynic acid: ototoxicity
aminosalicylic acid with aspirin: enhanced effect
androgens with estrogens: diminished effect
androgens with progestogens: diminished effect
anesthetics with reserpine: hypotension
antihistamines with MAO inhibitors: enhanced effect
cephalothin with barbiturates: IV solution incompatibility
cephalothin with erythromycin: IV solution incompatibility
cephalothin with tetracycline: IV solution incompatibility
chloramphenicol with diphtheria toxoid: decreased immune
    response

*The enhanced or diminished effect or toxicity referred to applies to the action of the
first drug of the pair.

chloramphenicol with tetanus toxoid: decreased immune response
cholinergics with iopanoic acid: enhanced effect
clofibrate with estrogens: diminished effect
clofibrate with progestogens: diminished effect
corticosteroids with antibiotics: diminished effect
corticosteroids with barbiturates: diminished effect
corticosteroids with phenytoin: diminished effect
digitalis preparations with calcium: enhanced toxicity
digitalis preparations with phenobarbital: diminished effect
digitalis preparations with reserpine: arrhythmias
digitalis preparations with thiazides: enhanced toxicity
guanethidine with amphetamines: enhanced effect
guanethidine with tricyclic antidepressants: diminished effect
haloperidol with epinephrine: hypotension
heparin with phenytoin: enhanced effect
levarterenol with reserpine: enhanced effect
levodopa with pyridoxine: action reversed
metaproterenol with guanethidine: diminished effect
metaproterenol with reserpine: diminished effect
MAO inhibitors with ethchlorvynol: enhanced effect
mercaptopurine with allopurinol: enhanced effect
mercurial diuretics with alkalizing agents: enhanced diuresis
mercurial diuretics with ammonium chloride: enhanced diuresis
narcotics with phenothiazines: enhanced effect
neomycin with ether: respiratory paralysis
neomycin with succinylcholine: respiratory paralysis
penicillin with probenecid: enhanced penicillin levels
phenytoin with folic acid: diminished effect
sulfonamides with aspirin: enhanced toxicity
sulfonamides with phenylbutazone: enhanced toxicity
tetracyclines with antacids: decreased absorption
tetracyclines with iron preparations: decreased absorption
tricyclic antidepressants with MAO inhibitors: enhanced toxicity
warfarin with milk of magnesia: increased warfarin absorption

5. Drugs with Possible Adverse Effects on the Fetus

Androgens	Masculinization
Anesthetic gases	Depressed respiration
Anticoagulants	Intrauterine bleeding, fetal death
Antineoplastics	Congenital anomalies
Aspirin	Neonatal bleeding
Barbiturates	Depressed respiration
Chloramphenicol	Gray syndrome
Chloral hydrate	Fetal death
Chloroquine	Thrombocytopenia
Chlorpromazine	Jaundice
Corticosteroids	Cleft palate
Dextroamphetamine	Transposition of vessels
Heroin	Fetal death
Iodides	Neonatal goiter
Isoniazid	Retarded psycomotor activity
Lithium	Neonatal goiter
Lysergic acid diethylamide (LSD)	Stunted growth
Methadone	Respiratory depression
Morphine	Respiratory depression
Nicotine	Small neonates
Nitrofurantoin	Fetal hemolysis
Phenylbutazone	Neonatal goiter
Phenytoin	Congenital anomalies
Phytonadione (vitamin K) ("megadoses")	Kernicterus
Propylthiouracil	Neonatal goiter
Quinine	Deafness
Reserpine	Nasal congestion
Streptomycin	Eighth cranial nerve damage

Sulfonamides	Kernicterus
Sulfonurea hypoglycemics	Prolonged neonatal hypoglycemia
Tetracyclines	Discolored teeth, micromelia, syndactyly
Thiazides	Neonatal thrombocytopenia
Vitamin A ("megadoses")	Congenital anomalies
Vitamin D ("megadoses")	Retardation

6. Drugs in Nursing Mothers

Most drugs will appear in the nursing mother's milk, but the effect on the infant depends on a number of variables, including type of drug, concentration, amount of milk ingested, and tolerance. Generally, the following drugs should not be given to nursing mothers:

atropine
anticoagulants
antithyroid drugs
antimetabolites
bromides
cathartics (except senna)
ergot preparations
iodides
mercurials
metronidazole
narcotics
tetracyclines

The following drugs are not contraindicated, but the infant should be watched carefully for adverse signs:

antibiotics
barbiturates
chlorpromazine
corticosteroids
diuretics
lithium
nalidixic acid
oral contraceptives
phenytoin
reserpine
salicylates
sulfonamides

7. Weights and Measures

The International System of Units

The International System of Units is the modernized version of the metric system established by international agreement. Officially abbreviated SI (from the French, Le Système International d'Unités), the system is built on a foundation of seven base units (plus two supplementary units). All other units are derived from these units, and multiples and submultiples are expressed decimally. The prefixes for these multiples and submultiples (and their symbols) are the same for all SI units. The base units and their derivatives of chief concern to everyday medicine and nursing are presented below.

Length and Area

Unit	Symbol	Value
meter	m	—
centimeter	cm	0.01 m
millimeter	mm	0.001 m
square meter	m^2	—

Weight (Mass)

Unit	Symbol	Value
kilogram	kg	1,000 g
gram	g	—
milligram	mg	0.001 (10^{-3}) g
microgram	μg	0.000001 (10^{-6}) g
nanogram	ng	0.000000001 (10^{-9}) g

Volume

Unit	Symbol	Value
liter	l (or L)	—
milliliter	ml	0.001 (10^{-3}) l
cubic millimeter	mm^3	0.001 (10^{-3}) m^3
cubic centimeter	cm^3 (or cc)	0.01 (10^{-2}) m^3

Useful Equivalents

1 inch = 2.5 cm = 25.4 mm
1 grain (gr) = 65 mg
1 ounce (avoir.) = 28.35 g
1 ounce (apoth.) = 31.1 g
1 pound (avoir.) = 7,000 gr (16 oz) = 453.59 g
1 pound (apoth.) = 5,760 gr (12 oz) = 373.24 g
1 fluidounce = 30 ml
1 quart = 0.946 l; 946 ml
1 meter = 39.37 in.; 3.3 ft; 1.1 yd
1 centimeter = 0.4 in.
1 millimeter = 0.04 in.
1 kilogram = 2.2 lb
1 gram = 15.4 gr
1 milligram = 1/65 gr
1 liter = 1.06 qt
1 milliliter = 16 minims

Household Equivalents

Measure	Apothecary	SI (metric)
1 drop (from eyedropper)	1 minim	0.06 ml
1 teaspoonful	1 fl dram	5 ml
1 dessertspoonful	2 fl dram	10 ml
1 tablespoonful	½ fl oz	15 ml
1 jigger	1½ fl oz	45 ml
1 cup (glassful)	8 fl oz	240 ml
1 pint	2 cups	480 ml
1 quart	2 pints	960 ml

8. Pediatric Drug Dosage

Young's Rule

$$\frac{age \times adult\ dose}{age + 12} = approximate\ dose$$

Example:

age of child 4; adult dose 20 mg

$$\frac{4 \times 20}{4 + 12} = \frac{80}{16} = 5\ mg$$

Cowling's Rule

$$\frac{age\ at\ next\ birthday \times adult\ dose}{24} = approximate\ dose$$

Example:

age of child 2; adult dose 16 mg

$$\frac{3 \times 16}{24} = \frac{48}{24} = 2\ mg$$

Clark's Rule

$$\frac{weight\ of\ child\ in\ pounds \times adult\ dose}{150} = approximate\ dose$$

Example:

child weighs 50 lb; adult dose 30 mg

$$\frac{50 \times 30}{150} = 10\ mg$$

Body Surface Area (BSA) Rule

$$\frac{body\ surface\ area\ of\ child\ (in\ m^2)^*}{body\ surface\ area\ of\ adult\ (1.73\ m^2)} \times 100 = \%\ of\ adult\ dose$$

*Obtained from nomogram (p. 580) by means of a straight-edge ruler connecting "height" and "weight," the surface area appearing at point where edge crosses middle column.

Body Surface Area of Children: Nomogram for Determination of Body Surface Area from Height and Weight*

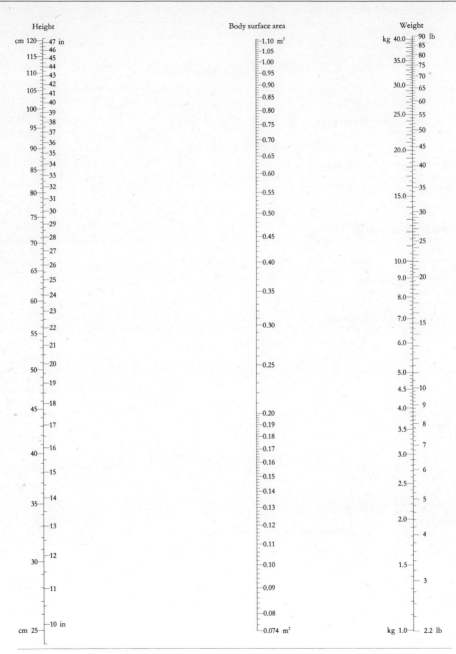

*Reproduced from *Documenta Geigy Scientific Tables,* 7th edition, 1970. Courtesy CIBA-GEIGY Limited, Basel, Switzerland. From the formula of Du Bois and Du Bois, *Arch. Intern. Med.,* 17, 863 (1916): $S = W^{0.425} \times H^{0.725} \times 71.84$, or $\log S = \log W \times 0.425 + \log H \times 0.725 + 1.8564$ (S = body surface in cm², W = weight in kg, H = height in cm).

580

9. Recommended Daily Allowances of Vitamins and Minerals*

	Males	Females	Pregnancy
Vitamins			
Vitamin A	5,000 IU	4,000 IU	5,000 IU
Ergocalciferol (vitamin D)	400 IU	400 IU	400 IU
Vitamin E	15 IU	12 IU	15 IU
Ascorbic acid (vitamin C)	45 mg	45 mg	60 mg
Folic acid	400 μg	400 μg	800 μg
Thiamine	1.4 mg	1 mg	1.3 mg
Riboflavin	1.6 mg	1.1 mg	1.4 mg
Niacin	18 mg	13 mg	15 mg
Pyridoxine (vitamin B_6)	700 μg	2 mg	2.5 mg
Cyanocobalamin (vitamin B_{12})	3 μg	3 μg	4 μg
Minerals			
Calcium	800 mg	800 mg	1.2 g
Iodine	130 μg	100 μg	125 μg
Iron	10 mg	18 mg	18+ mg
Magnesium	350 mg	300 mg	450 mg
Phosphorus	800 mg	800 mg	1.2 g

*For adults, ages 23–50. Values set forth by the Nutrition Board (1974), National Academy of Sciences-National Research Council.

10. United States Adopted Names (USAN) Assigned to Radioactive Pharmaceuticals*

The United States Adopted Names (USAN) applicable to radioactive pharmaceuticals are composed of the name of the basic compound serving as the carrier for the radioactivity, the symbol for the radioactive isotope, and the atomic weight (since several radioactive isotopes of a given element may be in use—see listing under iodine). The following listing of nonproprietary names (shown in boldface type) is arranged in alphabetical order according to the English name of the radioactive element. The isotopes of hydrogen are listed under their specific names, deuterium and tritium. Radioactive pharmaceuticals are often supplied by the manufacturers under a designation equivalent to the adopted nonproprietary name and are listed as such; specific trademarks are given in brackets when they exist.

^{74}As–**sodium arsenate As 74**

^{45}Ca–**calcium chloride Ca 45**

^{131}Cs–**cesium chloride Cs 131**

^{51}Cr–**chromated Cr 51 serum albumin** [Chromalbin–Squibb]; **chromic chloride Cr 51; chromic phosphate Cr 51; sodium chromate Cr 51** [sodium chromate Cr 51–Mallinckrodt; Chromitope Sodium–Squibb]

^{57}Co–**cobaltous chloride Co 57** [Cobatope-57–Squibb]; **cyanocobalamin Co 57** [Racobalamin-57–Abbott; cyanocobalamin Co 57–Mallinckrodt; Rubratope-57–Squibb]

^{60}Co–**cobaltous chloride Co 60** [Cobatope-60–Squibb]; **cyanocobalamin Co 60** [Rubratope-60–Squibb]

^{64}Cu–**cupric acetate Cu 64**

^{2}H–**deuterium oxide** (stable isotope)

^{67}Ga–**gallium citrate Ga 67** [gallium citrate Ga 67–New England Nuclear]

^{198}Au–**gold Au 198** [gold Au 198–Mallinckrodt; Aureotope–Squibb]

^{125}I–**diatrizoate sodium I 125; diohippuric acid I 125; diotyrosine I 125; human growth hormone I 125** [human growth hormone I 125–Abbott]; **insulin I 125; iodinated I 125 serum albumin** [Radioiodinated (I_{125}) Serum Albumin (Human) IHSA

*Reproduced from *J.A.M.A.* 235:296, Jan. 19, 1976. Copyright 1976, American Medical Association.

583

125–Mallinckrodt; Albumotope I-125–Squibb]; **iodopyracet I 125; iomethin I 125; iothalamate sodium I 125** [Glofil-125–Abbott]; **liothyronine I 125** [Triomet-125–Abbott]; **oleic acid I 125** [oleic acid I 125–Mallinckrodt]; **povidone I 125; sodium iodide I 125** [sodium iodide I 125–Mallinckrodt]; **thyroxine I 125** [thyroxine I 125–Mallinckrodt; Tetramet-125–Abbott]

[131]I–**ethiodized oil I 131; iodinated I 131 serum albumin** [Radioiodinated (I_{131}) Serum Albumin (Human) IHSA 131–Mallinckrodt; Albumotope I-131–Squibb]; **iodinated I 131 serum albumin aggregated** [Macroscan-131–Abbott; Aggregated Radioiodinated (I_{131}) Albumin (Human) MAA I 131–Mallinckrodt; Albumotope-LS–Squibb]; **iodipamide sodium I 131; iodoantipyrine I 131; iodohippurate sodium I 131** [Hippuran-131–Abbott; Hippuran I 131–Mallinckrodt; Hipputope–Squibb]; **iotyrosine I 131; rose bengal sodium I 131** [Sodium Rose Bengal I 131–Mallinckrodt; Robengatope–Squibb]; **sodium iodide I 131** [Oriodide-131, Oriodide-131-H, Radiocaps-131, Theriodide-131–Abbott; sodium iodide I 131–Mallinckrodt; Iodotope, Iodotope Therapeutic–Squibb]; **tolpovidone I 131; triolein I 131** [triolein I 131–Mallinckrodt]

[192]Ir–**iridium Ir 192**

[59]Fe–**ferric chloride Fe 59** [ferric chloride Fe 59–Mallinckrodt]; **ferrous citrate Fe 59** [ferrous citrate Fe 59–Mallinckrodt]; **ferrous sulfate Fe 59**

[85]Kr–**krypton clathrate Kr 85**

[197]Hg–**chlormerodrin Hg 197** [chlormerodrin Hg 197–Mallinckrodt; chlormerodrin Hg 197–Squibb]; **merisoprol Hg 197; merisoprol acetate Hg 197**

[203]Hg–**chlormerodrin Hg 203** [chlormerodrin Hg 203–Mallinckrodt]

[32]P–**chromic phosphate P 32** [chromic phosphate P32–Abbott; Phosphocol P32–Mallinckrodt]; **polymetaphosphate P 32; sodium phosphate P 32** [sodium phosphate P 32–Mallinckrodt; Phosphotope–Squibb]

[42]K–**potassium chloride K 42**

[86]Rb–**rubidium chloride Rb 86**

[75]Se–**selenomethionine Se 75** [selenomethionine Se 75–Mallinckrodt; Sethotope–Squibb]

[22]Na–**sodium chloride Na 22**

[85]Sr–**strontium chloride Sr 85; strontium nitrate Sr 85** [strontium nitrate Sr 85–Mallinckrodt; Strotope–Squibb]

^{35}S–**sodium sulfate S 35**

^{99m}Tc–**sodium pertechnetate Tc99m** [sodium pertechnetate Tc99m–Mallinckrodt; sodium pertechnetate Tc99m–New England Nuclear]; **technetium Tc99m** [Elutex–Abbott; Ultra-TechneKow/Ultra-Technekow FM Generator, Neimotec–Mallinckrodt; Technetope, Minitec–Squibb; Tc99m Generator–New England Nuclear]; **technetium Tc99m albumin aggregated; technetium Tc99m sulfur colloid** [technetium 99m sulfur colloid–Mallinckrodt; technetium 99m sulfur colloid–New England Nuclear; Collokit–Abbott]

^{3}H–**tritiated water**

^{133}Xe–**xenon Xe 133** [Xeneisol 133–Mallinckrodt]

^{169}Yb–**pentetate trisodium calcium Yb 169** [pentetate trisodium calcium Yb 169–Minnesota Mining & Mfg Co]

^{65}Zn–**zinc chloride Zn 65**

11. Latin Phrases and Abbreviations

aa; a̅a̅	ana	of each
a.c.	ante cibum	before meals
aq.	aqua	water
aq. dest.	aqua destillata	distilled water
b.i.d.	bis in die	twice a day
c.; c̄	cum	with
caps.	capsula	capsule
cochl. parv.	cochleare parvum	teaspoonful
dil.	dilue	dilute
elix.	elixir	elixir
et	et	and
ex	ex	from
ext.	extractum	extract
fld.	fluidus	fluid
gr.	granum	grain
gtt.	gutta(e)	drop(s)
h.	hora	hour
h.s.	hora somni	bedtime
M.	misce	mix
m	minimum	minim
non. rep.	non repetatur	not to be repeated
O.	octarius	pint
O.D.	oculus dexter	right eye
o.h.	omni hora	every hour
os	os	mouth
O.S.	oculus sinister	left eye
O.U.	oculus uterque	each eye
p.c.	post cibum	after meals
per	per	through
p.o.	per os	by mouth

p.r.n.	pro re nata	when required
q.h.	quaque hora	every hour
q.2h.	—	every 2 hours
q.3h.	—	every 3 hours
q.4h.	—	every 4 hours
q.i.d.	quater in die	four times a day
q.s.	quantum satis	as much as necessary
R$_\chi$, Rx	recipe	take
s; s̄	sine	without
Sig.; s.	signa	label
s.o.s.	si opus sit	if necessary
ss., s̄s̄	semis	one-half
stat.	statim	immediately
t.i.d.	ter in die	three times a day
tinct.; tr.	tinctura	tincture
uncia	uncia (℥)	ounce
ung.	unguentum	ointment
ut dict.	ut dictum	as directed

12. Pharmacologic Terms Defined

absorption: the movement of a drug from the site of application toward the systemic circulation

absorption, percutaneous: absorption through the skin

acetaldehyde: a metabolite of ethyl alcohol

acetate: a salt of acetic acid

acetylcholine: the neurohormone released at the endings of all cholinergic nerves

acid: a proton donor; reacts with bases to form salts and with alcohols to form esters

ACTH: andrenocorticotropic hormone

addiction: a state of periodic or chronic intoxication produced by repeated use of a drug and marked by psychological and physical dependence

ADH: antidiuretic hormone; vasopressin

adrenolytic: inhibiting the action of adrenergic (sympathetic) nerves; inhibiting the action of epinephrine

adsorbent: an agent that attracts other substances to its surface

adverse drug reactions (ADRs): toxic drug reactions that occur in therapeutic situations

aerosol: a solution of a drug that can be atomized into a fine mist

affinity: the propensity of a drug to bind with a given receptor

agonist: a drug that interacts with a cellular receptor and thereby elicits a response

albumin: a protein characterized by being soluble in water and coagulable by heat

alimentation: the giving of nutriment

alkali: a strong, soluble base (e.g., sodium hydroxide, NaOH); physiologically, any compound that neutralizes acid

alkali reserve: the total amount of alkali (namely, bicarbonate ions, HCO_3^-) utilizable in maintaining acid-base balance

alkalizer, urinary: an agent used to increase the pH of urine

alkaloid: one of a large group of nitrogenous organic bases of plant origin; typically, they are bitter, insoluble in water, and pharmacologically active, and they react with mineral acids to form water-soluble salts; major examples are atropine, caffeine, codeine, morphine, papaverine, quinine, nicotine, pilocarpine, reserpine, scopolamine, and strychnine

alkylating agent: any agent in a chemical reaction that transfers its hydrocarbon fragment onto another organic molecule

allergen: an agent that provokes hypersensitivity

allergy, drug: an altered response to a drug resulting from a previous sensitizing exposure; immediate drug allergies include anaphylaxis, urticaria, angioneurotic edema, drug fever, and asthma; delayed drug allergies include serum sickness, contact dermatitis, and certain hematologic disturbances

amebicide: an agent that inhibits or destroys amebae, especially *Entamoeba histolytica* (the cause of amebiasis)

amide: an organic compound derived from ammonia (by the substitution of an acyl radical for hydrogen) or from an organic acid by the substitution of an amino group ($-NH_2$) for $-OH$

amine: a compound formed from ammonia by the substitution of one or more organic radicals for one or more hydrogens

amino acid: an acid containing one or more amino ($-NH_2$) groups and one or more carboxyl ($-COOH$) groups

aminoglycoside: any of a group of antibiotics derived from various species of *Streptomyces* and characterized by an inositol substituted with two or more amino groups and with one or more sugars and amino sugars

amphetamine: adrenergic CNS stimulant; a term often applied to any drug related to amphetamine

ampul(e): a small glass container with sterile contents

analeptic: a restorative, especially an agent that counteracts respiratory depression

analgesic: an agent that allays pain without causing loss of consciousness

analogue: a structural derivative of a parent compound with similar or opposite pharmacologic action

anaphylaxis: a severe allergic reaction to a foreign substance

androgen: a male hormone

anesthesia: loss of sensation

anesthesia, basal: a state of narcosis produced by preanesthetic medication

anesthesia, caudal: anesthesia produced by injection of a local anesthetic into the caudal or sacral canal

anesthesia, epidural: anesthesia produced by injection of a local anesthetic into the extradural space between the vertebral spines

anesthesia, field block: regional anesthesia produced by injecting a local anesthetic into the area encompassing the operative field

anesthesia, general: the production of a state of unconsciousness with loss of sensation over the entire body

anesthesia, infiltration: local anesthesia produced by deposition of a drug in the area of terminal nerve endings

anesthesia, nerve block: regional anesthesia produced by injection of a local anesthetic in close proximity to the nerves supplying the area in question

anesthesia, regional: local anesthesia produced by interrupting the sensory nerve conductivity from a given region of the body; see anesthesia, field block and anesthesia, nerve block

anesthesia, saddle-block: anesthesia produced in a region roughly corresponding to the areas of the buttocks, perineum, and inner aspects of the thighs that encounter the saddle in riding

anesthesia, spinal: anesthesia produced by injection of a local anesthetic into the subarachnoid space around the spinal cord

anesthetic: an agent that abolishes pain

anesthetic, local: an agent whose action is limited to the area of the body to which it is applied or injected

anesthetics, halogenated: anesthetics containing one or more atoms of halogen (bromine, chlorine, fluorine, iodine) per molecule

angiography: roentgenography of blood vessels following injection of appropriate contrast medium

anhydrase, carbonic: an enzyme that catalyzes the breakdown of carbonic acid into carbon dioxide and water

anion: a negative ion

anodyne: a medicine that relieves pain

anorectic: inhibits or checks the appetite

antacid: an agent that neutralizes stomach acid

antacid, systemic: an antacid whose effects may include alkalosis (alkalemia)

antagonism, drug: interference in the action of one drug by another

antagonist: a drug that interacts with a receptor and in so doing prevents the action of the agonist

antarthritic: an agent that alleviates arthritis

anthelmintic: an agent used in the treatment of helminthiasis

anthelmintic, broad-spectrum: an anthelmintic effective against a variety of parasitic worms

antiadrenergic: an agent that inhibits the function of the sympathetic nervous system; also known as adrenergic blocking agent

antianemic: an agent that counteracts or prevents anemia

antiarrhythmic: an agent that relieves or prevents arrhythmias

antiasthmatic: an agent that relieves or prevents asthma

antibiotic: an agent produced by one microorganism that inhibits or kills other microorganisms

antibiotic, broad-spectrum: an antibiotic effective against a wide range of bacteria

antibiotic, fungistatic: an antibiotic effective against pathogenic molds and yeasts

antibody: a specific immune substance produced by the body in response to the presence of an antigen; almost all are plasma gamma globulins (immunoglobulins)

anticholinergic: an agent that inhibits the action of cholinergic (parasympathetic) nerves

anticoagulant: an agent that inhibits or prevents coagulation of the blood

anticoagulants, coumarin: anticoagulants derived from or related to coumarin (1, 2-benzopyrone)

anticonvulsant: an agent that relieves or prevents convulsions (especially epileptic seizures)

antidepressant: an agent that relieves or prevents depression

antidiabetic: an agent that counteracts or prevents diabetes

antidiarrheal: an agent that combats diarrhea

antidiuretic: an agent that inhibits or prevents the formation of urine

antidiuretic hormone: a hormone, produced by the anterior pituitary, that stimulates the absorption of water from the renal tubules

antidote: an agent that counteracts the effects of a poison

antiemetic (antinauseant): an agent that relieves or prevents nausea and vomiting

antiflatulent: an agent that relieves or prevents flatulence

antifungal agent: see fungicide

antigen: any agent that stimulates the formation of antibodies and specifically reacts with those antibodies

antihistamine: an agent that counteracts the action of histamine and is useful in certain allergies

antihypertensive: an agent that relieves or prevents hypertension

antihypotensive: an agent that elevates the blood pressure

anti-infective: an agent effective in the treatment and prevention of infection

antileprotic: an agent effective against leprosy

antilipemic: an agent that counteracts high levels of fat (and other lipids) in the blood

antimalarial: an agent used in the treatment and prevention of malaria

antimaniacal: an agent used in the treatment and prevention of mania

antimetabolite: an agent similar in chemical structure to one that is essential to normal physiologic function and that exerts its effects via molecular competition

antinauseant: see antiemetic

antimicrobial: an agent that destroys or inhibits the growth of microorganisms

antineoplastic: an agent that inhibits or checks the development of neoplasms or cancers

antiparkinsonic: an agent used in the treatment of Parkinson's disease

antiprotozoal: an agent that inhibits or destroys protozoa

antipruritic: an agent that relieves or prevents itching

antipsoriatic: an agent that relieves psoriasis

antipyretic: an agent that reduces fever

antischistosomal: an agent destructive to schistosomes

antiseptic: an agent that inhibits microorganisms

antiseptic, urinary: an agent used in the treatment of urinary tract infections

antispasmodic: an agent that relaxes muscle (especially smooth muscle)

antithyroid: an agent that inhibits the function of the thyroid gland, especially the synthesis of thyroid hormones

antitoxin: an antibody against a toxin (especially bacterial exotoxins)

antitrichomonal: an agent effective against *Trichomonas* species, especially *Trichomonas vaginalis* (the cause of trichomonas vaginitis)

antitrypanosomal: an agent used in the treatment of trypanosomiasis

antituberculotic: an agent used in the treatment of tuberculosis

antitussive: an agent that relieves or prevents cough

antivenin: a serum (containing antitoxin) used in the treatment of envenomation

antiviral: an agent that destroys or inhibits viruses

aortography: roentgenography of the aorta following the injection of appropriate contrast medium

APC: refers to a combination of aspirin, phenacetin, and caffeine

apothecary (apoth.): a system of weights and measures in which the pound contains 12 ounces or 5,760 grains (equal to 373.24 grams)

arteriography: roentgenography of an artery following injection of appropriate contrast medium

astringent: a topically applied agent that contracts epidermal tissue

atropinism: poisoning due to atropine or belladonna; applied generally to anticholinergic poisoning

avitaminosis: a vitamin deficiency

avoirdupois (avoir.): a system of weights and measures in which the pound contains 16 ounces or 7,000 grains (equal to 453.59 grams)

balsam, peruvian: a fragrant viscous juice (from *Myroxylon pereirae*) used topically as a protectant and counterirritant

barbiturate: any one of a class of sedative-hypnotics derived from barbituric acid

barbiturate, intermediate-acting: acts in 15 to 30 minutes and lasts for about 5 hours

barbiturate, long-acting: acts in 30 to 60 minutes and lasts for about 6 hours

barbiturate, short-acting: acts in 10 to 15 minutes and lasts for about 3 hours

barbiturate, ultrashort-acting: a barbiturate that acts in a few minutes; used as an IV anesthetic

base: a compound that reacts with acids to form salts

belladonna: the dried leaves and flowering tops of *Atropa belladonna*, the chief alkaloids of which include atropine, hyoscyamine, and scopolamine (hyoscine)

benzoin: a balsamic resin obtained from certain species of *Styrax*, a genus of shrubs and trees grown mainly in Java, Sumatra, and Thailand

bicarbonate: any salt containing the anion HCO_3^-

bioavailability: the relative amount of an administered drug that reaches the general circulation and the rate at which this occurs

bioequivalents: chemical equivalents that, when administered to the same individual in the same dosage regimen, result in equivalent concentrations of drug in blood and tissues

biological half-life: the time required for the amount of drug initially present in the system to be halved

biologicals: pharmaceutical products of biological origin

bolus: a rounded mass of a pharmaceutical preparation ready to swallow or a concentrated mass of a pharmaceutical preparation given IV

borate: salt of boric acid

BP: British Pharmacopoeia

brand name: trademark (see)

bronchodilator: an agent that dilates the air passageways of the lung

bronchoscopy: examination of the bronchial tree through the bronchoscope

BSA: body surface area

BSP: sulfobromophthalein sodium (Bromsulphalein®)

buccal: pertaining to the cheek or mouth; see tablet, buccal

buffer: a chemical system that resists a change in pH

BUN: blood urea nitrogen

calcitonin: a thyroid hormone that lowers plasma calcium and phosphate levels and inhibits bone resorption

calorie: small calorie (cal) is the amount of heat required to raise the temperature of 1 gram of water 1 degree Celsius; large calorie (Cal), or kilocalorie, is the amount of heat required to raise the temperature of 1 kilogram of water 1 degree Celsius

camphor: an antipruritic obtained from the plant *Cinnamomum camphora*

cannabis: the dried flowering tops of *Cannabis sativa,* the active principle of which is the hallucinogen tetrahydrocannabinol; also called hashish and marijuana

capsule: a soluble gelatinous sheath enclosing a dose of an oral medicine

carbohydrase: an enzyme that acts on a carbohydrate

carbohydrate: a class of organic compounds encompassing sugars and starches

cardiotonic: having a tonic effect on the heart

cardiotoxicity: having poisonous effects on the heart

carminative: an agent that relieves flatulence

cascara sagrada: the dried bark of the shrub *Rhamnus purshiana*; used as a laxative

catecholamine: a body amine (derived from catechol) having sympathomimetic action

cathartic: an agent that stimulates evacuation of the bowels

cation: a positive ion

caustic: corrosive or destructive to living tissues

cautery: a caustic agent or a very hot or very cold instrument used to destroy tissue

cellulose: a high-polymer carbohydrate and the main constituent of all plant tissues and fibers

cephalosporin: any of a group of broad-spectrum penicillinase-resistant antibiotics derived from the fungus *Cephalosporium*

ceruminolytic: an agent that dissolves earwax

chelate: a heterocyclic ring containing a sequestered metal ion

chelation: the incorporation of a metal ion into an organic ring

chemotherapy: the treatment of disease using highly specific drugs; commonly applied to drugs used to treat cancer

chemical equivalents: refers to preparations that contain the same active constituent in the dosage form and meet official standards

chloride (Cl): salt of hydrochloric acid

cholangiography: roentgenography of the biliary ducts

cholecystography: roentgenography of the gallbladder

cholepoiesis: production and secretion of bile salts

choleretic: an agent that stimulates the production of bile

cholesterol: a steroid alcohol that occurs mainly in bile, gallstones, the brain, blood cells, and plasma

cholinergic: an agent that effects parasympathetic action; also called parasympathomimetic and cholinomimetic

cholinesterase: an enzyme that effects the hydrolysis and deactivation of acetylcholine

cholinomimetic: cholinergic

cinchona: the crude drug derived from various species of *Cinchona* and serving as the source of the alkaloids quinine and quinidine

cinchonism: toxic condition (headache, tinnitus, deafness, cerebral congestion) caused by excessive use of quinine, quinidine, and related cinchona (see) alkaloids

citrate: salt of citric acid

CNS: central nervous system

coal tar: a viscous black liquid obtained by the destructive distillation of coal

cocaine: the narcotic alkaloid obtained from the leaves of *Erythroxylon coca;* used as a local anesthetic

coenzyme: a heat-stable organic molecule that must be loosely associated with an enzyme for the enzyme to function

colchicum: the dried seeds or corms of *Colchicum autumnale,* a source of colchicine

colloid: a physical system in which one substance is dispersed throughout another substance, such as an emulsion of "oil in water"

compendia, official: legally, the United States Pharmacopeia (USP) and National Formulary (NF)

compound: a chemical combination of two or more elements

concomitant: accompanying or together

congeners: closely related chemical compounds with similar or antagonistic pharmacologic action

conjugation: the joining together of two compounds, especially a drug or poison with another substance to form a nontoxic product (which is then excreted)

contraindication: a condition or situation in which a drug is not to be used

contrast medium: an agent used in roentgenography to render "soft structures" opaque to x-rays

corpus luteum: the yellow glandular mass (formed by ruptured ovarian follicle) that secretes progesterone and estrogens

corticosteroid: any of the hormones produced by the adrenal cortex or their synthetic congeners

corticotropin: see ACTH

counterirritant: an agent that induces local irritation to counteract general or deep irritation

cream: a semisolid emulsion of oil in water or water in oil that vanishes when rubbed into the skin

crisis, cholinergic: excessive or overwhelming cholinergic stimulation

curare: an extract of *Chondodendron tomentosum* containing the muscle relaxant tubocurarine

curariform: resembling curare

cyanide: a compound containing the —CN radical

cycloplegic: an agent that causes paralysis of accommodation

cystostatic: an agent that suppresses cell growth

cytotoxic: an agent toxic to cells

debridement: the removal of necrotic tissue

debridement, biochemical: debridement effected by the use of proteolytic enzymes

decongestant: an agent that reduces congestion or swelling

demulcent: any soothing application

dependence, drug: a state of psychological or physical dependence (or both) on a drug, arising in a person following administration of that drug on a periodic or continuous basis

desensitization: the process of rendering the body nonresponsive to a specific antigen

detergent: an agent that cleans

dextran: a water-soluble polysaccharide (obtained from sucrose) used as a plasma extender

dextro- (*d*- or +): denoting the dextrorotatory form of an optically active organic compound

dextrose: glucose

dialysis: the separation of a crystalloid and a colloid by means of a semipermeable membrane

dialysis, peritoneal: dialysis employing the peritoneum as the semipermeable or dialyzing membrane

dibasic: an acid with two replaceable hydrogen atoms

digestant: an agent that aids digestion

digitalis: the powdered leaves of *Digitalis purpurea* (purple foxglove); commonly applied to drugs (glycosides) derived from this plant or similar species

diluent: pharmaceutically, a liquid agent used to effect solution of a drug supplied in the solid state

disinfectant: a topical agent that destroys pathogens

diuretic: an agent that promotes the secretion of urine

diuretic, mercurial: a diuretic drug containing mercury

diuretic, potassium-sparing: a diuretic that enhances the excretion of sodium and inhibits the excretion of potassium

diuretic, thiazide: any of a class of diuretics related to chlorothiazide, the parent drug

dose: the amount of medication to be given at one time

dose, average: the amount of medication that usually produces the desired effect

dose, booster: an amount of vaccine or toxoid, usually smaller than the original dose, administered at an interval after primary immunization for the purpose of maintaining protection; called also booster shot

dose, lethal: the amount of a drug that will cause death

dose, toxic: the amount of a drug that usually produces untoward effects

dressing, occlusive: a dressing that seals the wound from contact with air or bacteria

drops: a topical pharmaceutical preparation for use in the ear, eye, or nose

drug: any agent used in the diagnosis, treatment, or prevention of disease, or to improve the condition of the body

drug, crude: the whole drug with all its ingredients, both active and inactive

ECT: electroconvulsive therapy

efficacy: the biological effectiveness per unit of drug-receptor complex

electrolyte: a chemical compound that dissociates into ions in solution

elixir: a clear, sweetened, hydroalcoholic solution of a medicament for oral use

emetic: an agent that induces vomiting

emollient: an agent that soothes or softens body surfaces

emulsion: a colloidal system of one liquid dispersed in another liquid

enteric-coated: a special coating of tablets or capsules that prevents disintegration in the stomach

enzyme: an organic catalyst

enzyme, proteolytic: an enzyme that hydrolyzes or digests proteins

epinephrine: a hormone secreted by the adrenal medulla in response to hypoglycemia and sympathetic stimulation; used as an adrenergic agent

ergot: the dried filamentous mass of the fungus *Claviceps purpurea;* it contains several alkaloids, including ergonovine and ergotamine

ergotism: poisoning from excessive or misdirected use of ergot or ergot alkaloids

ester: an organic salt formed from an alcohol and an acid

estrogen: any of several steroid hormones produced chiefly by the ovary and responsible for the development of female genitalia and secondary sex characteristics

excipient: an inert substance (e.g., petrolatum) used to confer a suitable consistency to a pharmaceutical preparation

exotoxin: a toxin released by a living bacterium

expectorant: an agent that promotes the expulsion of exudate from the bronchial tree and trachea

extract: a concentrated preparation of a vegetable or animal drug

factor VIII: a substance in the blood essential to the clotting process; a deficiency results in hemophilia A (classic hemophilia); also called antihemophilic factor

factor IX: a substance in the blood essential to the clotting process; a deficiency results in hemophilia B; also called Christmas factor

fat: a glyceryl ester of a fatty acid

ferric: iron at its plus three (Fe^{3+}) oxidation state

ferrous: iron at its plus two (Fe^{2+}) oxidation state

fluidextract: an alcoholic solution of a vegetable drug containing the equivalent of one gram in powdered form of the active principle in each milliliter

fluoride: a compound of fluorine and another element

fluoroscope: a fluorescent screen on which the internal structures of the body can be continuously viewed as shadows formed by differential transmission of x-rays

fructose: simple sugar derived via digestion from sucrose

fumarate: a salt of fumaric acid

fungicide: an agent that destroys fungi

gamma globulin: immunoglobulin

gastroscopy: inspection of the interior of the stomach by means of an endoscope (gastroscope)

gel: a jelly-like topical preparation

generic name: a drug name (often descriptive of its chemical class) not protected by a trademark

germicide: an agent used topically to kill pathogenic microorganisms ("germs")

GFR: glomerular filtration rate (see)

globulin, immune serum: a sterile solution of globulins containing many of the antibodies of adult human blood

glomerular filtration rate (GFR): an expression of the amount of glomerular filtrate formed each minute

glucocorticoid: any adrenocortical hormone or congener that stimulates glyconeogenesis

gluconate: a salt or ester of gluconic acid

gluconeogenesis: glyconeogenesis (see)

glucose: the chief end product in the digestion of carbohydrates; also called dextrose

glucose-6-phosphate dehydrogenase (G-6-PD): an enzyme that removes hydrogen from the substrate glucose-6-phosphate (an intermediate in carbohydrate metabolism)

glucoside: a glycoside in which the carbohydrate portion of the molecule is glucose

glycerine: glycerol

glycerol: a sweet, viscous alcohol with the formula $C_3H_5(OH)_3$

glyconeogenesis: the metabolic formation of carbohydrate from fats and proteins

glycoside: any compound containing a molecule of sugar, especially such a compound of plant origin with pharmacologic action

glycoside, cardiotonic: a glycoside acting on the heart

goitrogen: a goiter-producing agent; an antithyroid drug

gonadotropin: an agent having a stimulating effect on the gonads

G-6-PD: glucose-6-phosphate dehydrogenase (see)

habituation: psychological dependence on a drug

hallucinogen: an agent that induces hallucinations

HBr: hydrobromic acid; pharmaceutically, stands for "hydrobromide"

HCl: hydrochloric acid; pharmaceutically, stands for "hydrochloride" (e.g., tetracycline HCl)

hematinic: an agent that increases the hemoglobin level and number of red cells

hemodialysis: removal of wastes from the blood by means of a hemodialyzer or artificial kidney (see dialysis)

hemostatic: an agent that checks bleeding

hepatotoxicity: property of exerting a destructive or poisonous effect upon liver cells

5-HIAA: 5-hydroxyindoleacetic acid (a serotonin metabolite)

hippurate: a salt of hippuric acid

histamine: a biological amine occurring in a variety of tissues and postulated as a prime chemical factor in immediate hypersensitivity

hyaluronidase: an enzyme that dissolves intercellular cement

hydrate: any compound containing "water of crystallization"

hydrobromide (HBr): an addition salt of hydrobromic acid

hydrochloride (HCl): an addition salt of hydrochloric acid

hydrocholeretic: an agent that stimulates the production of watery bile

hydrolysates, protein: a mixture of amino acids prepared by chemical or enzymatic digestion (hydrolysis) of a protein

hydroxide: an inorganic base

hyoscyamus: the dried leaf of *Hyoscyamus niger* (henbane); it contains hyoscyamine, an anticholinergic related to atropine

hyperalimentation: the administration of a greater than usual amount of nutrients

hyperglycemic: an agent that raises blood glucose levels

hyperinsulinism: an excessive amount of insulin in the body, resulting in hypoglycemia and insulin shock

hyperkalemia: an abnormally high amount of potassium in the blood

hypersensitivity: a state of altered reactivity in which the body reacts with an exaggerated response to a foreign agent

hypertonic: a solution having greater tonicity (osmotic pressure) than other solutions with which it is being compared

hypnotic: a drug that induces sleep

hypodermic: given beneath the skin

hypodermoclysis: infusion of fluids subcutaneously

hypoglycemic: an agent that decreases blood glucose levels

hypotonic: a solution having lower tonicity (osmotic pressure) than another solution with which it is being compared

iatrogenic: occurring as a result of treatment

ichthammol: a brownish black viscous liquid prepared from a distillate of bituminous schists; used as an antiseptic and emollient

idiosyncrasy: an unexpected reaction to a drug

IM: intramuscularly

immunization: the process of rendering a subject immune

immunization, active: immunization effected by inoculation with a specific antigen

immunization, passive: immunization effected by administration of serum (or immunoglobulins) from immune individuals

immunoglobulin: a protein (globulin) of animal origin that functions as an antibody

immunosuppressive: an agent that effects immunosuppression

index, therapeutic: the maximal tolerated dose per kilogram of body weight divided by the minimal curative dose per kilogram of body weight; the larger the index, the greater the relative safety of the drug

injection: pharmaceutically, a solution or suspension suitable for parenteral administration

injection, intrathecal: injection into the subarachnoid space

inotropic: affecting the strength of muscle contraction

insulin: the pancreatic hormone produced by the beta cells of the islands of Langerhans; it regulates carbohydrate, lipid, and protein metabolism

interaction, drug: a situation in which the effectiveness or toxicity of a drug is modified by administration of a second drug; clinically significant interaction mechanisms relate to the delivery of a drug to the site of action and the altered response at the site of action

intra-articular: within a joint

intracutaneous: within the skin

intradermal: intracutaneous

intramuscular: within the muscle

intraperitoneal: within the peritoneal cavity

intraspinal: within the spinal or vertebral canal

intrathecal: intraspinal

intravascular: within a vessel or vessels

intravenous: within a vein

intrinsic factor: a glycoprotein secreted by gastric glands essential to the intestinal absorption of vitamin B_{12}; also called Castle's factor

iodide: a compound of iodine and some other element or radical

iodism: chronic iodine poisoning

ipecac: the dried roots of *Cephaelis ipecacuanha*; source of the alkaloid emetine

isotonic: a solution having the same tonicity (osmotic pressure) as another solution with which it is being compared

IU: a unit of biological material (such as enzymes or vitamins) established by the International Conference for Unification of Formulas

IV: intravenously

jelly: a semisolid, more or less translucent, pharmaceutical preparation

joule: international unit of work, energy, and quantity of heat; 4.2 joules equals 1 calorie (cal)

kaolin: a fine white to yellowish or grayish clay used as an adsorbent and in kaolin mixture with pectin (as in Kaopectate®)

keratolytic: an agent that promotes the softening and dissolution of the horny layer of the epidermis

lanolin: the purified fat-like substance from the wool of sheep *(Ovis aries)* mixed with 25 to 30% water; also called hydrous wool fat

laxative: a mild cathartic

LDH: lactic dehydrogenase

levo- (*l*-): a chemical prefix used to designate the levorotatory form of an optically active substance

levulose: fructose

liniment: a liquid preparation applied to the skin by rubbing as an anodyne or counterirritant

lipase: any enzyme that hydrolyzes (digests) fats

lipid: any organic fat-like substance that is insoluble in water but soluble in alcohol, chloroform, and ether

lipodystrophy: loss of subcutaneous fat

lipodystrophy, insulin: lipodystrophy (see) in a region due to repeated insulin injections

lotion: a suspension, usually aqueous, for external application; also, an oily emulsion used to cool and dry inflammatory and exudative lesions

lozenge: a medicated tablet or disk

LSD: lysergic acid diethylamide, a potent hallucinogenic compound

lyophilization: preparation of a biological product by rapid freezing and dehydration under high vacuum

maceration: the softening of a tissue by soaking

macrolides: antibiotics chemically characterized by the presence of a lactone ring

magma: a pharmaceutical preparation of finely divided material in water

mandelate: a salt of mandelic acid

MAO: monoamine oxidase

marijuana: the leaves and flowering tops of *Cannabis sativa,* the active principle of which is the hallucinogen tetrahydrocannabinol

materia medica: pharmacology

menthol: an alcohol obtained from oil of peppermint and certain other mint oils

metabolism: the sum total chemical processes of life

metabolite: any substance produced by metabolism

methemoglobin: a form of hemoglobin (produced by the action of certain poisons and drugs on hemoglobin) that does not combine with oxygen

metric system: a decimal system of weights and measures based on the meter as the unit of length and the kilogram as the unit of mass or weight

milliequivalent (mEq): the amount of an ion equal to its atomic weight in milligrams divided by its valence

mineralocorticoid: a corticosteroid that acts on the kidney to cause retention of sodium and loss of potassium

mineral oil: liquid petrolatum

miotic: an agent that constricts the pupil

molar: pertaining to moles per unit volume

mole: the gram molecular weight expressed in grams

monoamine oxidase: an enzyme that catalyzes the oxidation of certain neurohormonal amines

monobasic: an acid, such as hydrochloric acid, with only one replaceable atom of hydrogen per molecule

mucolytic: an agent that dissolves mucus

mydriatic: an agent that dilates the pupil

myelography: roentgenography of the spinal cord

narcotic: an agent that produces insensibility

nebulization: conversion into a spray; treatment by a spray

nephrotoxic: toxic or destructive to kidney cells

nerve block: see anesthesia, nerve block

neurohormone: a hormone released at a synapse or at a neuroeffector junction

neuroleptanalgesia: a state of altered awareness and analgesia produced by the administration of an analgesic and tranquilizer in combination

neuroleptic: a major tranquilizer chiefly affecting psychomotor activity

neurotoxicity: toxic or destructive to nervous tissue

NF: National Formulary; one of the two works (the other is the USP) recognized by the federal government as official pharmacologic compendia; both works provide standards of strength, quality, and purity for the drugs they describe

nitrate: salt or ester of nitric acid

nitrite: salt or ester of nitrous acid

norepinephrine: the neurohormone released at adrenergic nerve endings; called also noradrenalin and levarterenol (Levophed®)

normal saline: see saline

ointment: a semisolid topical medicament

oleate: an ester of oleic acid

ophthalmic: pertaining to the eye

opium: the air-dried exudate obtained by incising the unripe capsules of *Papaver somniferum;* it contains morphine, codeine, papaverine, and certain other alkaloids

osmolar: pertaining to the concentration of osmotically active solutes

OTC: over the counter; applied to medications that do not require a prescription

otic: pertaining to the ear

ototoxic: toxic to the inner ear or eighth cranial nerve

oxidation: the loss of electrons; the removal of hydrogen atoms

oxide: any compound of oxygen and another element or radical

oxytocic: an agent that stimulates contraction of the uterus

oxytocin: one of the two hormones secreted by the posterior pituitary; it acts as an oxytocic and also stimulates the release of milk

palliative: an agent or treatment that affords relief, but does not cure

palmitate: a salt or ester of palmitic acid

parasiticide: an agent that kills parasites

parasympatholytic: anticholinergic

parasympathomimetic: cholinergic (see)

paregoric: camphorated tincture of opium

parenteral: any route of administration other than oral, especially by injection

paste: a semisolid pharmaceutical preparation with a fatty, mucilaginous, or starch base; for topical use

PBI: protein bound iodine

pediculicide: an agent that destroys lice

penicillin: any of a group of bactericidal antibiotics having the 6-aminopenicillanic acid (6-APA) nucleus in common; naturally occurring penicillins (the most important of which is benzyl penicillin [penicillin G]) are produced by several species of mold; all other penicillins in common use are semisynthetic, obtained by substituting various side chains on 6-APA

penicillinase: an enzyme (produced by certain bacteria) that deactivates penicillin

petrolatum: a mixture of semisolid hydrocarbons (obtained from petroleum) used as an ointment base

petrolatum, liquid: mineral oil

petrolatum, white: purified petrolatum (also called petroleum jelly)

pH: a measure of hydrogen ion concentration in a scale ranging from 0 (pure acid) to 14 (pure base); pH 7 is neutrality

pharmaceutical: pertaining to pharmacy and drugs

pharmacodynamics: the study of the action of drugs on living systems

pharmacogenetics: pertains to genetic factors that create distinct populations in terms of drug response

pharmacognosy: the branch of pharmacology dealing with natural drugs, especially medicinal plants

pharmacokinetics: the study of the time courses of drug absorption, distribution, metabolism, and excretion

pharmacology: the science that deals with the action of drugs

pharmacopeia: a compendium of drugs (in the U.S., the USP and the NF)

pharmacotherapeutics: the study of the use of drugs in the treatment of disease

pharmacy: the preparing, compounding, and dispensing of drugs

phenothiazines: a chemical group of major tranquilizers

phosphatase, alkaline: a phosphatase active in alkaline medium

phosphate (PO_4): phosphate radical; salt or ester of phosphoric acid

pill: a small globular or oval pharmaceutical preparation to be taken orally

piperazine: a nitrogenous organic compound, several salts of which are used as anthelmintics

placebo: an inactive agent (e.g., "sugar pills") given to satisfy the patient; used in clinical pharmacology in the evaluation of new drugs

plasma: the fluid portion of the blood

plasma extenders: an intravenous fluid (supplemental to whole blood and plasma) used to maintain blood volume

plasmodicide: antimalarial (see)

plaster: a paste-like mixture for application to the skin

podophyllin: caustic resin obtained from rhizomes and roots of *Podophyllum peltatum*

poison: any substance that in relatively small amounts and acting chemically causes injury or an untoward reaction

polypeptide: a peptide composed of several amino acids

potassium (K^+): chief cation of the intracellular compartment

potentiation: synergism (see)

poultice: a soft, moist mass applied hot to a given area for the purpose of providing heat and counterirritation

powder: a drug used or dispensed in powdered form

powder, dusting: a fine powder used as a substitute for talc

precipitate: the substance formed in the process of precipitation

precipitation: the process through which a substance in solution is transformed into an insoluble form

precursor: any substance that gives rise to a more biologically active substance

prescription: a written instruction by a physician for the preparation and administration of a medicine; it consists of a heading or superscription "R_χ" (meaning take), inscription (the names and quantities of the ingredients), and signature ("S" or "Sig"), which gives the directions for the patient

progesterone: the female hormone secreted by the corpus luteum

progestogen: any drug possessing progestational activity; same as progestin

prophylaxis: preventive treatment

propionate: salt or ester of propionic acid

proprietary name: brand name

protectant: a topical agent used to protect the skin or mucous membranes

protein: any one of a huge class of organic polymers constituted by alpha amino acids in peptide linkage

proteinase: an enzyme that acts on protein

proteolysis: the splitting ("digestion") of proteins (via hydrolysis) into polypeptides and/or amino acids

proteolytic: pertaining to or promoting proteolysis

prothrombin: the blood plasma precursor of thrombin

psychotropic: an agent that affects the mental state or alters behavior

purgative: a powerful cathartic (see cathartic)

pyelography: roentgenography of the kidney and ureter employing an appropriate contrast medium

racemic (*dl-*): made up of equal parts of the dextro- and levo- isomers of an optically active substance

radiation, ionizing: high-energy radiation (namely, x-rays and gamma rays)

radioisotope: an isotope that is radioactive by virtue of its unstable nucleus

radiomimetic: effecting a response similar to x-rays or other ionizing rays

radiotherapy: treatment using ionizing radiation

rauwolfia: refers pharmaceutically to the Asiatic shrub *Rauwolfia serpentina,* the source of the alkaloids reserpine and rescinnamine

rebound: a reversed response on the withdrawal of a drug, e.g., acid rebound following the taking of sodium bicarbonate

receptor, drug: cellular constituent that mediates the action of a drug

receptors, adrenergic: receptor sites on effector organs innervated by adrenergic fibers (of the sympathetic nervous system); they are classified as alpha-adrenergic and beta-adrenergic receptors

receptors, alpha(α)-adrenergic: adrenergic receptors that respond to norepinephrine

receptors, beta(β)-adrenergic: adrenergic receptors responsive to epinephrine and inhibited by propranolol

receptors, cholinergic: receptor sites on effector organs innervated by cholinergic nerve fibers; they respond to acetylcholine secreted by those fibers

reconstitution: the preparation of an injection by the addition of diluent (see) to a sterile powder

reduction: the gaining of electrons or the removal of oxygen

resin: a solid or plastic complex organic substance derived from plants or produced synthetically

Rh factor: antigen(s) present on the surface of red blood cells

Rh-negative: the absence of the Rh factor

Rh-positive: the presence of the Rh factor

roentgenography: photography by means of roentgen rays (x-rays)

rubefacient: a topical agent that effects hyperemia and lessens pain

salicylate: salt or ester of salicylic acid

salicylism: the toxic effects resulting from overdosage of aspirin or other salicylates

saline: a salt solution; the term is usually applied to sodium chloride injection (isotonic sodium chloride, 0.9% NaCl; also called normal saline)

salt: a chemical compound of a metal in combination with a non-metal or radical; found in the reaction between an acid and base

SC: subcutaneous (see)

scabicide: an agent that destroys *Sarcoptes scabiei* (the cause of scabies)

schedule: the category to which a particular drug belongs in the Comprehensive Drug Abuse Prevention and Control Act of 1970

sclerosing agent: an agent used to obliterate varicose veins

sedative: an agent having a calming, soothing, and tranquilizing effect

senna: the dried leaves of *Cassia angustifolia* or *Cassia acutifolia*; used as a laxative

sensitivity, cross-: sensitivity to drugs of the same class

serotonin: a vasoconstrictor compound occurring throughout the body, especially in nervous tissue

serum: blood plasma minus fibrinogen

slurry: an aqueous suspension

solution: a clear, homogeneous mixture of one substance (the solute) dissolved in another substance (the solvent); typically a solid dissolved in a liquid

solution, dialyzing: a crystalloid solution used in peritoneal dialysis and hemodialysis

solution, nasal: a pharmaceutical preparation for instillation into the nose

solution, ophthalmic: a sterile pharmaceutical preparation for instillation into the eye

somnolence: sleepiness; unnatural drowsiness

spasmolytic: antispasmodic (see)

spermicide: an agent that destroys spermatozoa

steroid: a group name for a four-ring molecular system called cyclopentanoperhydrophenanthrene; synthetic and biological steroids include adrenocortical hormones, androgens, estrogens, progesterone, bile acids, and cholesterol

steroid, anabolic: a steroid (typically androgen) that promotes the synthesis of protein and new tissue

subcutaneous: under the skin

substrate: that upon which an enzyme acts

succinate: a salt or ester of succinic acid

sugar, invert: a mixture of equal parts glucose and fructose

sugars: crystalline, sweet, water-soluble carbohydrates

sulfa drugs: sulfonamides

sulfide: a compound of sulfur and another element

sulfonamide: any anti-infective chemically related to sulfanilamide, the parent molecule

sulfonate: salt or ester of sulfonic acid

sulfones: a chemical class of anti-infectives used in the treatment of leprosy

sulfonylureas: a class of oral drugs used in the treatment of diabetes mellitus

superinfection: a new infection arising in the course of antimicrobial therapy as a consequence of an invasion by pathogens resistant to the drug in use

suppository: an easily fusible medicated mass to be introduced into a body orifice, especially a rectal or vaginal suppository

surface tension: a stretched membrane effect at the surface of a liquid, arising from unbalanced molecular cohesive forces at the surface

suspension: a pharmaceutical preparation of a finely divided drug incorporated (suspended) in a suitable liquid vehicle

synergism: agents acting together in such a way that the combined effect is greater than the algebraic sum of their individual effects

syrup: an aqueous sugar solution, often containing one or more medicinal agents

systemic: affecting the entire body

tablet: a solid dosage form of a drug prepared by molding or compression

tablet, buccal: a small flat tablet to be held between the gum and cheek, permitting direct absorption via the mucosa

tablet, enteric-coated: a tablet coated with a substance that prevents disintegration in the stomach

tablet, hypodermic: a tablet used to prepare a solution for subcutaneous (hypodermic) injection

tablet, sublingual: a small flat tablet to be held beneath the tongue, permitting direct absorption via the mucosa

tachyphylaxis: rapidly developing tolerance to a drug

tannate: salt of tannic acid

teratogen: an agent that causes birth defects

test, glucose tolerance: a metabolic test of carbohydrate tolerance that measures active, available insulin

tetracyclines: a group of antibiotics closely related to and including the parent compound tetracycline

therapeutic: relating to therapeutics; curative

therapeutic equivalence: refers to chemical equivalents that, when administered to the same individual in the same dosage, provide essentially the same efficacy and/or toxicity

therapy: treatment

therapy, replacement: the use of natural body products or synthetic substitutes to correct a deficiency

threshold: that point at which a stimulus just elicits a response; or that concentration above which a substance appears in the urine

thrombin: a plasma enzyme in the coagulation process that converts fibrinogen into fiber

thromboplastin: one of the factors necessary in the formation of thrombin

thymol: a white, crystalline aromatic antiseptic derived from thyme oil

time, circulation: the time required for blood to flow between two points, e.g., arm-to-tongue time

time, coagulation: the time required for blood to clot in a glass tube

time, partial thromboplastin: a relatively sophisticated test for the detecting of certain defects in the coagulation system

time, prothrombin: the time required for clot formation after tissue extract and calcium have been added to blood plasma

tincture: an alcoholic solution of a nonvolatile drug

tolerance: a decreased response to a drug through continued use

topical: applied to the skin

toxicology: the study of poisons

toxin: a poisonous agent of plant or animal origin

toxoid: a neutralized exotoxin used to effect active immunity

trademark: a name (or symbol) officially registered and legally restricted to the use of the owner or manufacturer; called also brand name and trade name

tranquilizer: a drug that calms without affecting the essential quality of consciousness

tranquilizer, major: a tranquilizer used in the management of psychotic symptoms

tranquilizer, minor: a tranquilizer used in the management of anxiety and tension or psychoneuroses

transaminase: a transferase enzyme involved in the exchange of amino groups between keto acids and amino acids

transferase: an enzyme that catalyzes the transfer of a chemical group from one substrate to another

treatment, palliative: treatment designed to alleviate symptoms (but not intended to effect a cure)

trichomonacide: an agent that destroys protozoa of the genus *Trichomonas,* especially *T. vaginalis* (an important cause of vaginitis)

tricyclic: a type of antidepressant drug

triglycerides: fatty acid esters of glycerol

troche: a small circular lozenge

tryptophane: an essential amino acid and the precursor of serotonin

tyramine: a metabolite of tyrosine present in ergot and ripe cheese

tyrosine: the amino acid precursor of the catecholamines

undecylenate: salt of undecylenic acid

urate: any salt of uric acid, especially that of sodium; constituent of the urine, blood, and tophi

uricosuric: an agent that promotes the excretion of uric acid

urography: roentgenography of a part of the urinary tract employing an appropriate contrast medium

USAN: United States Adopted Name; a generic designation for a drug arrived at by the manufacturer in concert with the USAN council, which is jointly sponsored by the American Medical Association and American Pharmaceutical Association (see Appendix 10)

USP: the United States Pharmacopeia, one of the two recognized compendia of standards for drugs in the United States

vaccine: the causative agent of a disease so modified that it is incapable of producing disease while retaining its power to stimulate antibody formation

vaccine, bivalent: a vaccine prepared from two strains or species of microorganisms

vaccine, monovalent: a vaccine containing only one variety of microorganism

vaccine, polyvalent: a vaccine prepared from more than one strain or species of microorganism

vaccine, trivalent: a vaccine prepared from three strains or species of microorganisms

vasopressin: antidiuretic hormone (ADH)

vasopressor: an agent that constricts blood vessels and elevates the blood pressure

vehicle: an excipient (see)

vial: a glass container (with a rubber stopper) containing parenteral dose(s) of a drug

vitamin: an organic substance occurring naturally in plant and animal tissue essential (in very small amounts) for the control of metabolic processes

vitamin A: a fat-soluble vitamin occurring as retinol (A_1), dehydroretinol (A_2), and the precursor carotene; a deficiency results in night blindness, keratomalacia, xerophthalmia, and decreased resistance to infection

vitamin B_1: thiamine

vitamin B_2: riboflavin

vitamin B_6: includes pyridoxine, pyridoxal, and pyridoxamine

vitamin B complex: a group of water-soluble vitamins including thiamine, riboflavin, niacin (nicotinic acid), niacinamide (nicotinamide), pyridoxine, biotin, pantothenic acid, folic acid, choline, inositol, para-aminobenzoic acid, and cyanocobalamin

vitamin B_{12}: cyanocobalamin

vitamin C: ascorbic acid

vitamin D (calciferol): any of several compounds which have antirachitic properties, namely, ergocalciferol (D_2) and cholecalciferol (D_3)

vitamin E: alpha-tocopherol

vitamin G: riboflavin

vitamin K: a group of vitamins (namely, K_1, K_2, K_3) that promote the clotting of blood by increasing the synthesis of prothrombin

VMA: vanillylmandelic acid, an excretory end product of catecholamine metabolism

wetting agent: a substance that lowers surface tension of water and thereby promotes wetting

witch hazel: an alcoholic extract of the bark and leaves of the shrub *Hamamelis virginiana*

withdrawal symptoms: symptoms that follow sudden abstinence from a drug to which a person has become addicted

wool fat: anhydrous lanolin

wool fat, hydrous: lanolin (see)

xanthines: a class of drugs chemically related to xanthine, namely, caffeine, theophylline, theobromine, and aminophylline

zymogen: an enzyme precursor

13. Trademarked Dosage Forms

Abbojet®	Disposable prefilled syringe	Abbott Laboratories
Aspirol®	Crushable, fabric-coated ampul for inhalation	Eli Lilly and Co.
Bristoject®	Disposable prefilled syringe	Bristol Laboratories
Buccalet®	Buccal tablet	Ciba Pharmaceutical Co.
Caplet®	Capsule-shaped tablet	Ciba Pharmaceutical Co.
Carpujet®	Disposable prefilled syringe	Winthrop Laboratories
Chronosule®	Long-acting capsule	White Laboratories
Demilet®	Chewable pediatric tablet	Schering Corporation
Dospan®	Long-acting tablet	Merrell-National Laboratories
Dulcet®	Chewable tablet	Abbott Laboratories
Duratab®	Long-acting tablet	Cooper Laboratories, Inc.
Enduret®	Long-acting tablet	Geigy Pharmaceuticals
Enseal®	Enteric-coated tablet	Eli Lilly and Co.
Extentab®	Long-acting tablet	A. H. Robins and Co.
Filmtab®	Film-coated tablet	Abbott Laboratories
Glosset®	Sublingual tablet	Winthrop Laboratories
Gradumet®	Long-acting tablet	Abbott Laboratories
Gyrocap®	Long-acting capsule	Dooner Laboratories, Inc.
Hyporet®	Disposable prefilled syringe	Eli Lilly and Co.
Infatab®	Children's chewable tablet	Parke, Davis and Co.

Inlay-tab®	Long-acting tablet	Dorsey Laboratories
Juvalet®	Pediatric tablet	Dorsey Laboratories
Kapseal®	Hermetically sealed capsule	Parke, Davis and Co.
Lederject®	Disposable prefilled syringe	Lederle Laboratories
Linguet®	Sublingual tablet	Ciba Pharmaceutical Co.
Lontab®	Sublingual tablet	Ciba Pharmaceutical Co.
Lozi-tab®	Chewable tablet	Hoyt Laboratories
Medihaler®	Aerosol (oral) spray	Riker Laboratories, Inc.
Medule®	Long-acting capsule	Upjohn Co.
Mistometer®	Metered aerosol spray	Winthrop Laboratories
Ovoid®	Oval-shaped tablet	Winthrop Laboratories
Perle®	Soft gelatin capsule	Ciba Pharmaceutical Co.
Plateau Cap®	Long-acting capsule	Marion Laboratories, Inc.
Pulvule®	Bullet-shaped capsule	Eli Lilly and Co.
Repetab®	Repeat-action tablet	Schering Corporation
Respihaler®	Aerosol spray for oral inhalation	Merck Sharp and Dohme
Sequel®	Long-acting tablet	Lederle Laboratories
Singlet®	Long-acting tablet	Dow Pharmaceuticals
Spacetab®	Long-acting tablet	Sandoz Pharmaceuticals
Spansule®	Long-acting capsule	Smith, Kline and French Laboratories
Steri-vial®	Sterile vial of injectable medication	Parke, Davis and Co.
Supposicone®	Suppository	Searle Laboratories
Tabloid®	Tablet	Burroughs Wellcome Co.

Tembid®	Long-acting tablet	Ives Laboratories, Inc.
TenTab®	Long-acting tablet	National Laboratories
Timespan®	Long-acting tablet	Roche Laboratories
Tubex®	Disposable prefilled syringe	Wyeth Laboratories
Turbinaire®	Nasal aerosol spray	Merck Sharp and Dohme
Vaporole®	Crushable, silk-covered ampul for inhalation	Burroughs Wellcome Co.
Wyseal®	Long-acting capsule	Wyeth Laboratories

Bibliography

Bibliography

American Druggist Blue Book. New York: Hearst Corporation, 1977.

American Hospital Formulary Service. Washington, D.C.: American Society of Hospital Pharmacists, 1977.

Arndt, K. A. *Manual of Dermatologic Therapeutics* (2nd ed.). Boston: Little, Brown, 1978.

Brooks, S. M. *Basic Facts of Body Water and Ions* (3rd ed.). New York: Springer, 1973.

Brooks, S. M. *Basic Science and the Human Body.* St. Louis: C. V. Mosby, 1975.

Brooks, S. M. *Going Metric.* Cranbury, N.J.: A. S. Barnes, 1976.

Dorland's Illustrated Medical Dictionary (25th ed.). Philadelphia: W. B. Saunders, 1974.

Goodman, L., and Gilman, A. *The Pharmacological Basis of Therapeutics* (5th ed.). New York: Macmillan, 1975.

Goth, A. *Medical Pharmacology* (8th ed.). St. Louis: C. V. Mosby, 1976.

Levine, R. R. *Pharmacology: Drug Actions and Reactions* (2nd ed.). Boston: Little, Brown, 1978.

Manufacturers' labels and package inserts.

Martin, E. W. *Hazards of Medications.* Philadelphia: J. B. Lippincott, 1972.

The Merck Manual (13th ed.). Rahway, N.J.: Merck Sharp and Dohme Research Laboratories, 1977.

The National Formulary (14th ed.). Washington, D.C.: American Pharmaceutical Association, 1975.

The Pharmacopeia of the United States (19th ed.). Rockville, Md.: U.S. Pharmacopeial Convention, 1974.

Physicians' Desk Reference (32nd ed.). Oradell, N.J.: Medical Economics, 1978.

Notes